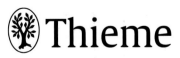

Peripheral Vascular Interventions:
An Illustrated Manual

Juergen Schroeder, MD
Associate Professor
Department of Diagnostic and Interventional Radiology
Diaconess Medical Center
Flensburg, Germany

573 Illustrations

Thieme
New York • Stuttgart

Library of Congress Cataloging-in-Publication Data

Schröder, Jürgen, 1938-
  [Trainer vaskuläre Interventionen. English]
  Peripheral vascular interventions : an illustrated manual /
Jörgen Schröder.
     p. ; cm.
  Includes bibliographical references and index.
  ISBN 978-3-13-169751-6
  I. Title.
  [DNLM: 1. Peripheral Vascular Diseases--surgery.
2. Radiography, Interventional--methods. WG 500]

  616.1'31--dc23
                        2012046150

This book is an authorized translation and update of the
1st German edition published and copyrighted 2011 by
Georg Thieme Verlag, Stuttgart, Germany. Title of the
German edition: Trainer Vaskuläre Interventionen.

Translator: John Grossman, Schrepkow, Germany

llustrator: Jürgen Schröder, Fockbek, Germany and
Malgorzata & Piotr Gusta, Paris, France

Important note: Medicine is an ever-changing science undergoing continual development. Research and clinical experience are continually expanding our knowledge, in particular our knowledge of proper treatment and drug therapy. Insofar as this book mentions any dosage or application, readers may rest assured that the authors, editors, and publishers have made every effort to ensure that such references are in accordance with **the state of knowledge at the time of production of the book**.

Nevertheless, this does not involve, imply, or express any guarantee or responsibility on the part of the publishers in respect to any dosage instructions and forms of applications stated in the book. **Every user is requested to examine carefully** the manufacturers' leaflets accompanying each drug and to check, if necessary in consultation with a physician or specialist, whether the dosage schedules mentioned therein or the contraindications stated by the manufacturers differ from the statements made in the present book. Such examination is particularly important with drugs that are either rarely used or have been newly released on the market. Every dosage schedule or every form of application used is entirely at the user's own risk and responsibility. The authors and publishers request every user to report to the publishers any discrepancies or inaccuracies noticed. If errors in this work are found after publication, errata will be posted at www.thieme.com on the product description page.

© 2013 Georg Thieme Verlag,
Rüdigerstrasse 14, 70469 Stuttgart, Germany
http://www.thieme.de
Thieme New York, 333 Seventh Avenue,
New York, NY 10001, USA
http://www.thieme.com

Cover design: Thieme Publishing Group
Typesetting by Maryland Composition, USA
Printed in Germany by Stürtz GmbH, Würzburg

ISBN 978-3-13-169751-6
eISBN 978-3-13-169761-5

Preface

It has been a mere 48 years since the first intervention in a pelvic artery - an incidental observation yet one that Charles Dotter pursued systematically and enthusiastically. This has since given rise to a major specialty that now boasts its own congresses, journals, and thousand-page textbooks. Scholars in this field will naturally be more interested in the broad and rapid increase in new scientific knowledge than in the description of the fundamentals, which have changed little since Dotter's time.

Vascular interventions have evolved from the technique of angiography. As recently as 20 years ago, every beginner in diagnostic angiography had ample opportunity to learn how to work with guidewire and catheter. Many of today's diagnostic studies require contrast but dispense with the catheter. At the same time, shrinking budgets for medical staff have made it far less common to find an experienced practitioner side by side with a beginner at the angiography table. Many of the details that were once conveyed in such a teacher-student relationship are difficult to present clearly in text alone, nor can they be demonstrated on standard angiographic images.

Abstract description will always be a roundabout way for imparting practical instructions for procedures performed primarily under visual control. The emphasis must be on visual representation. Since there is an obvious shortage in this respect, I have combined concise texts with numerous schematic diagrams in an attempt to illustrate what one needs to perform vascular interventions successfully.

This little book is hardly intended to replace one of the customary textbooks. Moreover, I have purposely omitted detailed descriptions of certain complex, high-risk interventions such as endovascular aortic prostheses or carotid artery stents. Whoever intends to attempt such procedures should no longer need this book.

There are some firm rules in interventional radiology that one may not disregard without endangering the patient. Yet many other precepts that are also accepted as rules are actually better described as conventions. Some originate from such simple considerations as the limited time available for performing the intervention. This does not mean that such rules should not become established. On the contrary, only the observance of rules generally accepted as binding can provide a basis for optimizing procedures according to empirical criteria. From this it also follows that such rules must continually be reexamined in the interest of further developing the methods.

You will occasionally find an instruction in this book that deviates from the customary recommendations. A review of the current literature will reveal that this is hardly unusual. Yet every such deviation must be based on logical reasoning and supported by one's own experience.

The allurement of interventional radiology is that it can often achieve maximum successes with minimal procedures. Its actual therapeutic tools are almost always simple. Interventional radiology is not magic. Its successes are largely the result of meticulous planning. And the fast interventionalist is one who understands how to reach their goal directly.

Winter 2012   *Jürgen Schröder*

Acknowledgments

I feel very grateful for many people. Above all to my wife Elisabeth and our children Hannah, Robert, and Ruth.

Walter Frommhold, Charles Dotter, and Josef Rösch were important teachers. Since the beginnings of interventional radiology, many have accompanied me in Tübingen, Heidelberg, Rendsburg, and Flensburg. I have learned from them and with them, and have acquired and evaluated experience together with them. I would expressly like to mention Gernot Bürkle, Ulrich Mittmann, Burckhard Terwey, Jens Allenberg, Christos Papachrysanthou, Bernd Glücklich, Issifi Djibey, Walter Müller, Ulrich Schroeder, Stefan Müller-Hülsbeck, Lothar Wöstenberg, Hedwig Horn, Klaus Graeber, Gudrun Petersen, Mathias Ehmke, Van Khiem Tran, and Karsten Schmidt.

I owe so very much to my mother Josefine Gieshoff who died at a young age. One gift of hers was the joy of drawing.

Glossary

"Glide" wire	Nitinol wire with hydrophilic coating
Ipsilateral	On the same side as the vascular access
Contralateral	On the opposite side
Overlay	Fluoroscopic image over an angiographic image
Primary patency rate	Percentage of patent vessels after one treatment
Roadmapping	Digital subtraction fluoroscopy
Secondary patency rate	Patency rate after the second or third intervention
Y prosthesis	Aortobifemoral or aortobiiliac bypass

Abbreviations

A.	Artery		**IM**	Intramuscular
Aa.	Arteries			
ABI	Ankle brachial index		**LAO**	Left anterior oblique
ACC	Acetylcysteine			
ACE	Angiotensin converting enzyme		**M**	Muscle
ADP	Adenosine diphosphate		**MRA**	Magnetic resonance angiography
ATA	Anterior tibial artery		**MRI**	Magnetic resonance imaging
AV fistula	Arteriovenous fistula			
			NaCl	Sodium chloride
C-arm	C-arm fluoroscopic image intensifier		**NFS**	Nephrogenic systemic fibrosis
CFA	Common femoral artery			
CFV	Common femoral vein		**OTW**	Over the wire (balloon catheter)
CIA	Common iliac artery			
CLI	Critical limb ischemia		**PA**	Posteroanterior (projection)
CO₂	Carbon dioxide		**PA**	Plasminogen activator
CT	Computed tomography		**PD**	Plantodorsal
CTA	CT angiography		**PTA**	Percutaneous transluminal angioplasty
			PTA	Posterior tibial artery
DES	Drug-eluting stent		**PTFE**	Polytetrafluoroethylene
DSA	Digital subtraction angiography		**PTT**	Partial thromboplastin time
			PVA	Polyvinyl alcohol
EIA	External iliac artery			
			RA	Renal artery
FMD	Fibromuscular dysplasia		**RAO**	Right anterior oblique
			RAS	Renal arterial stenosis
GFR	Glomerular filtration rate		**RDC**	Renal double curve
			RH	Rösch Hepatica
HIT	Heparin-induced thrombocytopenia		**r-tPA**	Recombinant tissue plasminogen activator
			RX	Rapid exchange
IA	Intra-arterial			
IIA	Internal iliac artery		**SFA**	Superficial femoral artery
IJV	Internal jugular vein		**SVC**	Superior vena cava
IV	Intravenous			
IVC	Inferior vena cava		**TIPS**	Transjugular intrahepatic portosystemic shunt
IU	International units		**TOS**	Thoracic outlet syndrome

Contents

1 General

Clinical Presentation of Peripheral Arterial Occlusive Disease

This book describes treatment methods that are used in the vast majority of cases of patients with peripheral arterial occlusive disease. It is not the task of this book to discuss this disease entity in its various manifestations. This chapter is a brief review of what the physician must be aware of when examining and treating a patient with peripheral arterial occlusive disease.

Peripheral arterial occlusive disease is in most cases a degenerative disorder that increases in severity with age and is promoted by various risk factors.

Risk factors:
- Age
- Smoking
- Diabetes
- Hypertension
- Hyperlipidemia
- Sedentary lifestyle

Every invasive therapy must therefore include consultation with the patient about how the further course of the disorder can be favorably influenced by avoiding or reducing these risk factors.

Recommendations:
- Quit smoking
- Reduce weight
- Treat hyperlipidemia
- Control diabetes
- Reduce hypertension
- Acetylsalicylic acid (aspirin)
- Exercise

Quitting smoking and losing weight are probably the most challenging tasks for patients, and most patients must seek professional help.

Hyperlipidemia can be very well controlled with medication in many patients, and treatment is inexpensive. It is interesting to note the result of a study on the effect of perfusion-stimulating medications on walking distance. Cholesterol synthesis inhibitors had the best *long-term effect* (Momsen et al 2009).

Diabetes must be rigorously treated. Hypertension is also usually controllable with medications (and by weight loss as well). Small doses of acetylsalicylic acid have long been recognized as prophylaxis against recurrence and possibly for primary prevention. Clopidogrel may be tried in those patients who do not tolerate aspirin. Finally, those who do not enjoy walking or cycling may consider finding a walking companion, adopting a dog, or joining an athletic club that features a coronary sports group.

Certainly there are few diseases that can be so extensively clarified by a thorough patient history as can early-stage peripheral arterial occlusive disease. The cardinal symptom is intermittent claudication. Typically this manifests itself as lower leg pain or cramps that occur after the patient walks a certain distance and disappear after a rest. Less often such cramps will occur in the thigh or buttocks. In such cases the cause is usually located in the iliac arteries.

Walking distance should be measured on a treadmill. There are numerous noninvasive diagnostic methods. The most important one is measuring systolic blood pressure in all four extremities to determine the ankle-brachial index (ABI), also referred to as the ankle-brachial pressure index (ABPI).

$$\text{ABI} = \frac{\text{Systolic pressure in distal posterior tibial or dorsalis pedis artery}}{\text{Systolic blood pressure in arm}}$$

Where pressure varies between the right and left arms, the higher value serves as reference. The ABI is determined for each leg. Unreasonably high ABI values are not uncommon in patients with diabetes. This is due to sclerosis of the arterial media, which reduces the compressibility of the arteries of the leg regardless of blood pressure.

> Normal values for the ABI lie between 1.1 and 1.0. An ABI < 0.90 at rest is regarded as abnormal; after exercise it can decrease by 15–20%.

This index is particularly suitable for documenting the success of treatment and evaluating the course of the disorder. The findings detected with the ABI become significantly more apparent with exercise (treadmill).

Table 1.1 Staging of peripheral arterial occlusive disease according to Fontaine and Rutherford

Fontaine's classification		Rutherford's classification		
Stage	Clinical aspects	Degree	Category	Clinical aspects
I	No symptoms	0	0	Asymptomatic
IIa	Claudication, walking distance > 200 m	I	1	Slight claudication
IIb	Claudication, walking distance < 200 m (moderate to severe claudication)	I	2	Moderate claudication
		I	3	Severe claudication
III	Ischemic pain at rest ("cold leg")	II	4	Ischemic pain at rest
IVa	Trophic changes, minor necrosis, and tissue loss	III	5	Minor tissue loss
IVb	Major tissue loss	III	6	Major tissue loss

The pressure drop along a stenosis is nearly proportional to the flow according to Poiseuille's law. Therefore, when blood flow increases with exercise, the pressure gradient must also increase.

Standardizing therapy and promptly agreeing on treatment options require that peripheral arterial occlusive disease be classified in defined stages (**Table 1.1**).

Staging According to Fontaine and Rutherford

For purposes of everyday clinical practice, Fontaine's classification is sufficient and more practicable:

Stage I: No symptoms = no treatment. Usually it is an incidental finding, for example, occlusion of the superficial femoral artery that is fully compensated for by collaterals of the deep femoral artery.

Stage IIa: Findings are compensated for at rest so that there is no absolute indication for treatment. Indications depend on lifestyle. A maximum walking distance of 200 m would render a postal delivery worker unfit for employment, whereas it hardly represents a significant restriction for an elderly retired person.

Stage IIb: Where the maximum walking distance is < 200 m, one will usually opt for invasive treatment if the anatomical situation so permits.

Stage III: Absolute indication for treatment. The leg is acutely at risk, for example, from thromboembolic occlusion of a major vessel.

Stage IV: Treatment is clearly indicated and depends on the extent of findings, the vascular situation, and comorbidities (very often diabetes mellitus).

Other Clinical Definitions

Critical Limb Ischemia

Critical limb ischemia (CLI), a common term, is defined as chronic pain at rest, ulceration, or gangrene secondary to peripheral arterial occlusive disease. It is important to distinguish this from acute ischemia (stage III, see below). CLI is a clinical category but should be corroborated by objective examinations (ulcers on the lower leg are usually caused by venous pathology, foot ulcers by arterial). Revascularization is the best therapy. Systemic antibiotic treatment is indicated in cases of infection.

Acute Ischemia ("Cold Leg"), Stage III

Causes:
- Arterial thrombosis (thrombosed bypass, thrombosed popliteal artery aneurysm)
- Embolism

Clinical symptoms:
- Pain
- Lack of pulse (confirmed by Doppler ultrasonography)
- Pallor
- Paresthesia
- Palsy

▷ **Important:** Cause must be identified immediately as irreparable damage could otherwise result. Angiography wherever possible. Anticoagulation (heparin).

Treatment options:
- Thrombolysis
- Aspiration thrombectomy

- Surgery (especially with proximal embolisms and in popliteal aneurysm)

Trans-Atlantic Inter-Society Consensus (TASC) II

In 2007, recommendations for defining the respective indications for open surgical and interventional treatment were published for the second time under the name TASC II (Norgren et al 2007).

Interventional treatment is recommended for a constellation of findings of type A and surgical treatment for type D. Findings of types C and D can be treated by surgical or interventional means, depending on the patient's general health and the experience of the attending physicians.

Aortoiliac Occlusive Disease

Type A:
- Unilateral or bilateral stenoses of the common iliac artery
- Unilateral or bilateral short stenoses (< 3 cm) of the external iliac artery

Type B:
- Short stenoses (< 3 cm) of the infrarenal aorta
- Unilateral occlusion of one common iliac artery
- Isolated or multiple stenoses of one external iliac artery with a total length of 3 to 10 cm and not extending into the common femoral artery
- Unilateral occlusion of the external iliac artery not extending to the origin of the common femoral artery

Type C:
- Bilateral occlusion of the common iliac arteries
- Bilateral stenoses of the external iliac arteries with a total length of 3 to 10 cm and not extending to the origin of the common femoral artery
- Unilateral stenosis of the external iliac artery extending into the common femoral artery
- Unilateral occlusion of the external iliac artery with involvement of the origin of the internal iliac or common femoral arteries or both
- Severely calcified unilateral occlusion of the external iliac artery with or without involvement of the origins of the internal iliac or common femoral arteries

Type D:
- Infrarenal occlusion of the aorta
- Diffuse bilateral disease of the aorta and iliac arteries requiring treatment
- Diffuse multiple unilateral stenoses of the common iliac, external iliac, and common femoral arteries
- Unilateral occlusion of the common iliac and external iliac arteries
- Bilateral occlusion of both external iliac arteries

- Stenoses of the iliac arteries in patients with an aortic aneurysm requiring treatment but unsuitable for an endoprosthesis, or with other disorders requiring open surgery of the aorta or iliac arteries

Occlusive Disease of the Leg Arteries

Type A:
- Isolated stenosis < 10 cm long
- Isolated occlusion < 5 cm long

Type B:
- Multiple stenoses or occlusions, each < 5 cm long
- Isolated stenosis or occlusion < 15 cm long without involvement of the distal popliteal artery
- Isolated or multiple lesions in the absence of continuous arteries of the lower leg suitable as recipient vessels for a distal bypass
- Severely calcified occlusion < 5 cm long
- Isolated popliteal artery stenosis

Type C:
- Multiple stenoses or occlusions > 15 cm total length with or without severe calcification
- Recurrent stenosis or occlusion requiring treatment after two endovascular interventions

Type D:
- Chronic total occlusion of the common femoral artery or superficial femoral artery > 20 cm and involving the popliteal artery
- Chronic total occlusion of the popliteal artery and the proximal arteries of the lower leg (trifurcation)

However, Sixt et al (2008) demonstrated in a study published in 2008 that the TASC II recommendations are not necessarily to be interpreted as binding guidelines. In 375 patients with aortoiliac disorders, nearly identical results were achieved for the four TASC II classifications (primary patency rates after 1 year were 89, 86, 86, and 85%). The conclusions drawn by Conrad et al (2009) for the arteries of the leg were very similar. Assisted patency after 3 years was 94.3% for TASC II categories A and B, and 89.7% for categories C and D.

In everyday practice one should invariably consult one's surgeon when deciding whether to opt for surgical or interventional treatment. Regular consultations conducted candidly and without regard for personal ambition will quickly give each individual a realistic idea of the other specialist's skills. This in turn will help one to decide which treatment is indicated. Familiarity with the TASC II recommendations makes it easier to define reasonable limits of one's capabilities with respect to the surgeon and also with respect to patients' expectations.

It is wise to avoid the pitfall of viewing the surgeon as a rival. When in doubt self-restraint may be the best policy. It is a bitter setback when to fail after having argued in favor of treating a specific patient. The converse is true when one overcomes one's own hesitation and complies with a colleague's request that one treat a difficult case.

The literature documents the following trends over the last 10 to 15 years:

- Even in the arteries of the leg (especially in the thigh), endovascular procedures have become established as the treatment of choice.
- They are employed early and are often combined with endovascular interventions at other levels (pelvis and lower leg). This is presumably the reason for a decrease in the rate of amputation by 25 to 38% over 10 years (Egorova et al 2010, Goodney et al 2009).

- In the superficial femoral artery the primary patency rates are significantly worse than in the iliac arteries. However, good middle-term results have been achieved with second interventions.
- As expected, the results correlate with the TASC categories, although the differences are small (DeRubertis et al 2007).
- In contrast to the coronary arteries the processes that lead to recurrent stenosis in the arteries of the leg are not complete within 6 months (Shammas 2009). Optimal results require the following:
  - Excellent angiographic results of intervention with little dissection and residual stenosis
  - Protection of the arteries of the lower leg and reduction in the growth of smooth muscle cells by means of pharmacological intervention

Consultation with the Patient

It is a privilege to be able to conduct the consultation with the patient prior to obtaining informed consent. It is one of the most noble tasks the physician performs. Only this consultation can create the trust the patient needs to believe or even to know for certain that one can help, that one is the right physician to perform this intervention. For the physician as well it is of great importance to know that he has gained the patient's trust. This person believes in the chances of improvement and is not terrified of all the possible complications described in the patient handout.

Naturally the patient must be informed about possible risks, and patient handouts are clearly helpful in listing them comprehensively. Yet one shudders at the thought that patients should simply sign a form relinquishing all control to a physician they have never met. This reflects poorly on those physicians who never took the opportunity to place the long list of risks in perspective and to kindle their patient's trust in the far greater chance of improvement or healing.

Whenever possible, one should not leave it to the family doctor, the attending physician on duty on the ward, or a younger colleague to discuss the procedure with the patient and obtain informed consent.

Just do it yourself! One should speak so the patient will understand. And above all, one should listen and have the patient describe his or her complaints. One should ask questions in a way that leads the patient to those details that are of importance. In simple words one should describe what can presumably be done to address these complaints, and describe how it all works. If there is anything left to the patient handout let it be all the rare complications.

The patient is supposed to relinquish all control, and one will be doing something to the patient that he or she is unfamiliar with and barely understands. Therefore one must make a concerted effort to win the patient's trust. The patient must believe that what one will do will be helpful and necessary and that one can do it well. If this trust is gained, one will rarely find it necessary to prescribe preoperative sedatives.

Is it possible to imagine that any surgeon would fail to visit his or her patients on the afternoon or evening after their operation? The same applies to radiologists if they are to be perceived as responsible physicians. This is also the only way to establish a good working relationship with the ward. Nurses learn what specific aftercare radiological procedures require, how to recognize complications requiring treatment, and how to distinguish them from harmless findings. For example, a little blood seeping from the needle path into the bandage after closure of the artery with Angio-Seal (Kensey Nash, Exton, PA, USA) does not represent postprocedure bleeding.

Those radiologists who visit their patients after the procedure will experience some of life's most beautiful moments!

One other important thing develops from these interpersonal contacts: Coworkers and patients will experience one as a good physician in whom they can confide. Colleagues in one's own department and in the vascular surgery department are best able to evaluate how well one performs one's interventions. Others can only assess one's performance by how humanely one deals with patients (and coworkers) and by how one involves everybody at the workplace and on the ward with whom one shares the responsibility of caring for patients.

Everyone who shares with the responsibility for caring for one's patients should know that those patients are in good hands. They will pass this confidence on to patients in many ways. And in their anxiety and doubt, patients are thankful for every sign that shows them the right physician is treating them.

Preparing the Patient

A history is obtained and clinical findings documented before it is determined that intervention is indicated. Here it is especially important to identify high-risk patients. As a rule this will be done by another physician. One will see that patient on the day before the intervention, if not earlier, and have the patient describe his or her complaints and discuss with the patient which, if any, particular risks to be alert to.

To ensure the intervention proceeds smoothly it is important to verify at this stage that all necessary documentation is on hand or will be available the next day at the latest. At a minimum this includes the international normalized ratio (INR) value and serum creatinine level. However, it should also include findings and images of any previous angiographic examinations and interventions, computed tomographic (CT) and magnetic resonance imaging (MRI) studies, and ultrasonographic findings.

Coagulation
The INR value is routinely determined before every intervention. INR values of up to ~2.0 are usually regarded as harmless unless obesity or hypertension renders treatment of the access site more difficult. In patients who depend on INR values in the therapeutic range, oral anticoagulation must be gradually substituted by heparin prior to the intervention. During the procedure, all patients are regularly given unfractionated heparin.

Platelet Aggregation Inhibitors
At least 2 hours before the intervention each patient receives 100 mg of oral acetylsalicylic acid or 500 mg intravenously. Where a stent is implanted, the patient receives clopidogrel for 6 weeks. An initial saturation dose of 300 mg is administered on the first day and a daily dose of 75 mg thereafter. If placement of a stent is planned from the outset, then the saturation dose is administered on the day before the procedure.

Impaired Kidney Function
Serum creatinine is routinely determined before contrast administration. Note that a normal value does not exclude renal functional impairment. Serum creatinine increases over the normal value of 1 to 1.1 mg/dL only when the glomerular filtration rate (GFR) drops to 50%.
- With **slight renal insufficiency** (creatinine 1.0 to 1.5 mg/dL) have the patient drink a lot of fluids: 1 L before and after the intervention.

- With **moderate or severe renal insufficiency** (creatinine > 1.5 mg/dL), administer 0.9% saline solution 1 mL/kg body weight/h 12 hours before and 12 hours after the intervention.

In the presence of simultaneous heart failure, a 5% glucose solution is administered in place of the saline solution, and the infused fluid may be balanced against the volume of urine. Contrast should be used extremely sparingly and replaced with CO_2 wherever possible. Diuretic agents should be discontinued wherever possible.

> In patients with renal insufficiency do not administer contrast again for the next 2 days.

Diabetes
Diabetics receiving metformin must discontinue the medication on the day of treatment and not resume until 24 hours after contrast administration. With diabetics, one should carefully consider the possibility of renal insufficiency and should keep the contrast dose as low as possible.

Hyperthyroidism
Where there is the slightest suspicion of thyroid dysfunction, one should determine the thyroid-stimulating hormone (TSH) level to exclude latent hyperthyroidism. In cases of elevated TSH consultation with an endocrinologist is recommended.

Adverse Reaction to Contrast Agents

> **Important:** It is not the iodine but the organic carrier molecule that is responsible for adverse reactions that may occur. If a patient did not tolerate a certain contrast agent in a previous examination, then a different preparation must now be selected to minimize the risk of a second reaction.

Naturally, prophylactic administration of cortisone and antihistamines is indicated in any patient with a history of previous contrast intolerance. The patient is given 30 to 50 mg of oral prednisolone on the evening before and 2 hours before the procedure, and antihistamines shortly before the intervention: slow intravenous injection (sequentially, not mixed together) of one ampoule each of Fenistil (dimethindene maleate, H1 receptor blocker) (Novartis, East Hanover,

NJ, USA) and Tagamet (cimetidine, H2 receptor blocker) (GlaxoSmithKline, Research Triangle Park, NC, USA).

In patients with a history of severe reaction to a contrast agent, one should consider whether it is possible to dispense with contrast agents entirely and use carbon dioxide instead.

On the Day of the Examination

When one receives the patient on the day of the examination one should briefly recapitulate the most important points of the previous day's discussion. As soon as the patient is on the examining table, one should check the peripheral pulses and examine the planned site of the approach in particular, using fluoroscopy with a metal object to determine the access site. Also a possible alternate site should be identified. Then venous access is established in the arm and local anesthesia is applied for the arterial access. It is generally sufficient to use 10 mL of a 1% local anesthetic.

Radiation Protection

In no other radiologic specialty are physicians and their assistants exposed to as much ionizing radiation as in interventional radiology. This makes information about how to minimize unnecessary exposure all the more important.

Make it a rule to work with pulsed fluoroscopy, using the lowest possible pulse frequency that provides sufficient image quality. It goes without saying that each use of fluoroscopy and every imaging series should be no longer than absolutely necessary. The influence of **collimation** is even more important. Failing to limit the fluoroscopic field to the smallest possible area can easily double the radiation dose for both patient and physician. This also decreases image quality significantly.

> One must always remember this: Collimation is the most important factor in the following:
> - Radiation protection
> - Image quality

Most units are designed so that the X-ray tube is located beneath the patient and the image intensifier is above the patient. The exit dose on the patient (above) is only ~1% of the entrance surface dose (below). This means that the physician and assistants will be exposed to significantly more intense radiation in the lower half of their body than in the upper half unless steps are taken to block this scattered radiation. For this reason the examining table is equipped with lead curtains containing a thicker layer of lead than that in the protective apron worn on the body.

Upper body structures that require particular protection include the lenses of the eyes and the thyroid gland. Therefore one should never work without both lead-glass spectacles (which include side protection) and a thyroid shield. Alternatively or in addition, one may use a lead-glass shield suspended from the ceiling on a mobile mount and draped in a sterile fashion.

The examiner's hands are often very close to the fluoroscopic field. This makes narrow collimation particularly important. With a very small fluoroscopic field, one should switch off the automatic dose regulation with the lock-in function before collimating. The hand should not be placed in the path of the beam unless it is unavoidable. One should consider beforehand how to minimize radiation exposure in this situation. Finger exposure can be checked with a personal dosimeter worn regularly on a finger ring.

For most patients, especially older ones, the risk of radiation exposure involved in an intervention is a secondary consideration. Protection of the gonads is recommended in patients of reproductive age. When working in the vicinity of the gonads, the physician should carefully collimate the beam to keep the gonads out of the fluoroscopic field.

Erythema has occasionally been observed. However, this damage occurred only where the beam remained focused on a certain area for an extremely long time without changing direction. This is hardly ever the case in peripheral endovascular interventions.

References

Conrad MF, Kang J, Cambria RP, et al. Infrapopliteal balloon angioplasty for the treatment of chronic occlusive disease. J Vasc Surg 2009;50(4):799–805.e4

DeRubertis BG, Pierce M, Chaer RA, et al. Lesion severity and treatment complexity are associated with outcome after percutaneous infra-inguinal intervention. J Vasc Surg 2007;46(4):709–716

Egorova NN, Guillerme S, Gelijns A, et al. An analysis of the outcomes of a decade of experience with lower extremity revascularization including limb salvage, lengths of stay, and safety. J Vasc Surg 2010;51(4):878–885, 885.e1

Goodney PP, Beck AW, Nagle J, Welch HG, Zwolak RM. National trends in lower extremity bypass surgery, endovascular interventions, and major amputations. J Vasc Surg 2009;50(1):54–60

Momsen AH, Jensen MB, Norager CB, Madsen MR, Vestersgaard-Andersen T, Lindholt JS. Drug therapy for improving walking distance in intermittent claudication: a systematic review and meta-analysis of robust randomised controlled studies. Eur J Vasc Endovasc Surg 2009;38(4):463–474

Norgren L, Hiatt WR, Dormandy JA et al. Inter-Society Consensus for the Management of Peripheral Arterial Disease (TASC II). Eur J Vasc Endovasc Surg 2007;33 (Suppl 1):S1–S75

Shammas NW. Restenosis after lower extremity interventions: current status and future directions. J Endovasc Ther 2009; 16(Suppl 1):I170–I182

Sixt S, Alawied AK, Rastan A, et al. Acute and long-term outcome of endovascular therapy for aortoiliac occlusive lesions stratified according to the TASC classification: a single-center experience. J Endovasc Ther 2008;15(4):408–416

2 Material

Size Specifications for Cannulas, Guidewires, Catheters, and Sheaths

The unit "gauge" for cannulas (referring to the outer diameter) corresponds to the number of processing steps required to produce wire of the same diameter. Thus thick cannulas have low gauge numbers and thin cannulas high ones. The diameter of guidewires is specified in thousandths of an inch (1 in. = 2.54 cm). Sizes of catheters and sheaths are specified using the French scale (one French unit = 0.33 mm in diameter).

> **Note:** The catheter size refers to the **outer diameter**, whereas the sheath size refers to the **inner diameter:** A 5 French catheter fits into a 5 French sheath, which in turn has an outer diameter of ~7 French, depending of course on the material. This occasionally causes some confusion, such as when the recommended material for an intervention includes a 6 French guiding sheath or, alternatively, an 8 French guiding catheter.

Cannulas

Vascular access to an artery or a deep vein is best established with a simple open 18 gauge cannula measuring 7 or 9 cm in length (**Fig. 2.1**). A 19 gauge, thin-walled cannula is sufficient for 0.035 in. wires. The cannula must be sharp; a blunt cannula compresses the vessel instead of passing through the proximal wall into the lumen.

For a long time three-piece **Seldinger cannulas** were used. A double mandrin sealed the lumen of the cannula during the puncture. Because no blood escaped, it was impossible to determine when the tip of the needle had entered the vascular lumen. Often the needle was advanced through the distal wall of the vessel as well. This was nearly unavoidable because the cannulas were almost invariably blunt; they were reused time and again and only occasionally resharpened. Finally the double mandrin was removed and the cannula withdrawn until blood flowed. The puncture of the distal wall that usually occurred was both unnecessary and harmful. Thankfully, this puncture technique has largely fallen from favor.

Some physicians use cannulas with plastic sheathing. This puncture technique is really only suitable for superficial vessels that can be punctured at a very acute angle.

In deeper vessels it is often necessary to shift the cannula to a more acute angle once it enters the vascular lumen. This makes it easier to advance the guidewire into the vessel. Naturally this cannot be done with a plastic cannula.

In small superficial arteries (brachial and radial arteries), one may prefer not to use the comparatively large 18 or 19 gauge cannulas. Alternatively, one may make the puncture with a small cannula (21 gauge = 0.8 mm outer diameter, preferably only 4 cm long) and insert a 0.018 in. wire. The track is then expanded with the dilator of the appropriate sheath to permit insertion of catheters of 5, 6, or 7 French diameter depending on the sheath size (e.g., the Cook KCFN [Cook Medical, Bloomington, IN, USA], **Fig. 2.2**). The advantage of this technique is that it requires significantly less force to insert the cannula through the wall of the vessel. This means that the artery is less likely to slip away from the cannula, it will not collapse as easily before the cannula, and perforation of the distal wall may be more easily avoided.

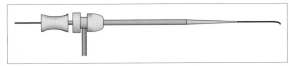

Fig. 2.2 Sheath of 5, 6, or 7 French diameter with a dilator for a 0.018 in. nitinol wire that fits a 21 gauge cannula (Cook Medical).

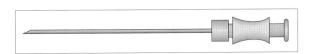

Fig. 2.1 Angiography cannula.

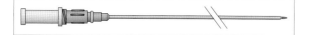

Fig. 2.3 Catheter cannula, 18 gauge, with a length of 18 cm (Cook Medical).

An 18 gauge catheter cannula 18 cm long (**Fig. 2.3**) can be very helpful in various situations: not the metal cannula but the plastic sheathing that has the same diameter as the customary puncture cannulas but is longer and more flexible. (A 4 French dilator may used in a similar manner. It is only slightly thicker, although less flexible.) Following are three examples:

- A **vessel wall is so hard** that it is impossible to introduce a sheath over the normal wire. This is almost always remedied with the aid of an Amplatz guidewire (Boston Scientific, Natick, MA, USA). Introduce the long plastic cannula over the normal wire and then insert the Amplatz guidewire through this cannula.

- In **antegrade catheterization** the wire comes to rest in the deep femoral artery. Before a larger hole is opened in the artery it should be determined whether the puncture has come too close to the deep femoral artery or has even punctured that artery. Switch to the long flexible plastic cannula. It is now possible to verify correct access far more reliably than with the rigid metal cannula.

- When a patient has **trophic changes** in one or both feet (stage IV occlusive disease according to Fontaine), it is important to determine whether stenoses or occlusions of the arteries of the leg are present and require treatment. When the inguinal pulses are strong and there is no other sign of iliac arterial stenosis, the examination can be limited to angiography of the lower legs using an antegrade approach in anticipation of possible intervention:
  - Perform the puncture with the normal steel cannula.
  - Then switch to the plastic cannula over a short wire.
  - Perform angiography.
  - Determine whether intervention is indicated.

Guidewires

The guidewire acts as the "rail" over which the catheter (according to Seldinger 1953) or sheath is introduced into the vessel (see Chapter 3). It allows curved and straight catheters to glide through vessels while preventing the catheter tip from injuring the vascular wall. Catheters or sheaths can be guided around curves and across bifurcations only with the aid of guidewires. They are the most important instrument in the interventional management of stenoses and occlusions.

Every guidewire is composed of a **metal core** that determines its stiffness and **flexible cladding**. This is because a bare steel wire 0.9 mm in diameter would be far too stiff for most functions. The 0.035 in. wire (see **Table 2.1** for units) is the most common wire thickness used in peripheral vessels today. Its core is a steel wire with a diameter between 0.35 and 0.44 mm (**Fig. 2.4**). It achieves its diameter of 0.9 mm because an outer wire 0.23 to 0.27 mm in diameter is wrapped around the core much like on the string of a guitar or piano. This type of wire is referred to as spring wire. Most wire designs have a fine straplike "safety wire" running longitudinally beneath the spring coil. This safety wire is fused to the spring coil at both ends and to the core as well at the back (proximal) end. This is necessary because the soft tip of the wire usually projects beyond the distal end of the core and is only held by this safety wire.

The surface of the steel wire is usually covered with a thin coating of Teflon. This coating doubles the lubricity of the wire when moistened (Schröder 1993c). In between these normal spring wires and the extremely stiff

Table 2.1 Comparison of the customary size specifications for cannulas, guidewires, and catheters

mm	Cannulas (gauge)	Guidewires (inches)	Catheters (French)
0.3		0.012	
0.36		0.014	
0.46		0.018	
0.5	25		
0.8	21		
0.9	20	0.035	
1.0		0.038	3
1.1	19		
1.2	18		3.6
1.33			4
1.67			5
2.0			6
2.33			7
2.67			8
3.0			9

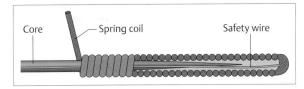

Fig. 2.4 Normal spring wire.

but rarely used wires (such as Back-up Meier [Boston Scientific] or Lunderquist [Cook Medical]) there is a third class of wires known as Amplatz wires. This type is used when a particularly stiff wire is needed. Here the core is wrapped not with a round wire but with a flat steel band that allows a thicker core to be used with the same outer diameter (**Fig. 2.5**).

> A 0.035 in. Amplatz wire with a 0.55 mm core is six times as stiff as a standard wire with a 0.35 mm core. Stiffness is directly related to the **4th power** of the core diameter (Schröder 1993a).

In the very slender catheter systems initially developed for cardiology and now increasingly used in peripheral interventions the wires must be correspondingly thin. Their stiffness need no longer be reduced artificially by wrapping. An 0.018 in. wire of this sort with a diameter of 0.46 mm is as stiff as the average 0.038 in. spring wire. A 0.014 in. wire with a diameter of 0.35 mm corresponds to a 0.035 in. spring wire. Yet even these wires are wrapped. This wrapping is at the tip, which has the desired flexibility only when the core is drawn out very thinly and therefore must be protected by a spring coil or plastic sheathing.

A very soft tip is desirable where the wire's only function is to guide a catheter through open or possibly stenosed vessels atraumatically. This can be different where a wire with a straight tip (and therefore with the least possible resistance) is needed to guide a catheter through an occluded segment of a vessel (see Chapter 5, Superficial Femoral Artery, p. 159, and Arteries of the Lower Leg, p. 184). For this reason 0.014 in. wires are now supplied with varying tip thicknesses (such as the Cook CMW–14 Series, 6–25 G). They are each designed for a

different "tip load," meaning the maximum resistance (gram) the straight wire can encounter without bending.

Even more important is the design of the transition between the soft tip and the stiff shaft. Wires that have no such transition are nearly useless (see Chapter 3, Crossover Catheterization, p. 60).

Here is an **example** for the effect of the gradual transition from a soft tip to a stiff shaft: Assume the curved end of a catheter has been introduced from the right iliac arteries across the bifurcation into the left common iliac artery. To advance the catheter further requires one to first advance a wire into the left iliac arteries. The soft tip of the wire follows the curvature of the catheter. If the stiff shaft of the wire then follows without any transition (**Fig. 2.6a**), the catheter will kink, and both catheter and wire will advance into the aorta.

However if the wire only gradually becomes stiffer, then the wire can continue to follow the curvature of the catheter (**Fig. 2.6b**). Gradually it will expand this into a wider arc that even the increasingly stiff shaft of the wire can follow. This arc will finally become so wide that it will no longer fit into the aorta. Consequently, the wire (and the catheter) will only be able to advance into the contralateral iliac arteries (**Fig. 2.6c**).

The length of this transition should be no less than 5 cm for standard wires. Significantly longer transitions (e.g., Bentson, long taper) are helpful for passages through certain difficult curves.

Example: When one wants to use such a wire to guide a catheter across the aortic bifurcation, there is often a mismatch between the stiffness in the part that has passed the curve and the part being flexed in the bifurcation. The part of the wire that has passed the curve must continue to support the path around the curve. It may prove too soft to do this if the area of increasing stiffness is limited to just a few centimeters. The problem can be avoided by using a wire with a much longer transition (e.g., Bentson, long taper). However, there is often not enough space for this beyond the curve (e.g., in a renal artery).

The obvious solution is to design the wire so that the core diameter (which determines stiffness) increases linearly from the tip to the shaft. This is exactly how most guidewires are designed. This design overlooks one thing: It results in stiffness that increases as the 4th power of the distance from the tip, which is certainly not optimal for every application.

For such cases it may be best to have a wire in which it is not the core diameter (**Fig. 2.7a**) but the stiffness that increases linearly from the tip (**Fig. 2.7b**). Then the cross section of the wire in the transitional segment would have the shape of a parabola (4th power). The diameter of the core would be proportional to the 4th power root of the distance from the tip of the wire:

$$D \sim \sqrt[4]{x} \text{ (distance from tip)}$$

Of course intermediate forms between these two extremes are conceivable.

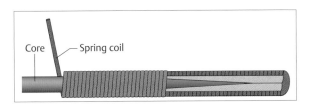

Fig. 2.5 Amplatz wire (Boston Scientific).

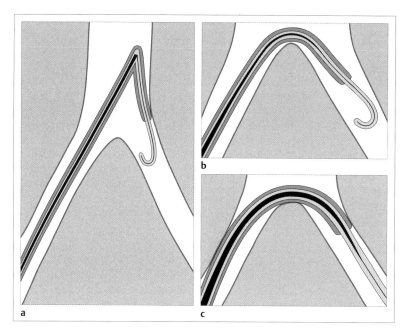

Fig. 2.6 Transition between soft tip and stiff shaft.
a Wire with abrupt transition to stiff segment.
b Wire with gradual transition to stiff segment.
c Later phase of catheterization using wire with gradual transition to stiff segment.

It is easy to put a bend in the tips of thin 0.014 or 0.018 in. steel wires (see **Fig. 2.10**). However, the tip can just as easily deform when it encounters resistance, which can quickly render such a wire unusable. A few special wires, such as the ones included in a puncture set for the radial artery or thin wires for catheterizing peripheral vessels (e.g., Terumo Glidewire Advantage, Terumo Interventional Systems, Somerset, NJ, USA) have a tip with a nitinol core, which is much more resistant to deformation (see below).

"Glide" Wires

Terumo introduced a completely different type of guidewire in the late 1980s. Its core is not made of steel but of nitinol, an alloy of nickel and titanium. Instead of being wrapped the wire has plastic sheathing with a hydrophilic outer coating, giving it excellent lubricity. Wires of the same material are now available from other companies as well.

A **nitinol wire** is significantly less stiff (by a factor of 4, Schröder 1993a) than a steel wire of the same core diameter. This can be good or bad depending on the application. One clear **advantage** is that the wire is largely resistant to kinking. The greatest advantage is the hydrophilic coating. Wires with this coating have three times the lubricity of Teflon-coated wires when moistened (Schröder 1993c). That makes this "glide" wire the instrument of choice for catheterizing high-grade stenoses or occluded segments of vessels. It is also very helpful when guiding catheters or sheaths around difficult curves or across bifurcations.

One **disadvantage** of glide wires is their vulnerable surface. For this reason one should avoid using them in combination with sharp cannulas when establishing vascular access. As the wire is withdrawn through the cannula, the cannula could cut into the wire's plastic sheathing.

The statement that nitinol wires are not deformable overlooks one interesting possibility: If one sharply

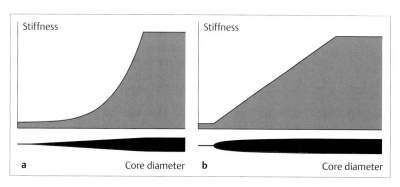

Fig. 2.7 With a linear increase in core diameter, stiffness increases as the 4th power of the distance from the tip of the wire. To achieve a linear increase in stiffness, one needs a core with a diameter that increases as the 4th power root of the distance from the tip of the wire.
a Linearly increasing core diameter.
b Linearly increasing stiffness.

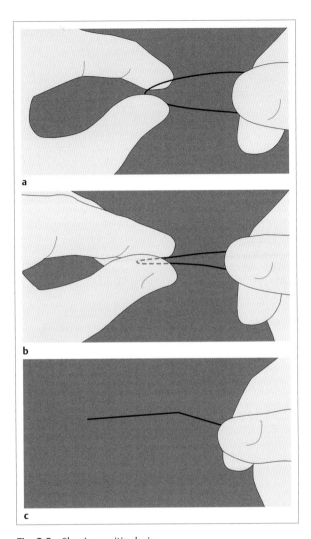

kinks the wire, the wire will no longer be perfectly straight at that point (**Fig. 2.8**). A slight kink will remain, which will then be as stable as the wire's previous straight shape (**Fig. 2.8c**, Schröder 1993b). Several such kinks create a **bend**. This can be very useful in certain situations, such as when guiding a balloon catheter past the deep femoral artery into the superficial femoral artery in crossover catheterization (see Chapter 3, Crossover Catheterization, p. 60). This method is also useful when you want to steer a bent glide wire from the brachiocephalic trunk into the right subclavian artery. In this case the original bend in the wire will often be too slight compared with the diameter of the brachiocephalic trunk (**Fig. 2.9**).

Glide wires are usually available as straight wires or slightly curved at the tip. Aside from the standard type there is also a stiff version. With a core diameter of 0.7 mm this wire is 5 times as stiff as the standard version with a core diameter of 0.46 mm (Schröder 1993a).

Wires for Steering Around Curves

Balloon catheters are almost always straight and can only be steered around curves or selectively introduced into certain branches with the aid of guidewires. This selective catheterization requires a wire with a suitable bend at its tip and rotational stability (**Fig. 2.10**).

The spring wires typically do not have a solid connection between their wrapping and core and are therefore not suitable for actively steering around certain curves. However, this works very well with all wires that are not wrapped with a spring. Such wires include the thin steel wires (0.018, 0.014, and 0.012 in.) and glide wires.

Fig. 2.8   Shaping a nitinol wire.
a Shaping a nitinol wire by putting a sharp bend in it.
b Continuation of **a**.
c Slight bend that keeps its shape: result of **a** and **b**.

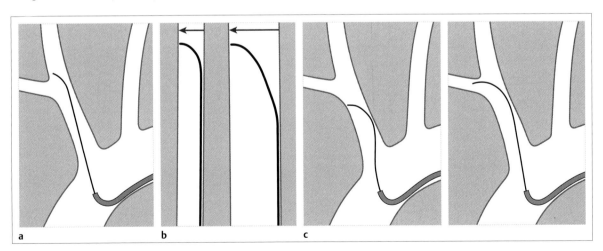

Fig. 2.9   Catheterizing the right subclavian artery.
a At first it is not possible to catheterize the subclavian artery from the brachiocephalic trunk.
b Additional bend in the glide wire.

c A more pronounced bend causes the tip of the wire to enter the right subclavian artery.

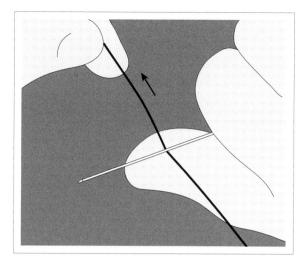

Fig. 2.10 To shape the tip of a steel wire, draw it between your thumb and a tightly held cannula. The greater the pressure, the more pronounced the bend.

> Like stiffness, the rotational stability of a wire is also proportional to the 4th power of its diameter (Schröder 1993a).

An 0.018 in. wire has nearly 3 times the rotational stability of a 0.014 in. wire. The thin steel wires are usually supplied with a twist grip that makes it far easier to steer the wire precisely.

> Every wire in its tube should be moistened with saline solution prior to use.

Inserting a curved guidewire into a cannula or catheter is greatly facilitated by the introducer supplied with every curved-tip catheter. It is usually very tightly inserted in the wire tube (see **Fig. 2.12**). When it is pulled out, it often comes out of the tube and off the wire all at once, so that one has to reinsert the curved tip. To avoid this, one should first withdraw the wire 10 to 15 cm out of the tube and then pull the introducer out of the tube. Then the introducer is pushed to the tip of the wire to extend the curve. When inserting the wire into a cannula or catheter, one grasps the wire a few centimeters behind the introducer (**Fig. 2.11**). This way one can bring the extended wire into a sufficiently stable position within the cannula or catheter in a single motion without having to change one's grip on the wire (**Fig. 2.11b**).

There are two types of **introducers:**

- Those whose proximal end lies **within** the wire tube have a narrow lumen that is in contact with the wire along its entire length. When one inserts the wire through the valve of a sheath with this device, there is only slight blood loss.

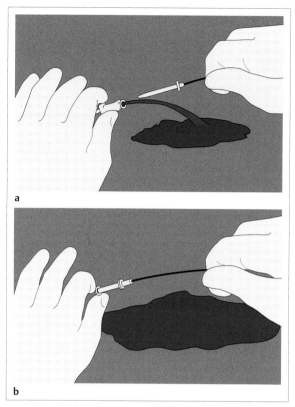

a

b

Fig. 2.11 Inserting the wire with an introducer.
a Grasp the wire a few centimeters behind the introducer.
b Insert the extended wire into the cannula or catheter in a single motion without changing your grip.

- The glide wires usually come with an introducer whose proximal end lies **over** the end of the wire sleeve. This model is wide at its proximal end and narrows toward its tip like a funnel (**Fig. 2.12**). When one inserts the wire through the valve of a sheath with this device, the resistance to retrograde blood flow is significantly less and blood loss is greater.

The elastic J tip in curved spring wires is created by a bend in the safety wire. The curvature also requires a little play between the coils of the wrapping. The safety wire is 1.5 to 2 mm longer than the tightly wound wrapping. This ensures the necessary play for the curvature (**Fig. 2.13**). Pulling apart the wrapping at another place on the wire will push the tip together and extend the curve. This

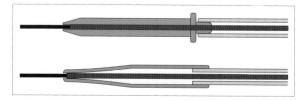

Fig. 2.12 Introducers for spring wires (top) and glide wires (bottom).

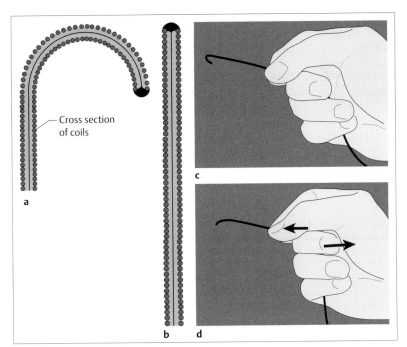

Cross section
of coils

a

b d

c

Fig. 2.13 Extending the end curve of a J wire.
a Curved J wire: play between the coils of the wrapping.
b J wire with tip extended.
c To extend the J wire, it is grasped between the fingers.
d The wrapping is spread apart by moving the fingers in opposite directions.

means that, to insert the wire into a catheter without an introducer, one spreads the wrapping apart between the fingers (**Fig. 2.13d**). This will make the tip nearly straight.

Following are common names for a few special guidewires:

Bentson: long soft tip (6 cm and long transition to stiff shaft [16 cm]).

Long taper: similar characteristics to Bentson.

Rosen: J wire with tight end curve, radius of curvature 1.5 mm, relatively stiff.

Amplatz (Boston Scientific): stiff wire, see earlier discussion.

Terumo (Terumo Interventional Systems): the original glide wire.

Sheaths

A sheath is not generally required for simple angiography using only one catheter. This assumes that the tip of the catheter is in close contact with the guidewire so its passage into the vessel is relatively atraumatic (see Chapter 3, Angiography, p. 80, and **Fig. 3.76**, p. 84). Use of a sheath is recommended where one plans to change catheters several times or where one expects to encounter a very hard vascular wall. A sheath is absolutely indicated to protect the vascular wall in every intervention with a balloon catheter, stent, or similar device.

The sheath is a thin-walled catheter with a valve and a lateral connection at its proximal end. The sheath is introduced into the vessel via a dilator that slides along the guidewire (**Fig. 2.14**). The most important **quality criteria** are smooth transitions with steps as little as possible between guidewire and dilator and between dilator and sheath. This requires a very strong material that retains its strength even when extruded to a thin layer and that will not crack upon encountering the resistance of a hard vascular wall. For the same reason the tip of the sheath

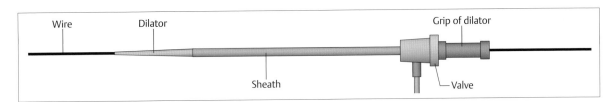

Wire   Dilator   Grip of dilator

Sheath   Valve

Fig. 2.14   Sheath.

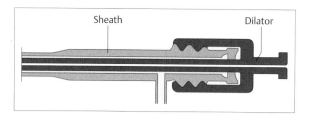

Fig. 2.15 Schematic diagram of a threaded connection between the sheath and dilator (Boston Scientific).

must be in close contact with the dilator. The fact that it has a sharp distal end does not pose a problem. This is because the sheath is only advanced with the dilator in place within it.

There must also be a reliable connection between the sheath and dilator. Otherwise the resistance of the vascular wall upon entering the vessel could cause the dilator to be pushed out of the sheath: One would push the sheath but the resistance would act on the dilator. The press fit connection between dilator and sheath that most sheaths have is not always sufficient for this task. Only a threaded connection between the two components is reliable (**Fig. 2.15**).

"Soft tip" sheaths (**Fig. 2.16**) should not be used. They have a higher step-off between dilator and sheath tip, making it hard to push them through a hard vascular wall. And because they are also soft they can become significantly deformed, tearing an unnecessarily large hole in the vascular wall.

The **valve** prevents blood from escaping when there is no catheter in the sheath. It also seals the sheath against the catheter or guidewire. The sheath is flushed through the lateral connection. This connection also allows injection of contrast agent or medications. However, forceful injection can cause part of the fluid to spray out through the valve. This situation can be avoided by introducing the dilator or catheter and injecting through its lumen.

Size Specifications for Catheters and Sheaths

Catheters are specified by their outer diameter but sheaths by their inner diameter (i.e., according to the catheter that fits in the sheath). A 6 French sheath is ~2.2 mm wide. Its outer diameter depends on the wall thickness but will usually be around 2.8 mm (8.3 French). Sheaths with a length of 9 to 11 cm are customarily used in daily routine. The length of 11 cm has an advantage over 9 cm because, in antegrade catheterization of the common femoral artery, it will better ensure a stable position within the superficial femoral artery.

Sheaths for Specific Tasks

Sheaths are available in various shapes and sizes for specific tasks. Balloon-expandable stents in particular are most securely placed when they are advanced to the stenosis within a sheath. Treating iliac arterial stenosis in this manner requires a sheath 25 cm in length.

Sheaths with a length of 40 cm are customarily used in crossover interventions. The sheath must have the following characteristics to be advanced across an acute-angle bifurcation (**Fig. 2.17**):

- Either the dilator and sheath have a suitable bend (e.g., Cook Medical's Balkin sheath, **Figs. 2.17** and **2.18**),
- or a flexible dilator projects a few centimeters beyond the tip of the sheath. The dilator is first advanced across the bifurcation. It splints the bifurcation so the stiffer sheath can be advanced. (This is the principle of gradually increasing stiffness, as with the guidewires, e.g., the Arrow sheath [Arrow International, Inc., Reading, PA, USA]; **Figs. 2.17** and **2.19**).

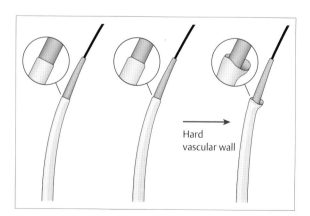

Fig. 2.16 Normal sheath (left) and soft-tip sheath (center and right).

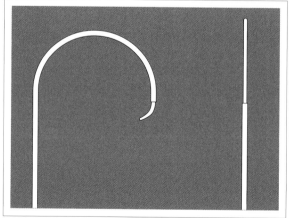

Fig. 2.17 Balkin sheath (Cook Medical, left) and Arrow sheath (right).

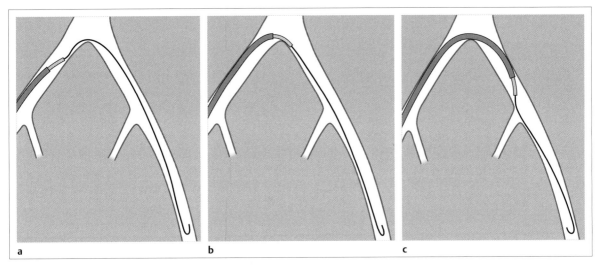

Fig. 2.18 Crossover catheterization with the Balkin Up and Over sheath from Cook Medical.
a The wire lies deep within the contralateral iliac arteries.
b The curved dilator follows the wire across the bifurcation.
c The bend in the sheath facilitates advancing it into the contralateral iliac arteries.

Because of their tendency to kink at a bifurcation, crossover sheaths usually have a spiral metal reinforcement in their wall. This makes them relatively stiff but also makes it easier to put a bend in them prior to insertion (even without steam heating) that will facilitate crossing the bifurcation.

Sheaths of 6 French diameter were originally common for crossover catheterization. Now sheaths of suitable length are also available in 5 and 4 French diameters. These of course are more easily advanced across an acute-angle bifurcation.

Sheaths 40 cm in length are normally used for interventions in the arteries of the lower leg. Guiding sheaths with various curvatures are supplied for interventions in the renal arteries (see Chapter 4, Renal Arteries, p. 121). The width and curvature of the aorta are the decisive criteria for adapting the sheath to the angles of the renal artery origins.

Aspiration thrombectomy, at least when performed with a simple aspiration catheter, requires a sheath with a removable valve. Such sheaths are supplied in the appropriate length by OptiMed, Ettlingen, Germany; Angiomed GmbH, Baden-Würtemberg, Germany; or Terumo.

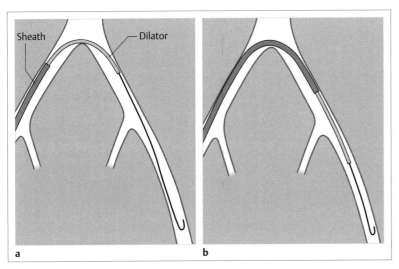

Sheath — Dilator

Fig. 2.19 Crossover catheterization with the Arrow sheath (Arrow International) or OptiMed Epsylar.
a The flexible dilator follows the wire across the bifurcation.
b The dilator splints the bifurcation so the shealth can be advanced.

Angiography Catheters

The catheter is the most important instrument in every vascular intervention: It transports contrast agent. Together with the guidewire it provides an access path through almost every curve and bifurcation. And it acts as the carrier for balloons, stents, and other instruments.

For nearly 3 decades angiography was performed without sheaths. For this reason it was only natural that the catheter tip was in close contact with the wire to ensure atraumatic entry into the vessel. Sheaths came into regular use only with the advent of interventional radiology. They would not normally be required for simple angiography if every manufacturer were to pay more attention to an optimally shaped catheter tip (see **Fig. 3.76**), and if every catheter had a tip like the pediatric catheter, the "self-dilating tip" of which is explicitly mentioned in the catalog. Note that a 4 French sheath creates an opening in the vascular wall twice as large (in terms of area) as the one a 4 French catheter alone would require.

General

Transport of Contrast Agent

Manufacturers often specify possible flow rates of contrast agent (mL/s). This will depend on the following catheter characteristics:

- Inner diameter
- Length
- Pressure-bearing capacity of the catheter wall

All other conditions being equal, Poiseuille's law indicates that the possible flow rate of contrast agent is directly related to the 4th power of the inner diameter. This means that doubling the inner diameter would allow a 16-fold increase in the flow rate. When the catheter length is doubled, the possible flow rate decreases by half, all other conditions being equal. (The flow rate can also be significantly increased by warming the contrast agent to body temperature and thus decreasing its viscosity.)

Digital subtraction and the option of increasing contrast electronically have made it possible to work with significantly lower contrast flow rates than were required earlier in analog imaging. For this reason the maximum possible contrast flow rate only becomes a problem in very narrow catheters.

Rotational Stability (Torsional Strength)

The diagnostic and therapeutic instruments are steered through the vascular system using curved catheters and with the aid of guidewires. This is only possible where the curve at the distal tip of the catheter can be steered in a certain direction by rotating the proximal end of the catheter. This in turn assumes that the catheter has sufficient rotational stability (torsional strength). Rotational stability (torsional strength) is primarily a function of catheter diameter. It is approximately proportional to the 4th power of the outer diameter (more precisely as the difference between the 4th powers of outer and inner diameter, $Do^4 - Di^4$).

The material also plays a role. Older measurements have shown that the rotational stability (torsional strength) of Teflon, polyethylene, and nylon is approximately in the proportion of 1:2:4 (Schröder and Weber 1992). The same study revealed that wire reinforcement in the catheter wall can increase rotational stability (torsional strength) by a factor of 3.

Catheter Shape

One material-related characteristic of catheters that has very important practical implications is the stability of the bends that are used to determine the catheter's path through the vessel. These bends become less pronounced when the catheter is kept extended for a long time. Warming also has an unfavorable effect. On the other hand, one can use heat (steam) to change the shape of this thermoplastic material (see later discussion).

Catheters for Aortography

The key quality criteria for a general aortogram include good contrast with minimal use of contrast agent and unobscured visualization of the vascular anatomy.

Renal arterial stenosis is the most important example. It is often associated with impaired kidney function that can be exacerbated by large quantities of contrast agent.

Therefore the contrast agent should be very selectively injected into the short segment from which the renal arteries (or other aortic branches of interest) arise. One should take particular care to prevent part of the contrast agent entering the aorta superior to the renal arteries. There are two reasons for this. First, it avoids a loss of contrast. Second, it also avoids contrast entering the superior mesenteric artery where it could obscure segments of a renal artery within the region of interest.

The pigtail catheter most often used for this purpose (**Fig. 2.20a**) fails to fulfill these requirements satisfactorily. The end of its distal circular curve through which 30 to 50% of the injected contrast agent exits is directed cranially on most catheters. This results in loss of

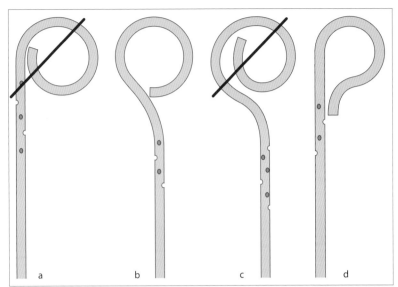

Fig. 2.20 Catheters for aortography.
a Pigtail catheter.
b Racket catheter with end hole in favorable position.
c Racket catheter with end hole in unfavorable position.
d Catheter with a 180° bend.

concentration and obscured anatomy. Part of the contrast agent is separated from the rest of the bolus so that the maximum possible contrast is not achieved.

Some "tennis racket" catheters avoid this problem, some do not. The racket, or tennis racket, catheter shown in **Fig. 2.20b** has a suitable shape: The hole at the distal end emits the contrast agent at the same level as the side holes. **Fig. 2.20c** on the other hand shows the end hole in the same position as on most pigtail catheters. All catheters with a 180° bend (**Fig. 2.20d**) reliably avoid this problem. Such models include Sos Omni Flush (AngioDynamics, Latham, NY, USA), ContraFlush (Boston Scientific), Universal Flush (Cordis, Miami, FL, USA), and VCF (Cook Medical). (The author has described a catheter that can be used to precisely inject contrast agent in the direction of the renal arteries in German Registered Design No. 20 2009 011 942.4.)

Modern digital subtraction angiography systems are able to generate a single summation angiogram from a series of sequential images (see **Fig. 3.72**). This means it is no longer necessary to fill a 30 or 40 cm segment of the aorta completely. In the interest of using contrast agent sparingly it is best to follow Sos and Trost's recommendation (Sos and Trost 2008) by reducing the number of side holes and concentrating on a short segment (**Fig. 2.21b**).

A pigtail catheter is not suitable for precision steering around curves such as from right to left at the aortic bifurcation or from the left subclavian artery into the descending aorta. This is because the tip of the pigtail catheter points straight ahead in most cases (**Fig. 2.22**). The pigtail opens only when a stiff segment of the wire lies within the curve. And by then the wire is so far into the aorta that it can no longer be used to guide the catheter across the bifurcation or into the descending aorta.

So-called **sizing catheters** (**Fig. 2.23**) are used wherever precise measurements of vascular diameter and the length of certain segments of the vessel are needed. These are usually aortography catheters bearing metal markings on their shaft at precisely defined intervals.

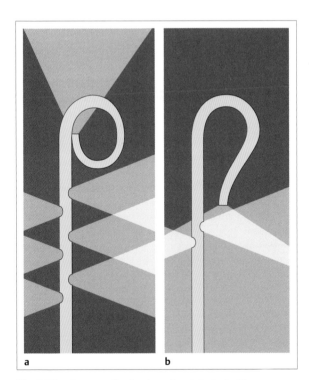

Fig. 2.21 Contrast distribution when injected with:
a Pigtail catheter.
b Sos Omni Flush catheter (AngioDynamics): its backward facing end hole and fewer side holes concentrate the contrast agent within a short segment.

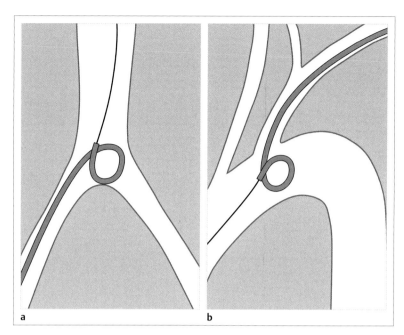

Fig. 2.22   The pigtail catheter is poorly suited for steering at these sites:
a At the aortic bifurcation.
b Within the aortic arch.

Incorrect measurements can result when the catheter segment with the graduations does not lie parallel to the entrance plane. Another type of sizing catheter is used to determine what length of endovascular aortic prosthesis to implant. This type may have 20 markings at intervals of 1 cm.

Practical tip: Pigtail and similar catheters are regularly supplied with a tube for extending the tip to facilitate slipping the catheter over a wire. With many catheters this will be easier if one grasps the very tip of the catheter and pulls it onto the wire. The catheter will then extend by itself (**Fig. 2.24**).

stability already discussed plays a crucial role in steering a curved catheter. The wire reinforcement that increases the rotational stability usually ends short of the curved segment.

Catheters today are supplied with a wide variety of shapes (**Figs. 2.25** and **2.26**). Identical or very similar shapes are often listed under different names in suppliers' catalogs. It is a good idea to look through the catalogs at regular intervals to discover new catheter shapes that will suit specific needs.

The **simple hook** is suitable for catheterizing the branches of the abdominal aorta (different radii of

Catheters for Selective Catheterization

It is now possible to catheterize nearly any artery of the body from an inguinal artery or an artery of the arm. We essentially owe this capability to the use of curved catheters in conjunction with guidewires. The rotational

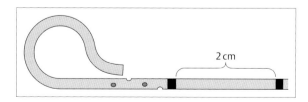

Fig. 2.23   Sizing catheter with two platinum rings on its shaft.

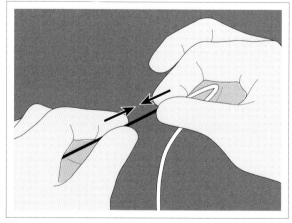

Fig. 2.24   Slipping a curved-tip catheter over a wire: grasp the very tip of the catheter and push the wire into it.

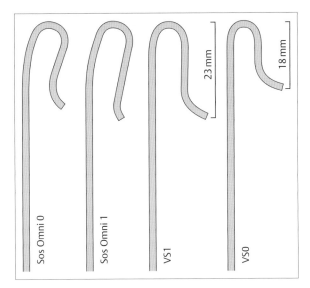

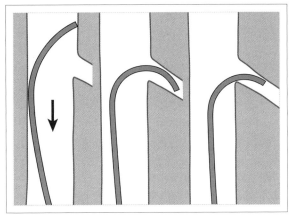

Fig. 2.27 Introducing a hooked catheter into an aortic branch artery.

Fig. 2.25 Catheters for visceral and crossover catheterization (left AngioDynamics, right Cook Medical).

curvature for different widths of the aorta; **Fig. 2.27**). The smallest hook (Rösch Inferior Mesenteric [RIM]; Cordis); see **Fig. 2.26**) is intended for angiography of the inferior mesenteric artery, best performed by catheterization via the left inguinal region.

Catheters whose gradually decreasing curvature continues into the shaft are better than simple hooks if the catheter is to be advanced farther into an aortic branch artery. The best known example by virtue of its unique name is the **cobra catheter** (**Fig. 2.28**). Yet this design has one bend too many. Such a configuration may be necessary for a rising cobra to keep its balance. Yet in the aorta, which is not exactly straight, it interferes with steering the catheter.

Typical problem: In an infrarenal aorta with a leftward bend, the tip of the cobra catheter will spontaneously veer to the left. The superfluous secondary bend makes it difficult or even impossible to catheterize the right renal artery (**Fig. 2.29**).

Therefore a catheter with a straight shaft proximal to the main bend is usually better. Such a design is available from various suppliers under the name **Levin** or **Lev** (see **Figs. 2.26** and **2.28**). The medium size (Lev 2) is suitable for most patients.

The branch arteries of the abdominal aorta that arise in caudal direction at an acute angle pose a problem. They can often only be catheterized from an inguinal approach with catheters with such a pronounced bend that their tip points backward (**Fig. 2.30**). The longer the inferiorly angled distal segment at its tip, the more stable will be the catheter's seating in the branch artery. However, when the distal segment is pulled into the aortic branch

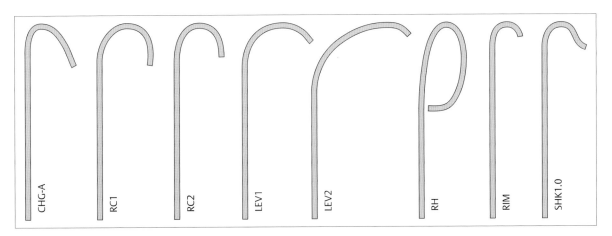

Fig. 2.26 Selection of Cook catheters for the aortic branch arteries.

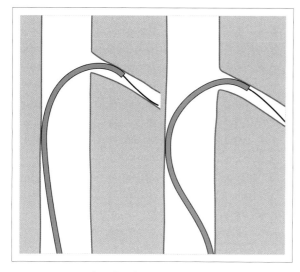

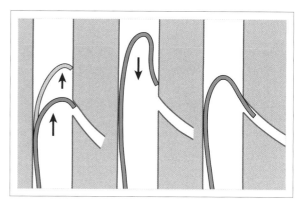

Fig. 2.30 Aortic branch artery arising at an acute angle.
a Attempted insertion of Levin catheter.
b Insertion of SIM1 catheter.

Fig. 2.28 Examples of catheters whose gradually decreasing curvature continues into the shaft: Levin catheter (left) and cobra catheter (right).

artery, it can easily be pressed tightly against the inferior vascular wall if the artery describes a lateral or superior arc distal to its origin.

The diagram in **Fig. 2.31** is drawn nearly to scale. It illustrates the relationship between the diameter of the aorta and the length (4 cm) of the backward facing distal segment of the SIM1 catheter (Cook Medical). The celiac trunk and renal arteries often exhibit a superior bend just distal to their inferiorly angled origin. A 4 cm distal segment can often impinge against the wall nearly perpendicularly. When the catheter is then drawn inferiorly without gliding farther into the branch artery, it

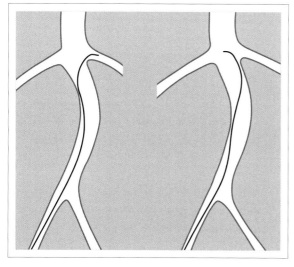

Fig. 2.29 Cobra catheter in a curved aorta: here the secondary curvature prevents catheterization of the right renal artery.

impinges against the contralateral wall of the aorta. This forces the catheter into the branch artery with a strong thrust against its tip. To avoid injury to the vascular wall, one should take care to use a soft wire to guide the catheter. However, it is better to use a catheter with a shorter distal segment and possibly even with an outward bend at its tip.

Many variants of such catheters are supplied with a distal segment just long enough so it can be turned inferiorly in the upper abdominal aorta or thoracic aorta with relative ease. Many also have a pronounced outward bend at their tip. This makes it easier to "hook into" an aortic branch artery and negotiate a superior arc further into the vessel.

The tip of this type of catheter will spontaneously point backward as soon as the diameter of the aorta exceeds the length of the downward-pointing distal segment. Where the aorta is not quite so wide, one can successfully turn the catheter tip backward by rapidly advancing the catheter while giving it a turn. The tip will impinge somewhere along the wall, and the bend will then be pushed past it (**Fig. 2.32**). If you then pull the backward angled tip downward, the tip will likely catch in a minor aortic branch artery or impinge on an irregularity in the vascular wall. The gentlest way to avoid this is to insert a wire with a long soft end (Bentson, long taper) into the catheter (**Fig. 2.33**). Alternative: Carefully withdraw the catheter under continuous fluoroscopic control. Continuously rotating the catheter can also prevent impingement.

In interventional radiology this problem is most often encountered in crossover catheterization of the contralateral iliac arteries. The curve in the catheter must be sufficient to permit advancing an increasingly stiff wire into the contralateral vessels. Where the catheter is to be advanced into the external iliac artery for angiography, it should not have any pronounced outward bend at its tip. Otherwise the tip of the extended catheter could be pressed against the vascular wall (**Fig. 2.34**).

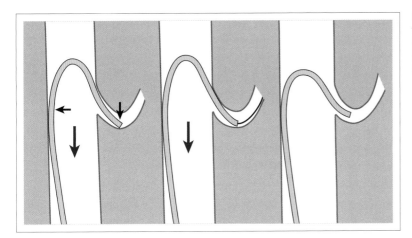

Fig. 2.31 Where the distal segment is too long, it can injure the vascular wall (**a**). Protect the catheter wall with a wire (**b**) or use a catheter with a shorter distal segment (**c**).

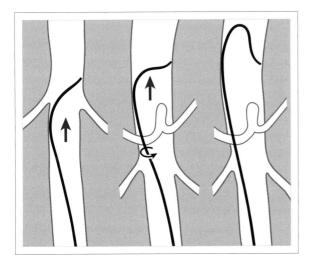

Fig. 2.32 Turning the tip backward by rapidly advancing and turning the catheter.
a Advancing the catheter.
b Rapidly advance and turn.
c Redirected catheter.

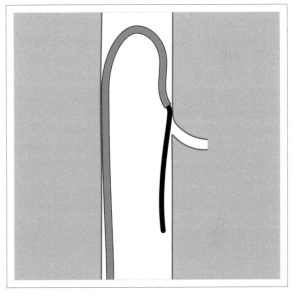

Fig. 2.33 A wire with a soft tip prevents the catheter from "hooking into" the wrong branch artery as it is drawn in a caudal direction.

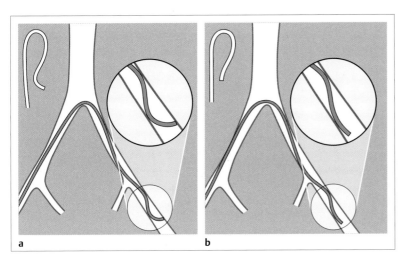

Fig. 2.34 Crossover catheterization of the iliac arteries.
a A pronounced outward bend at tip of the catheter makes it easier to insert into the contralateral iliac artery. However, the tip impinges against the wall of the external iliac artery.
b A catheter tip with only a slight outward bend is not as easily inserted into the contralateral artery. However, once it passes into the external iliac artery, the catheter tip will be better centered within the lumen.

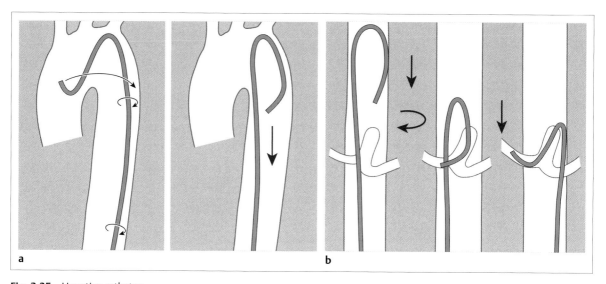

Fig. 2.35 Hepatica catheter.
a Turning the catheter within the aortic arch by rotating it clockwise.

b Catheterizing the celiac trunk and hepatic artery.

Josef Rösch described a very elegant catheter design, the RH (Rösch Hepatica, Cook Medical), for catheterizing the celiac trunk, common hepatic artery, and even the superior mesenteric artery where indicated. The main bend in the catheter angles a 4 cm segment downward. A segment ~1.5 cm long extends rightward from the plane of this bend. When the catheter is at least 80 cm long, its tip can be turned backward within the aortic arch by rotating the catheter clockwise. Then the tip will point in an anterior direction when it lies to the left of the ascending shaft of the catheter. And the origin of the celiac trunk usually lies to the left of the midline. Once the catheter tip has entered the ostium, one pulls it with a slight counterclockwise twist into the origin of the common hepatic artery (**Fig. 2.35**). It is very stable in this position and will not dislodge back into the aorta even at high-contrast flow rates. This is a very reliable approach for chemoembolization of the liver also.

A longer distal segment (SIM1−4) requires a special maneuver to bring it into an inferior position. Usually one enters the left subclavian artery and secures this position by advancing a wire into the subclavian artery (not the vertebral artery!). Then the catheter is advanced into the subclavian artery until its bend lies just proximal to the vessel's origin. The wire is withdrawn to below this bend, and the catheter is pushed backward out of the subclavian artery with a slight twist (**Fig. 2.36**).

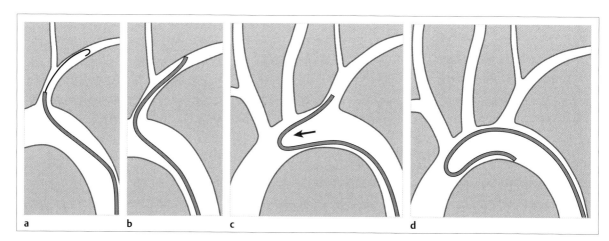

Fig. 2.36 Turning a SIM2 catheter at the left subclavian artery.
a The wire is advanced deep into the left subclavian artery.
b The catheter is advanced until its bend lies just proximal to the origin of the artery.

c The wire is withdrawn to below this bend, and the catheter is pushed backward out of the subclavian artery with a slight twist.
d The redirected catheter lies within the aortic arch.

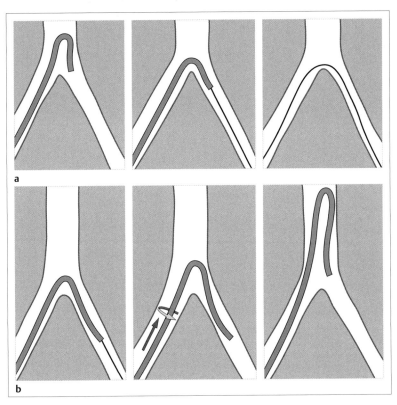

Fig. 2.37 Turning a SIM catheter at the aortic bifurcation.
a A wire is advanced to the contralateral side through a catheter with a short bend.
b Then the SIM catheter is advanced over the wire, the wire is withdrawn, and the catheter is pushed superiorly while being given a slight twist.

Naturally one can also turn a SIM or Hepatica catheter at the aortic bifurcation using the technique shown in **Fig. 2.37**: The contralateral iliac arteries are catheterized with a suitable catheter and guidewire. Then this catheter is exchanged for the catheter with its long distal segment, which is now advanced over the guidewire into the contralateral side up to its main bend. Then the wire is withdrawn and the catheter is pushed backward into the aorta with a slight twist. This is a very safe and reliable technique. However, the catheter with the short distal segment is needed as well for the crossover catheterization.

Cope et al (1990) described a very interesting alternative (see also Stavropoulos et al 2006): A 4° plastic suture with a knot at its end is fed backward into the tip of the catheter. From the other end, a guidewire is pushed through the catheter so that it blocks the tip sufficiently to prevent the knot from being pulled out of the catheter (**Fig. 2.38**). Then the catheter with wire and suture is inserted through a sheath. In the upper abdominal aorta, the tip of the catheter with the suture is held back as the catheter is advanced (**Fig. 2.39**). Once the bend in the catheter is fully developed, the wire is withdrawn to release the suture from the catheter. This technique has the advantage of avoiding every risk of complication in the branches of the aortic arch. Cope's technique can also be used with a Hepatica catheter.

A SIM2 or SIM3 catheter (for an elongated aortic arch) is almost always suitable for catheterizing the branches of the aortic arch (brachiocephalic trunk, right common carotid artery, left common carotid artery, and left subclavian artery). Once the tip has been turned backward one can effortlessly draw this catheter into any of these branch arteries (**Fig. 2.40**).

In approximately one quarter of all cases, the left common carotid artery arises from the brachiocephalic trunk. To catheterize the left carotid artery in this situation, first advance the catheter into the brachiocephalic trunk. Then, giving it a counterclockwise twist to rotate

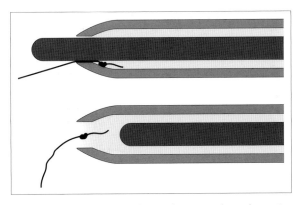

Fig. 2.38 The wire holds a knotted suture in the catheter tip. Withdrawing the wire releases the suture.

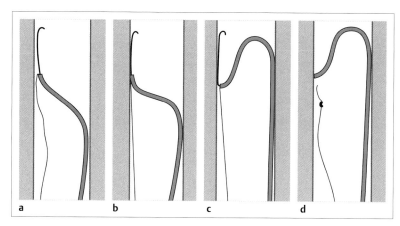

Fig. 2.39 Cope's method of turning a catheter using a suture.
a The suture holds back the catheter tip in the upper abdominal aorta.
b The catheter is advanced.
c Once the bend in the catheter is fully developed, the wire is withdrawn to release the suture from the catheter.
d Redirected catheter.

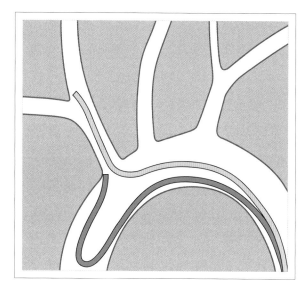

Fig. 2.40 Size issues with a SIM2 catheter: the length of the distal segment is not always sufficient to ensure reliable placement within the right common carotid artery.

the catheter tip into an anterior position, slowly push it back out until the tip drops into the origin of the left common carotid artery. Then pull it into the left common carotid artery.

Catheterization of the right subclavian and right or left internal carotid arteries is best performed with soft 4 French catheters having a short curve at the tip and a large bend in the opposite direction. The large bend fits the aortic arch and reliably aligns the curved tip superiorly, facing the branches of the aortic arch (e.g., JB2, JB3; **Fig. 2.41**, see also **Fig. 2.8** and **Fig. 2.9**). Such a catheter can be hooked into each of the aortic branch arteries. One can advance a curved glide wire into the desired branch artery and then push the catheter in over it.

Catheters for Interventional Manipulations

With the development of interventional radiology, a group of catheters have been described whose primary

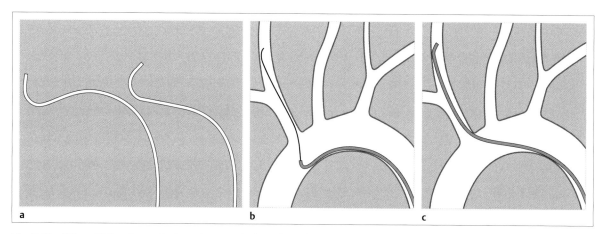

Fig. 2.41 JB2 and JB3 catheters for insertion into the branches of the aortic arch using a curved glide wire.
a JB2 and JB3 catheters.
b Glide wire inserted.
c Catheter advanced over the wire.

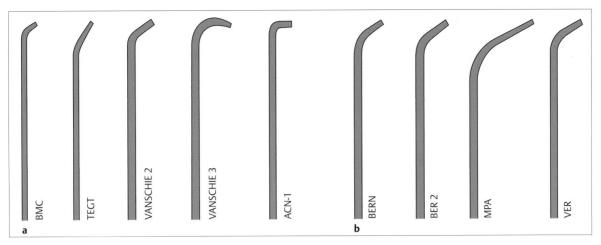

Fig. 2.42 Examples of catheters for manipulation.

a Cook.
b Cordis.

function is less to catheterize the aortic branch arteries than to change direction within a vessel or choose between two branches of a vessel. This is done in part with the aid of steerable guidewires also. Such catheters have a straight shaft and an angled tip (**Fig. 2.42**). The available catheter shapes often vary only slightly. So-called **support catheters**, straight or slightly angled, are used in combination with special guidewires to recanalize occluded artery segments. They have an increased pushability and a tapered low-profile tip for ease of lesion entry.

Changing the Shape of the Catheter

The available catheters or guiding sheaths do not always have the precise shape needed for a specific task. In such cases, it is good to have an electric kettle at hand. It can produce steam with just a little water in a few minutes. One can then heat up the catheter in the steam, bend it to the needed shape, and quickly quench it in a cold sterile saline solution (**Fig. 2.43**). The important thing is to hold the catheter in the steam and cold saline solution long enough for the entire catheter wall to assume the temperature. The process can be repeated to properly define the desired shape. It is not always easy to hold the catheter in the desired shape in the steam without burning one's fingers. One trick is to insert a sterile copper wire into the catheter and shape them both together. One can also use a guidewire inserted backward into the tip of the catheter.

Guiding sheaths can be shaped in steam just like catheters. The spiral metal reinforcement in the wall of the sheath will facilitate this process. When one bends the sheath while cold, the metal will retain this shape for a while. The shape can then be stabilized in the steam.

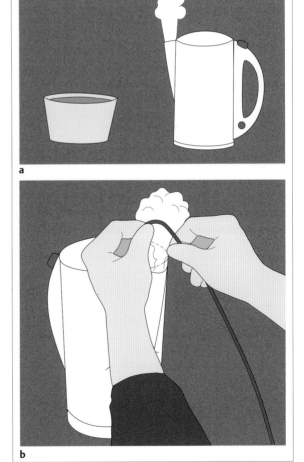

Fig. 2.43 Shaping a catheter.
a Electric kettle and bowl of cold sterile water.
b Shaping the catheter in steam.

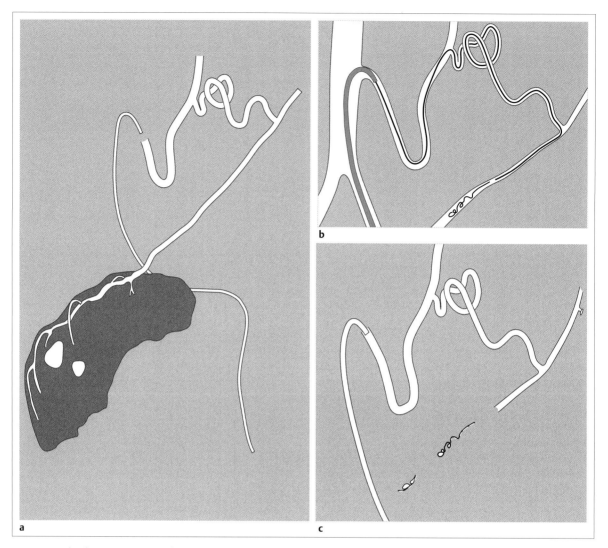

Fig. 2.44 Bleeding recurrent rectal carcinoma embolized with minicoils placed via microcatheter.
a Angiography via the inferior mesenteric artery.   **c** Minicoils occlude the bleeding branch.
b Microcatheter in bleeding branch, embolization.

Microcatheters for Embolization

Embolization of small vascular branches with minicoils or particles is performed with microcatheters introduced coaxially through catheters of 4 or 5 French diameter. These microcatheters are very flexible and can be steered with a very fine wire (0.010, 0.012, 0.014, 0.016, or 0.018 in.). The outer diameter of the microcatheters ranges between 1.5 and 2.8 French; the proximal end is usually thicker to facilitate steering.

The target vessel is first catheterized with an angiography catheter, which is advanced as far as possible. The fine guidewire used with the microcatheter usually requires a slightly curved tip. A twist grip is attached to the proximal end of the wire to steer it. The actual catheterization

procedure involves introducing the wire into the desired branch and then, once the wire has achieved a sufficiently stable position, advancing the microcatheter over it. If necessary this process is repeated several times until the catheter tip has reached the desired position (**Fig. 2.44**).

When a catheter lies within a sheath, the space between the catheter and sheath is open to the vessel; it is sealed off from the outside by the valve of the sheath. If one places a smaller catheter such as a microcatheter within the catheter, one can seal the space between the two catheters with a **hemostatic valve** attached to the outer catheter.

Wherever this sort of seal must be adapted to widely varying catheter sizes or wires or must withstand

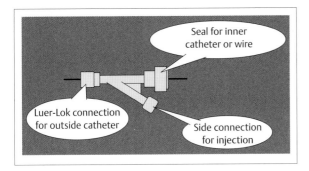

Fig. 2.45 Tuohy-Borst adapter.

higher pressure, a so-called **Tuohy-Borst adapter** is used. This device has an adjusting screw over the valve that can be used to vary the width of the valve (**Fig. 2.45**).

Special catheters for local thrombolysis (pulse-spray lysis) and thrombus aspiration are discussed in Chapter 3 (Local Thrombolysis, p. 97; Aspiration of Thrombus, p. 105).

Balloon Catheters

The treatment of stenosis or occlusion first described by Charles Dotter in 1964 consisted of dilation with the aid of a system of telescoping catheters. This procedure had two essential drawbacks: The dilation produced strong shear stresses in the vascular wall, and the vascular lumen achieved by the treatment could never be larger than the access opening in the vascular wall. Only the balloon catheters developed by Grüntzig and Hopf and available since 1975 have made **genuine dilation** possible. This means introducing a narrow instrument into the vascular lumen and expanding the vessel by applying a force only perpendicular to the vascular wall. An equally important factor was that it now became possible to obtain a lumen several times the size of the access opening.

Balloon catheters vary according to the following parameters:
- Width of the balloon
- Length of the balloon
- Length of the catheter
- Caliber of the catheter (balloon segment and catheter shaft) or required sheath size
- Thickness of the guidewire over which the catheter is advanced

Slender systems with 0.018 or 0.014 in. guidewires and catheters of 3 or 4 French diameter are usually marketed as "low profile" systems.

Balloon catheters are invariably introduced through sheaths and over guidewires. The sheath is necessary to prevent injury to the vascular wall because after dilation the balloon will never be as neatly and smoothly folded as it was when introduced into the vessel.

Over the Wire and Monorail

The traditional "over the wire" (OTW) catheters are the most common. They have two lumens, the larger one for the guidewire and the smaller one for inflating and deflating the balloon. The guidewire lumen extends the full length of the catheter from its tip to its proximal hub. This lumen is also used for injecting contrast agent, saline solution for flushing, or medications (**Fig. 2.46**).

In the newer "monorail" or "rapid exchange" (RX) system, the guidewire lumen extends proximally only a short distance from the catheter tip and balloon. The wire inserted into the catheter tip exits from the catheter right behind the balloon segment so that the long

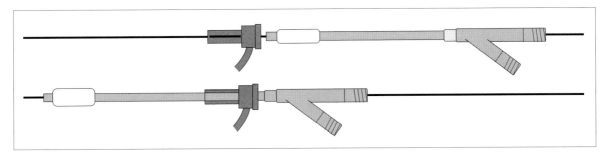

Fig. 2.46 Over the wire catheter (OTW).

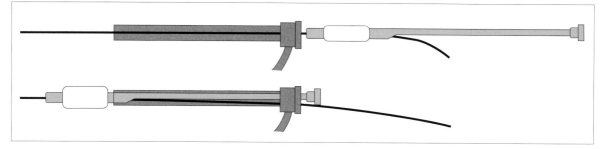

Fig. 2.47 "Monorail" or "rapid exchange" (RX) catheter.

catheter shaft needs only a single lumen through which the balloon is inflated and deflated (**Fig. 2.47**).

This system has its advantages, particularly in situations where the vessel to be treated is far away from the access site and the balloon catheter is introduced over a wire that already lies within the stenosis. In such cases a monorail system can be used with a shorter wire. This means the wire need not be long enough to cover the entire distance within the vessel plus the length of the catheter outside the body. It is also easier to hold the wire in a certain position.

The monorail system originally used in cardiology can also be used to advantage in other vessels, for example, in the renal arteries. Yet, because the wire in a monorail catheter no longer stabilizes the catheter shaft, less shear force can be applied to the catheter tip. Therefore it is recommended to use monorail systems only with long sheaths or guiding catheters.

OTW balloon catheters with a shaft diameter of 4 to 5 French and the balloon segment of which will fit through a 5 French sheath are now commonly used for routine procedures in the arteries of the pelvis and thigh. They are introduced over 0.035 in. wires and are therefore relatively easy to handle. They are also reasonably priced. However, it is not uncommon to encounter stenoses in the superficial femoral and popliteal arteries that are too narrow to allow passage of a 5 French catheter. For this purpose (possibly only for preliminary dilation), for arteries of the lower leg, and for the renal arteries in most cases, one will need narrower catheters whose shaft and balloon segment do not exceed 3 or 4 French. These catheters always require a thinner wire (0.018 or 0.014 in.).

Balloon Catheters with "Compliance"

An obvious basic requirement for percutaneous transluminal angioplasty (PTA) is that balloons must be made of a material that can withstand very high pressure. This will ensure that the balloons will maintain a reliably defined constant diameter over a relatively broad range of pressure (between 4 and 10 bar). This applies to the majority of available catheters.

There are also balloons with so-called compliance, whose diameter varies by ∼10% with pressure. Such a balloon may be, say, 6 mm in diameter at 8 bar but 6.5 mm in diameter at 14 bar (a table included in the package will show the degree of variation with pressure). This is a very useful characteristic for everyday routine practice. If the results of percutaneous transluminal angioplasty are unsatisfactory, one can repeat the dilation with the same catheter and a higher pressure. This saves one from having to introduce a second catheter with a larger balloon several times (**Fig. 2.48**).

Balloon Rupture

The manufacturer usually specifies a maximum pressure that may not be exceeded so as to reliably exclude the risk of the balloon bursting. Knowing this pressure is of interest when dilating a particularly obstinate stenosis, such as in a stenosed dialysis shunt.

Previously it was recommended to test the strength of every balloon prior to introducing it into the patient. This recommendation is no longer current. The quality of balloons today is such that leaks have become exceedingly rare.

A clear argument against testing the balloon is the fact that, once unfolded, the balloon can never be repacked as tightly as when it left the factory. The test inflation causes the balloon to lose its relatively smooth surface, which can make it more difficult to catheterize a narrow stenosis. This may also increase the risk of dislodging occlusive material from the vascular segment being treated. Such material might then be carried into the periphery by the bloodstream.

If the balloon slowly loses pressure, then a fine hole is probably the cause. This is a rare occurrence and is probably the result of the balloon having been punctured by a sharp calcification. Larger tears in the balloon are far less common. A balloon that has sustained a longitudinal tear can be easily withdrawn through the sheath and replaced with a new one. This maneuver may become difficult only

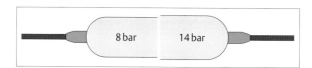

Fig. 2.48 Balloon catheter with compliance.

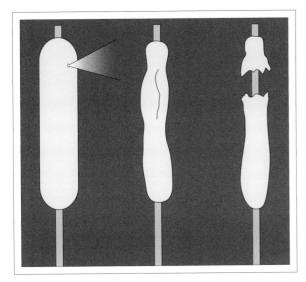

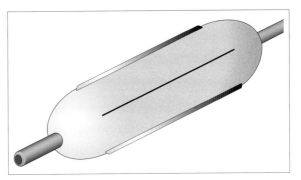

Fig. 2.50 Cutting balloon (Boston Scientific).

The balloon consists of an elastic latex skin (**Fig. 2.51**). Occlusion balloons are filled with dilute contrast agent at low pressure under fluoroscopic control.

Manometer Syringes

One can easily verify that with a good quality 10 mL syringe and moderate effort one can generate ∼10 bar of pressure.

If one uses a 5 mL syringe, the same effort will generate significantly higher pressure!

As an alternative to a strong hand, manufacturers supply syringes with an integral manometer that generates pressure with the aid of a screw thread (**Fig. 2.52**). These syringes have decisive advantages over uncontrolled manual pressure:

- Pressure can be increased gradually (this prevents unnecessary dissections).
- Pressure can be correctly adapted to the balloon used and the vessel caliber.
- A specified pressure can be more easily maintained over an extended period of time (often leading to better results).

Manometer syringes are disposable instruments. It is possible to cut the cost of one nearly in half by avoiding the most common, elaborate, and relatively convenient designs and opting instead for a very simple model (such as the LeVeen inflator from Boston Scientific).

Fig. 2.49 Types of balloon damage. Only the third form poses problems.

when the balloon has sustained a transverse tear (**Fig. 2.49**). Failure to draw the balloon into the sheath while rotating it will necessitate consultation with a vascular surgeon.

Other Special Balloon Catheters

Balloon Catheters with a Coated Surface
Like many other catheters, balloon catheters are also available with a hydrophilic coating. This can be helpful in catheterizing narrow stenoses and negotiating difficult curves.

The beneficial effect of a cytostatic agent (paclitaxel) applied to the vascular wall in preventing recurrent stenosis now appears to have been conclusively demonstrated, even for a single application during dilation. This is done using balloons the surface of which has been treated with the cytostatic agent (Kedhi et al 2008, Tepe et al 2010).

Cutting Balloons
The effect of simple dilation of a stenosis may be augmented by making incisions in the stenosing plaque. Special cutting balloons with four low longitudinal blades on their surface have been developed for this purpose (**Fig. 2.50**). The blades are hidden under the folds of the deflated balloon. When the balloon is inflated, the blades project from its surface and make four fine incisions in the thickened vascular wall wherever the blades come into contact with it.

Occlusion Balloons
Occlusion balloons are rarely used in endovascular interventions. They may be helpful in therapeutic embolization with an embolic liquid. They differ from Fogarty catheters in that they have a second lumen for the guidewire or for transporting the embolic liquid.

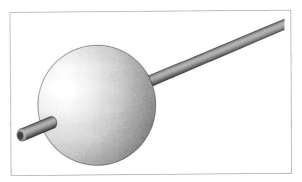

Fig. 2.51 Occlusion balloon.

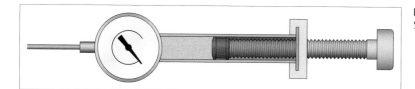

Fig. 2.52   LeVeen Inflator (Boston Scientific).

Stents

Stents are tubular metal meshes that maintain the patency of the vascular lumen when placed in a stenosis. Stents were introduced in everyday practice around 1990, following a long period of development. This may even be regarded as the decisive breakthrough that established interventional radiology as a discipline on an equal footing with vascular surgery. Before this, there had been many cases in which we could only hope that residual stenoses and dissections would not lead to recurrent occlusion. Now we could complete the treatment of such cases with a genuinely impressive result.

Yet there is one obvious limitation: The initial gain in lumen diameter is indeed greater than with simple balloon dilation. Yet stents lead to greater intimal cellular proliferation, meaning that over time the initial advantage can be partially reversed (the "late lumen loss" described by Kedhi et al 2008).

Occasionally it has been recommended to dilate a stenosis prior to planned stent implantation. This only serves a purpose where the results of PTA will determine whether additional placement of a stent is indicated. Otherwise the only plausible case would be where the stenosis is so narrow and rigid as to prevent the passage of a sheath or the application system for the stent. Where primary stent implantation is feasible, it is the quickest and cheapest solution, and it also diminishes the risk of thrombus material from the occluded segment entering the bloodstream. As soon as it is unfolded, the stent's mesh restrains all coarse thrombus material that might otherwise be mobilized.

We differentiate two classes of stents according to their material, function, and area of application:
- Balloon-expandable stents
- Self-expanding stents

Although commonly used, the expression "self-expandable" is semantically incorrect. The suffix "-able" denotes a passive process, whereas the stent **actively** expands itself as a result of its intrinsic elasticity.

Balloon-Expandable Stents

The vast majority of balloon-expandable stents are made of stainless steel, a few of cobalt-chrome alloy. Steel tubes of the proper size are cut with a laser to create a **slotted tube** (**Fig. 2.53**) that can be expanded into a tubular mesh.

This simple design has two disadvantages: It shortens when expanded, and it cannot adapt to any bend.

The relatively complex patterns in common use today serve several purposes:
- They prevent shortening when expanded.
- They allow the stent to adapt to a curved vascular segment.
- They maximize radial force.
- They cover the inner surface of the diseased vessel as uniformly as possible.

Fig. 2.54 shows an example (drawn according to the Express Vascular LD from Boston Scientific) of how shortening of the stent can be avoided: The longitudinal connections remain aligned parallel to the longitudinal axis of the vessel, and they each connect two points that move in the same manner.

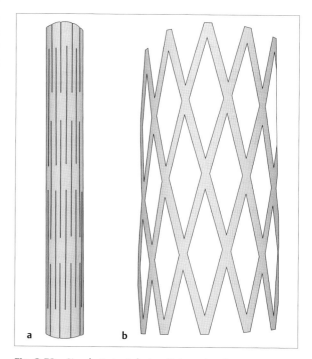

a   b

Fig. 2.53   Simplest stent design (Palmaz type).
a Initial state (slotted tube).
b After expansion: tubular mesh.

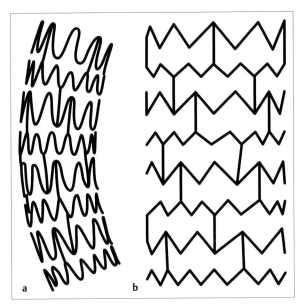

Fig. 2.54 Balloon-expandable stent (Express Vascular LD, Boston Scientific).
a Initial state (can be guided around curves).
b Expanded stent: the stent's longitudinal connections remain aligned parallel to the longitudinal axis.

Balloon-expandable stents generally have the following advantages:

- With their high radial strength they have very good chances of maintaining patency even in hard stenoses.
- They can be placed with greater precision.

Ideal **indications** for balloon-expandable stents are therefore stenosis and occlusion in the proximal iliac arteries, where there is minimal motion and significant calcifications may be expected, and renal arterial stenosis, where very precise placement is crucial.

Balloon-expandable stents are usually supplied attached to balloons of the appropriate size. They are introduced through sheaths and brought into the proper position with an overlay, using "road mapping," under angiographic control, or according to reliable anatomical landmarks such as bone margins or mural calcifications. Once in position, they are pressed against the vascular wall by the inflated balloon (**Fig. 2.55a**).

Wherever residual stenosis is present or the stent is not in contact with the wall at every point, a larger balloon should be used to further expand the stent over its entire length (**Fig. 2.55b**) or in the affected segment (see **Fig. 3.88**).

Ready-to-use stents mounted on balloons are available for vessel diameters of 2 to 10 mm. Larger stents, such as for the lower abdominal aorta, are supplied separately and must be fit over a balloon of the appropriate size by the attending physician. This procedure is not recommended for anyone who lacks extensive experience in dealing with stents. Good alternatives are available: a Wallstent (Boston Scientific) or nitinol stent of the appropriate size.

Balloon-expandable stents are supplied in lengths of 12 to 57 mm.

Self-Expanding Stents

The Wallstent, the first self-expanding stent, was introduced at about the same time as the Palmaz stent (Palmaz Scientific, Dallas, TX, USA). It consists of a tubular, self-expanding mesh of fine steel wire (**Fig. 2.56**). Today it is primarily used in the carotid arteries and wide-lumen vessels such as the infrarenal abdominal aorta or superior vena cava. These stents are flexible and have relatively high radial strength, and they uniformly

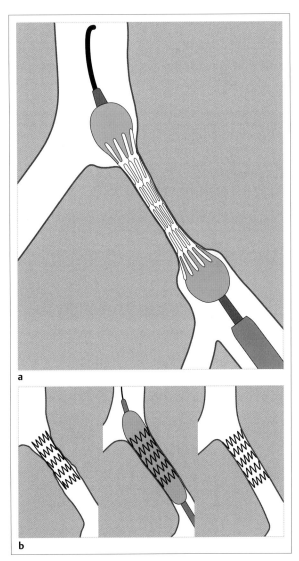

Fig. 2.55 Placing a balloon-expandable stent.
a Balloon and stent begin to expand.
b A stent that does not uniformly cover the vascular wall must be further expanded by a larger balloon.

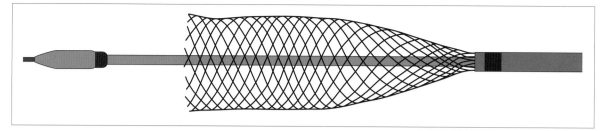

Fig. 2.56 Wallstent (Boston Scientific): self-expanding stent of elastic steel wire.

cover the vascular wall with a narrow mesh (closed cell design). However, when implanted they shorten by between 6 and 20% depending on vessel diameter. This is always a disadvantage where precision placement is crucial.

The vast majority of self-expanding stents are made of nitinol, an alloy of nickel and titanium. Most nitinol stents are cut with laser beams from tubes of the proper length and diameter. They are supplied on application systems in which they lie on an inner catheter covered by a thin-walled outer catheter.

Once they have been introduced through a sheath and brought into the correct position, the outer catheter is withdrawn to deploy the stent (**Fig. 2.57**).

> **Important:** In this maneuver the inner catheter must not be moved and the outer catheter must not be immobilized (**Fig. 2.58**)!

In the case of some products, the outer catheter is withdrawn by turning a wheel or actuating a slide device on a grip on the hub of the instrument. This neither simplifies the process nor does it exclude the risk of inadvertently immobilizing the outer catheter instead of the grip.

Once deployed, the stent will assume its set width after a slight delay. The radial force with which it presses itself into the vascular wall reaches its maximum only under the influence of body temperature; the material has a "memory effect," the memory of a programmed diameter. Often the strength of the stent will be insufficient to eliminate the stenosis completely. However, in most cases the residual stenosis can be eliminated by additional balloon dilation.

Nitinol stents up to 12 mm in diameter are available for use in the arteries of the pelvis and legs. To ensure that the stent is reliably pressed against the vascular wall, one should always select the nominal stent size 1 mm larger than the vessel diameter measured.

> Subsequently inflating a balloon cannot expand a nitinol stent any further. For this reason it is not possible to use balloon dilation to fix in place a stent that has insufficient contact with the wall.

Nitinol does not show up as well as steel on radiographs. Therefore it is recommended, especially in the iliac arteries, to use only stents with markings of gold, platinum, or tantalum on both ends. The essential advantage of nitinol

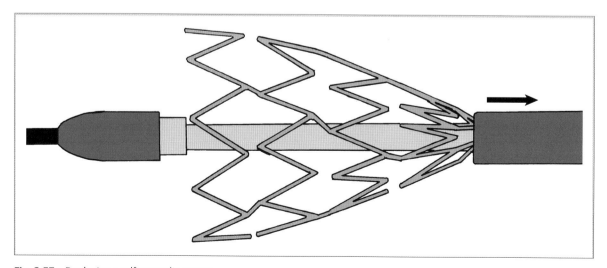

Fig. 2.57 Deploying a self-expanding stent.

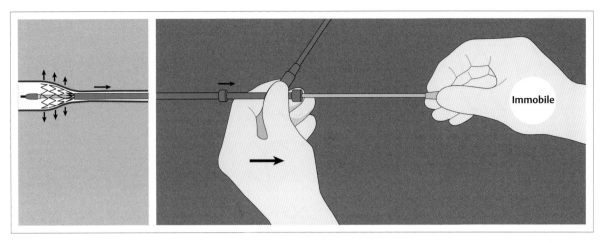

Fig. 2.58 Deploying a self-expanding stent: inner catheter must not be moved and outer one must not be immobilized.

stents lies in their flexibility. They can better adapt to vessels of varying caliber than steel stents. This assumes that one selects a sufficiently large stent.

The SUPERA stent (IDEV Technologies, Webster, TX, USA) is a unique design, consisting of 2×6 elastic nitinol wires arranged in a spiral pattern resembling crisscrossed left-handed and right-handed threading. The wires are interwoven but only fused together at the ends of the stent (**Fig. 2.59**). This structure gives the stent extraordinary flexibility. At the same time, this stent has several times the radial strength of standard nitinol stents. The SUPERA stent shortens greatly when it is unfolded in the vessel. Yet this effect is only possible when the stent is pushed out of the applicator when deployed. This is done with the aid of a pusher on the grip of the applicator under continuous fluoroscopic control. The stent will unfold correctly only when the vessel has been previously dilated to the outer diameter of the stent ($\sim$10% > than the specified stent size).

Stent Design

A stent's characteristics depend not only on its material but also on its design. A Palmaz stent (see **Fig. 2.53**) consisting of interconnected rhombic cells lacks flexibility and cannot adapt to any curve in the vessel. Because it is essentially the ring-shaped elements of the stent that maintain patency, some of the longitudinal connections between the circular "modules" can be removed to make the stent flexible. A stent consisting of circular zigzag struts interspersed with individual longitudinal connections is referred to as a **modular design**.

Eliminating longitudinal connections increases the size of the cells, creating what are referred to as **open cells**. Stents with open cells have the advantage of flexibility but do not cover the vascular wall as uniformly as

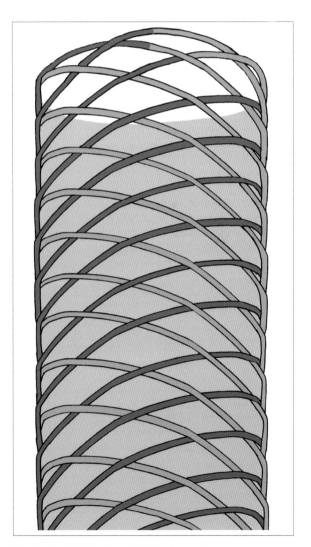

Fig. 2.59 SUPERA stent (IDEV Technologies).

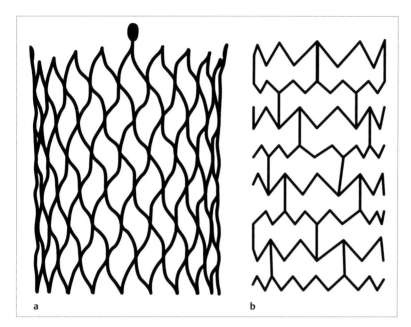

Fig. 2.60 Stent design.
a Closed cell (Sinus stent, OptiMed): nitinol with tantalum markers.
b Open cell (Express, Boston Scientific): steel.

other designs and are therefore less stable (**Fig. 2.60b**). Stents with **closed cells** are less flexible but very stable. They cover the inner surface of the vessel relatively uniformly (see **Fig. 2.56** and **Fig. 2.60a**). The SUPERA stent (see **Fig. 2.59**) is a stent that combines semiclosed cells with extreme flexibility and extraordinarily high radial strength.

A typical **indication** for a closed cell stent is an abdominal aorta with a hemodynamically significant stenosis. The vessel usually courses in a straight line, and a relatively high strength stent will be required to maintain a patent lumen. Because the inner surface is often severely fissured (rugged), uniform stent coverage is desirable. In this case, a closed cell design would be the optimal solution. On the other hand, a stent with an open cell design would be better adapted to a curved external iliac artery. A longer stenosis is best treated with a single long stent. Where several stents must be placed in succession, they should overlap by at least 5 mm.

Covered Stents (Stent Grafts)

In the vast majority of cases it is sufficient when the stent simply maintains patency without sealing the vascular wall. Sealing a mural tear or perforation or eliminating an aneurysm requires a stent combined with a closed membrane. This is referred to as a covered stent, stent graft, or endoprosthesis.

In its simplest form (e.g., Jostent, Abbott Vascular, Temecula, CA, USA), it consists of a tubular polytetrafluoroethylene (PTFE) sleeve between two balloon-expandable stents (**Fig. 2.61**). Self-expanding stents on

the other hand are integrated into the fabric of a vascular prosthesis. The endovascular aortic prosthesis represents the most important area of application for this. The Viabahn series (W. L. Gore & Associates, Flagstaff, AZ, USA) includes flexible and elastic vascular prostheses up to 25 cm long for use in the arteries of the

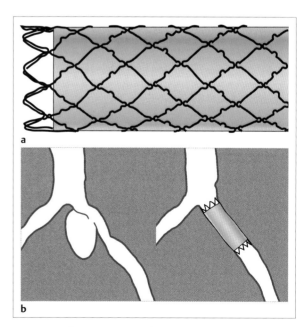

Fig. 2.61 Eliminating a pseudoaneurysm with a Jostent (Abbott Vascular).
a Tubular polytetrafluoroethylene sleeve between two balloon-expandable stents.
b Stent covers the mouth of the aneurysm.

pelvis and thigh. These are intended to function like an endovascular bypass.

Although it may be difficult to decide which model of covered stent to use, it is a good idea to keep a few covered stents on hand for emergencies. The most important example of such an **emergency** is the rupture of a blood vessel. This can occur with dilating abdominal arteries, a renal artery, an iliac artery, or the abdominal aorta.

Eliminating an aneurysm with covered stents is usually an elective procedure for which the specific material can be ordered in advance.

Drug-Eluting Stents

In recent years the possibility of coating stents with medications or radioactive substances has been the subject of extensive research and discussion. In such cases the surface of the stent is coated with a carrier layer that gives off the active ingredient into the vascular wall over an extended period of time.

So far, published results have largely been encouraging. However, these stents have not yet come into widespread clinical use, due in part to their high cost.

Contrast Agents

Radiologic interventions are controlled by fluoroscopy and angiography. There is no discernible difference in the radiodensity of the vascular contents and that of the surrounding soft tissue. Therefore, blood vessels can be visualized only by altering the radiodensity of the blood by adding a fluid of higher radiodensity (positive contrast) or by injecting gas in place of the blood (negative contrast).

There is very little bonding of contrast agent to plasma protein. As a result, and according to its low molecular weight, contrast agent is excreted by the kidneys by means of glomerular filtration and renal tubular resorption does not occur. The half-life of excretion is ~2 hours with normal kidney function. Slower excretion via the liver (according to the proportion bonded to plasma protein) may occur where kidney function is severely impaired.

Characteristics of Iodine-Containing Contrast Agents

The positive contrast agents used today are almost exclusively organic iodine compounds. Iodine (atomic number 53, atomic weight 127) is responsible for the high absorption of X-rays. It is bound, enveloped, and rendered tolerable by an organic carrier molecule. Each molecule of contrast agent includes one benzene ring on which iodine atoms have been substituted at three positions, alternating with strongly hydrophilic groups at the other three positions. These **hydrophilic groups** are what differentiates the various commercially available contrast agents.

The great majority of contrast agents in use today are monomers with one benzene ring and three iodine atoms per molecule. There is only one dimeric contrast agent with six iodine atoms per molecule on the market (iodixanol). This dimeric contrast agent is iso-osmolar with blood. Monomeric contrast agents are slightly hyperosmolar and tend to be more or less so depending on their concentration.

The heat and pressure sensations that can accompany injection of contrast agent occur only with hyperosmolar agents. Therefore, using a dimeric contrast agent is recommended when imaging particularly sensitive regions of the body such as the hands and face. A few studies suggest that the dimeric contrast agent iodixanol may also be more tolerable for the kidneys. However, these findings apparently require definitive confirmation.

Side Effects

There are no significant differences among the various nonionic agents with respect to their suitability as contrast agents. It is important to understand that **adverse reactions to contrast agents** are not caused by the iodine but by the organic carrier molecule. When a patient did not tolerate a certain contrast agent, then a different preparation must be selected for any subsequent examination. This will minimize the risk of a second reaction. Therefore the name, concentration, and quantity of the contrast agent used should be documented in every report of findings.

> Referring to an "iodine allergy" is incorrect. Whoever documents an iodine allergy in a report of findings commits an act of negligence because this makes it much harder to avoid an incident in subsequent applications of contrast agent.
> Aside from dictating the use of a different contrast agent, any history of adverse reaction to contrast agent means that the customary prophylaxis with cortisone and antihistamines is indicated.

The more moderate adverse reactions were far more common with the ionic contrast agents used in Germany into the 1980s, and in some other countries into the 1990s, especially for excretory urography.

Therefore, when an older patient reports having had an adverse reaction during a kidney examination performed at this time, it is unlikely that a reaction to a nonionic contrast agent for angiography will also occur.

Contrast agents invariably contain trace amounts of **free iodine (iodide)**. This is stored in the thyroid gland and in certain metabolic situations (increased TSH level) can lead to hyperthyroidism or trigger a thyrotoxic crisis (see Chapter 1, Preparing the Patient, p. 5).

All contrast agents are supplied in different concentrations (150 to 400 mg of iodine/mL). A concentration of 300 mg of iodine/mL is usually used for endovascular interventions.

Gadolinium-Containing Contrast Agents

For several years patients with severely impaired kidney function were given gadolinium contrast agents as an alternative to iodine-containing substances. This practice was discontinued when it was revealed that gadolinium agents pose a specific risk of causing nephrogenic systemic fibrosis. This is an occasionally fatal disease that manifests itself primarily in the skin and for which there is no known treatment. The use of gadolinium contrast is not advisable in patients with a glomerular filtration rate (GFR) less than 60 mL/min/1.73 m^2 (normal value: 100–160 mL/min/1.73 m^2, Miki et al 2009).

Other disadvantages of gadolinium include its comparatively low contrast density and the need to limit the dose to 40 mL.

CO$_2$ as a Contrast Agent

CO$_2$ is the best alternative to iodine-containing contrast agents in patients with hyperthyroidism, patients who have experienced a previous adverse reaction, and especially patients with impaired kidney function. However, its use requires special equipment, including the following:
- A pressurized container with medical grade CO$_2$
- A reducing valve for low pressure
- A bacterial filter
- Two connecting tubes with a special three-way stopcock
- A 50 mL syringe connected to the tubes via the three-way stopcock

- A program in the angiography system (digital subtraction angiography) that can generate a single screen image from a series of individual exposures (**Fig. 2.62**).

In any case it is a good idea to keep everything needed for CO$_2$ angiography on hand.

The **pressurized container** with CO$_2$ must never be directly connected to the catheter leading to the patient. The pressure is reduced to a low value (0.3 bar), and the gas is then fed through the bacterial filter and conducted from there to the three-way stopcock. The stopcock should not allow a direct connection to the catheter but should only conduct the gas into the injection syringe (**Fig. 2.63**). The gas may only be injected into the catheter from the syringe after the stopcock has been turned.

> The syringe may only be filled passively by the pressure of the CO$_2$. Actively drawing in the gas risks contaminating it with air.

Before the catheter is connected, CO$_2$ is used to **flush** the system repeatedly. The system is filled with CO$_2$, which is then released into the atmosphere. This bleeds any residual air out of the system (remember to close the stopcock to seal the exit line after each flushing). Oxygen and nitrogen must not be allowed into the vascular system because they are far less soluble than CO$_2$ and could therefore block small vessels.

Before beginning any CO$_2$ angiography, flush any residual saline solution or blood out of the catheter by slowly injecting 3 to 5 mL of CO$_2$. If this is not done, injection under pressure will cause the CO$_2$ to shoot out of the catheter explosively as soon as the catheter is free of fluid. The volume of CO$_2$ is adapted as follows to the respective vessel examined:
- Aorta 50 mL
- Iliac arteries 30 to 40 mL
- Single leg 20 to 30 mL (when injected into the external iliac artery)

Raising the leg 20 to 30° will improve the filling of the arteries of the leg. This also reduces the tendency of the CO$_2$ bolus to fragment (**Fig. 2.64**). The relatively high contrast of severe mural calcifications can diminish the

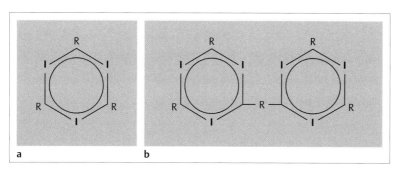

Fig. 2.62 Structure of nonionic iodine-containing radiologic contrast agent. I, iodine; R, hydrophilic group.
a Monomeric contrast agent.
b Dimeric contrast agent.

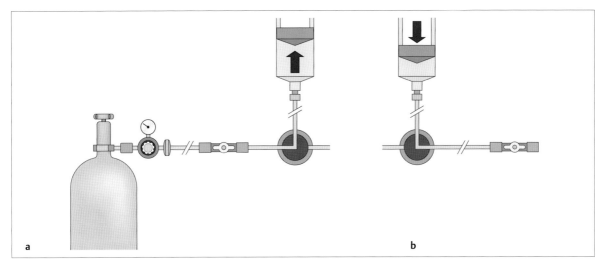

Fig. 2.63 Pressurized container with CO_2, reducing valve, bacterial filter, special three-way stopcock that does not allow CO_2 to flow directly into the catheter.
a Filling the angiography system with CO_2.
b CO_2 injection for angiography.

quality of the angiography. This is particularly true of the arteries of the lower leg, which are narrow and as a result provide poor contrast.

In large vessels such as the aorta, blood can easily **flow deep to** the CO_2 bolus, preventing contrast filling of the posterior branch arteries. To visualize the renal artery of one side, the patient should be placed in a lateral position on the contralateral side. The angiography is then performed as a cross-table examination with a horizontal beam (**Fig. 2.65**). Selective injection of CO_2 with the patient in the same position is recommended to alleviate unsatisfactory image quality.

Even **interventions** such as PTA and stent implantation can be performed using CO_2 as a contrast agent. Because of its low viscosity, the gas is particularly well suited for demonstrating intestinal bleeding.

In patients with **renal insufficiency** it can be helpful to use a small amount of iodine-containing contrast agent to visualize the decisive findings while using CO_2 for everything else. This is especially true for the small vessels of the lower leg.

> Restrictions on the use of CO_2: Because of its potentially toxic effect on cerebral tissue, CO_2 angiography should only be performed below the diaphragm!

Injection of the gas into peripheral vessels can cause discomfort or even severe cramping pain. These symptoms are presumably attributable to ischemia or hypoxemia. Therefore it is recommended to administer oxygen via a nasal tube during the examination. It may also become necessary to administer strong pain medication.

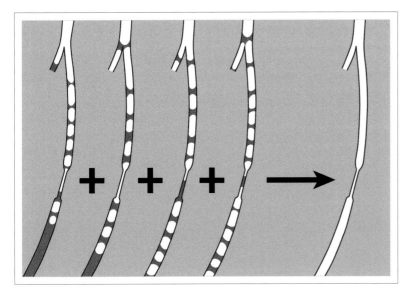

Fig. 2.64 Fragmentation of the bolus occurs easily with CO_2. The image processor generates a single composite image from a series of individual exposures.

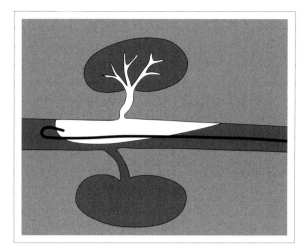

Fig. 2.65 Cross-table CO_2 angiography of a kidney with a horizontal beam and the patient in a lateral position.

(Of course raising a leg tends to promote ischemic pain.) In any case one should allow an interval of 2 to 3 minutes between two injections. No serious side effects in peripheral vessels have been reported.

OptiMed supplies a complete system for CO_2 angiography with the following standardization: A syringe with variable volume settings between 20 and 100 mL is filled at a CO_2 pressure of 1.3 bar and then opened to the catheter. The pressure differential causes the CO_2 to flow into the vascular system without having to press the plunger. A long, very thin connection to the catheter prevents the syringe from being emptied too rapidly (2 to 3 seconds for 20 mL, > 10 seconds for 100 mL).

The CO_2 dissolved in the blood is excreted by the lungs. Pulmonary insufficiency can therefore constitute a contraindication to CO_2 angiography.

Prophylaxis and Treatment of Reactions to Contrast Agents

Prophylaxis
The first important thing is the prophylactic treatment of patients who have experienced adverse reactions during previous interventions or who show signs of allergic diathesis. Because the anaphylactic reaction occurs in response to the organic carrier molecule and not the iodine, the first step in case of a previous reaction is as follows:
- Use a different agent than in the previous examination. This will greatly reduce the likelihood of another reaction.

Nevertheless, every patient with such a previous history should be given the following:
- An oral corticosteroid (such as 30 to 50 mg of prednisolone) 12 to 24 hours before the intervention and on the day of the intervention

- Antihistamines shortly before the intervention: slow intravenous (IV) injection (sequentially, not mixed together) of one ampule each of Fenistil (dimethindene maleate, H1 receptor blocker; Novartis, East Hanover, NJ, USA) and Tagamet (cimetidine, H2 receptor blocker; GlaxoSmithKline, Research Triangle Park, NC, USA)

Treatment
Adverse reactions to contrast agents can vary greatly in their nature and severity.
- **Urticaria:** Mild forms often do not require treatment. Where symptoms are more severe, slow IV injection of an H1 receptor blocker (such as Fenistil) possibly supplemented by an H2 receptor blocker (such as Tagamet) is indicated. Of course an IV corticosteroid is also very effective.
- **Vasovagal syncope** can be caused by a variety of stimuli including contrast agent. Have an assistant elevate the patient's legs and then promptly initiate volume replacement with an infusion of isotonic saline solution. At the same time administer oxygen via a nasal tube and possibly 0.5 mg of IV atropine (contraindicated in patients with glaucoma).
- **Nausea:** This usually occurs with the initial contrast bolus and usually subsides spontaneously within a short time. For persistent nausea, inject an antiemetic such as dimenhydrinate (Vomex A).

An **anaphylactic reaction** is associated with vasodilation and severe interstitial fluid loss (Schild 1996). Volume replacement and treatment with vasopressors are therefore important.

Treatment:
- Oxygen via nasal tube or mask (3 L/min)
- Prompt infusion of isotonic saline solution
- Epinephrine administered slowly by IV injection or subcutaneously; where peripheral perfusion is intact, subcutaneous administration is safest (0.3 to 0.5 mL of 1:1,000 solution, maximum 2 mL). In severe shock with peripheral circulatory collapse, administer 0.1 mg of epinephrine (1 mL of a 1:10,000 solution slowly by IV injection; high risk in patients with coronary insufficiency; Kessel and Robertson 2005).
- Administer an H1 receptor blocker (such as Fenistil 0.1 mg/kg) and an H2 receptor blocker (such as Tagamet 300 mg) by slow IV injection.
- For bronchospasm, administer a β2-antagonist as an inhalational aerosol (such as Salbutamol).
- Administer hydrocortisone or methylprednisolone (500 to 1,000 mg) slowly by IV injection.

It is important to call in an anesthesiologist or other colleagues with the necessary experience at the first signs of serious complications. One should immediately document every serious complication and discuss it candidly with the patient.

Medications

Sedatives

A patient who thoroughly understands what to expect rarely requires a sedative. If the patient remains restless and anxious in spite of this, then midazolam (Dormicum) may be administered. First give the patient 1.5 to 2.5 mg slowly by IV injection. If that is not sufficient, increase the dose to as much as 5 mg. **Caution:** In addition to the 5 mg ampoules there are also ones with 15 and 50 mg. To avoid any confusion you should not store these in your medicine cabinet.

Possible side effect: respiratory depression. For patients over 70 years of age diazepam (2 to 10 mg administered slowly by IV injection) may be more suitable because its effect varies less with age. However, the effect also takes longer to taper off. Sedated patients require monitoring of their blood pressure, pulse, and oxygen saturation (pulse oximetry).

When in doubt, ask an anesthesiologist!

Analgesics

▷ Pain is rare in peripheral endovascular interventions. When a dilation becomes painful, it is an important warning sign not to increase the pressure. This especially applies to percutaneous transluminal angioplasty of abdominal vessels such as the renal arteries, aorta, or iliac arteries. It would be a mistake to reduce the sensitivity to this kind of pain with medications.

Various unspecific pains, such as back pain that prevents the patient from lying relaxed, can usually be treated sufficiently with 20 to 30 drops of oral metamizol (Novalgin) or 1000 mg administered slowly by IV injection.

One situation regularly requires an opioid analgesic for severe pain: When a vessel is reopened by thrombolysis or aspiration thrombectomy after acute occlusion, sensitivity usually returns before the ischemic pain subsides. Here one must expect a brief period of extremely severe pain which must be immediately relieved with an appropriate analgesic, such as piritramide (Dipidolor) (7.5 to 15 mg slowly by IV injection).

Similar pain can occur with the embolization of organ arteries, for example, preoperative or palliative embolization of a renal artery. The intensity of the pain increases the more healthy tissue is affected.

Platelet Aggregation Inhibitors

Acetylsalicylic acid (aspirin) causes irreversible damage to thrombocytes. After the medication is discontinued, coagulation will normalize within about a week after new thrombocytes have formed in sufficient quantities. For this reason aspirin must be discontinued 1 week prior to planned surgery. However, inhibition of platelet aggregation is desirable for endovascular interventions. All patients with peripheral arterial occlusive disease should take aspirin at a dose of 75 to 100 mg daily if they tolerate it. The main risk is bleeding from ulcers. Clopidogrel may be tried as an alternative in patients who do not tolerate aspirin.

The mechanism of action of clopidogrel (Plavix, Bristol-Myers Squibb/Sanofi, New York, NY, USA) (or ticlopidine) is a different one; it selectively inhibits the binding of adenosine diphosphate (ADP). With a half-life of 8 days, clopidogrel's effect also subsides only gradually. The most important side effects include neutropenia and thrombopenia. These occur only very rarely and more often with ticlopidine than with clopidogrel.

At least 2 hours before an endovascular intervention each patient receives 100 mg of oral acetylsalicylic acid or 500 mg intravenously. Where a stent is implanted, the patient also receives clopidogrel (or ticlopidine) for 6 weeks. An initial saturation dose of 300 mg is administered on the first day and a daily dose of 75 mg thereafter. If placement of a stent is planned from the outset, then the saturation dose is administered on the day before the procedure.

Anticoagulants

Heparin is a fast-acting medication for inhibiting coagulation, and its short half-life of ~60 minutes makes it easy to control.
- Measurement of partial thromboplastin time (PTT) allows evaluation of the effect of the heparin.
- For endovascular interventions it is desirable to have an elevated PTT 2 to 2.5 times the normal value of <36 seconds. This means a value between 70 and 90 seconds.
- At the beginning of the intervention, a patient of normal weight is given 5,000 IU of unfractionated heparin (the dose may be reduced to as little as 3,000 IU for small and slender patients).
- In longer interventions ~1,000 IU per hour must be subsequently administered. This is usually done as perfusor-controlled infusion, with the dosage adjusted according to repeated measurements of PTT.

Heparin can be neutralized by injecting protamine: 1 mg of protamine for 100 IU of heparin (maximum 50 mg, administered very slowly by IV injection). Severe allergic reactions are encountered relatively often, especially in patients with a fish allergy. In practice protamine is very rarely needed; this author has never used it.

Whereas unfractionated heparin is used throughout the intervention, low molecular weight heparin is easier to handle during aftercare (Uflacker 2006).

Heparin-induced thrombocytopenia (HIT) is a rare but very serious immune reaction that occurs within 5 to 14 days of the onset of heparin therapy and is clinically characterized by thrombocytopenia and thromboses (Uflacker 2006). It is important to immediately discontinue heparin and switch to an alternate anticoagulant.

As prophylaxis against thromboembolic complications, patients with prosthetic heart valves and patients with deep venous thrombosis and pulmonary embolism receive long-term therapy with an oral anticoagulant such as phenprocoumon (Marcumar). The effectiveness is evaluated by monitoring the international normalized ratio (INR) value (1.0 is normal). The therapeutic range lies at ~2.5 to 4.5. Prior to endovascular interventions, Marcumar usually has to be replaced by heparin (PTT 60 to 80 seconds). This requires close monitoring of the coagulation values, which is best accomplished on the ward.

Thrombolytic Agents

Streptokinase, the first thrombolytic agent available for clinical use, is hardly used today. Urokinase was very well tolerated by patients but had to be taken off the market in 1999 due to problems with production in the United States. Since then it has never regained the position it once held.

Today the vast majority of medications used are tissue plasminogen activators produced by genetic engineering (such as alteplase, reteplase, tenecteplase; see also Chapter 3, Local Thrombolysis, p. 97).

Vasodilators

- Nitroglycerin in a dose of 0.1 to 0.2 mg administered intra-arterially rapidly produces vasodilation and is suitable for treating vasospasms.
- As prophylaxis one may administer the longer-acting verapamil (3 to 5 mg intra-arterially), for example, in the arteries of the arm, lower leg, or kidney.
- Sublingual administration of 10 mg of nifedipine (Adalat; Bayer Pharmaceuticals, Berlin, Germany) is recommended prior to interventions in the arteries of the lower leg, also as prophylaxis against vasospasm.

Emergency Medications

See the section on contrast agents (p. 35).

Recommended technique: When a medication is passed to the physician in a sterile area, it is regularly

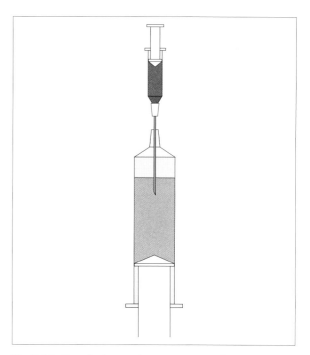

Fig. 2.66 Transferring medication into a sterile syringe. To avoid foam, dip the tip of the cannula into the saline solution.

dissolved in a small volume of fluid. To ensure that none of this volume is lost during injection (remaining in the catheter or sheath) it should be diluted. This means transferring it to a larger syringe (e.g., 20 mL). This can easily produce foam that one cannot inject. This problem can be avoided by dipping the tip of the cannula into the saline solution when one is transferring the fluid (**Fig. 2.66**).

References

Cope C, Burke DR, Meranze SG. Atlas of Interventional Radiology. Philadelphia, PA: Lippincott; 1990:7:18

Kedhi E, Tanguay JF, Bilodeau L. Pathophysiology of restenosis. In: Heuser RR, Henry M, eds. Textbook of Peripheral Vascular Interventions. 2nd ed. London; Informa Healthcare; 2008: 763–769

Kessel D, Robertson I. Interventional Radiology: A Survival Guide. London: Elsevier; 2005:23–32

Miki Y, Isoda H, Togashi K. Guideline to use gadolinium-based contrast agents at Kyoto University Hospital. J Magn Reson Imaging 2009;30(6):1364–1365

Schild H. Kontrastmittel. In: Günther RW, Thelen M, eds.(Hrsg.). Interventionelle Radiologie. Stuttgart, New York: Thieme; 1996: 55–60

Schröder J. The mechanical properties of guidewires. Part I: Stiffness and torsional strength. Cardiovasc Intervent Radiol 1993a;16(1):43–46

Schröder J. The mechanical properties of guidewires. Part II: Kinking resistance. Cardiovasc Intervent Radiol 1993b;16(1): 47–48

Schröder J. The mechanical properties of guidewires. Part III: Sliding friction. Cardiovasc Intervent Radiol 1993c;16(2):93–97

Schröder J, Weber M. Rotational stability of angiography catheters [in German]. Z Kardiol 1992;81(10):538–542

Seldinger SI. Catheter replacement of the needle in percutaneous arteriography; a new technique. Acta Radiol 1953;39(5): 368–376

Sos TA, Trost DW. Renal angioplasty and stenting. In: Kandarpa K, ed. Peripheral Vascular Interventions. Philadelphia, PA: Lippincott Williams & Wilkins; 2008

Stavropoulos SW, Rajan D, Cope C. Catheters, methods, and injectors for superselective catheterization. In: Baum S, Pentecost MJ, eds. Abrams Angiography, Interventional Radiology. 2nd ed. Philadelphia, PA: Lippincott Williams & Wilkins; 2006: 152–168

Tepe G, Zeller T, Albrecht T, et al. Lokale Applikation von Paclitaxel zur Prävention der Restenose bei peripherer arterieller Verschlusskrankheit. Persistierender Effekt der medikamenten-beschichteten Ballons auch nach zwei Jahren. Berlin: Deutscher Röntgenkongress; 2010

Uflacker R. Interventional therapy of pulmonary embolism. In: Baum S, Pentecost MJ, eds. Abrams Angiography, Interventional Radiology. 2nd ed. Philadelphia, PA: Lippincott Williams & Wilkins; 2006:965–990

3　Methods

Retrograde Catheterization of the Common Femoral Artery

Common Femoral Arterial Puncture

No endovascular intervention is possible without an arterial or venous puncture. A puncture at the wrong site can lead to serious complications. This means that any puncture must be meticulously planned and carefully performed.

Arterial access can be difficult to establish, and it is no cause for alarm if one only succeeds on the fifth attempt. Concentration increases after several attempts, or it can be achieved earlier, with the first attempt or after the first unsuccessful attempt.

The pulsation of the artery is best palpated where it courses over the femoral head. This also makes it easier to obtain effective compression after completion of the examination.

Many physicians have an exaggerated fear of puncturing the artery superior to the inguinal ligament and choose a site too far distal. Possible sequelae include insufficient compression and subsequently a large hematoma, pseudoaneurysm, or arteriovenous fistula.

The author now anticipates the possibility of intervention even in cases where only diagnostic angiography is planned. For this reason, a suitable site should permit use of a vascular closure system.

This makes it all the more important to establish access between the inguinal ligament and the origin of the deep femoral artery (distal to that site only in those rare cases where clearly indicated). The origin of the deep femoral artery usually lies at the level of the inferior contour of the femoral head (above it in 25% of all cases). It is very difficult to locate, especially in an obese patient. Therefore, **fluoroscopy** is highly recommended for determining the level of the puncture relative to the femoral head (**Fig. 3.1**): Place a metal object over the planned puncture site, and view the fluoroscopic image (lock in and collimate the beam).

If the puncture site is too high, withdraw the cannula and compress the site for a few minutes. Then puncture again, even if this requires reapplying local anesthesia and making a second skin incision. The skin incision for a retrograde procedure must lie distal to the planned vascular puncture site (and proximal to it for an antegrade procedure). The magnitude of the correction is determined by the thickness of the subcutaneous fatty tissue and the angle of entry (**Fig. 3.2**).

Local Anesthesia, Skin Incision, and Puncture

Material:
- 10 mL of a 1% solution of local anesthetic
- 12 gauge cannula, extra long in obese patients

First an intradermal skin wheal of anesthetic is raised at the site of the planned incision, possibly with an extra 25 gauge needle (this is important because the skin is

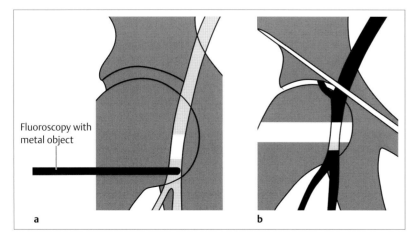

Fluoroscopy with metal object

a　　　　　　　　　　　　　　　　b

Fig. 3.1　Using fluoroscopy and a metal object to determine the puncture level. The target area distal to the center line of the femoral head is marked in white.
a Fluoroscopy with a metal object.
b Distance to the inguinal ligament.

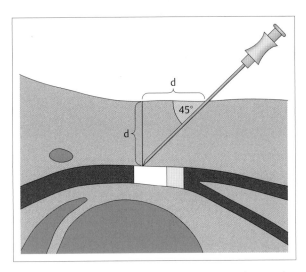

Fig. 3.2 Retrograde puncture. The target area in the vessel distal to the femoral head is marked in white. The light gray area would still be acceptable.

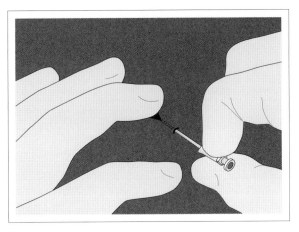

Fig. 3.4 The cannula is directed toward the strongest pulse.

much more sensitive than the subcutaneous tissue). Then the planned needle track is infiltrated down to the vicinity of the vessel (**Caution:** Puncturing the artery will lead to a hematoma!). In the supine patient, the arterial pulsation will be palpable exactly perpendicular to the horizontal plane of the skin (**Fig. 3.3**).

Make the **skin incision** above and perpendicular to the artery. Then insert the cannula and advance it toward the artery at an angle of ~ 45° (see **Fig. 3.2**). Make sure that the opening of the cannula is pointing in the direction in which the wire should run. Concentrate fully on where the pulse can best be felt beneath the finger. Then aim at the point where the pulse can be felt most clearly (it can help to close one eye to do this) and align the cannula precisely in this direction (**Fig. 3.4**).

Next, **slowly advance** the cannula until the pulsation of the artery can be felt through it as well. The vessel

wall is best anesthetized through the puncture cannula itself. Upon feeling the resistance of the vessel wall, apply a small amount of anesthetic to the wall and into it as the cannula enters (**Fig. 3.5**). The patient will be grateful for this; introducing the vascular closure system with insufficient anesthesia can be very painful. This small injection also ensures patency of the cannula as it enters the vessel. Now increase the pressure on the cannula as it passes through the vessel wall until the resistance decreases. Now the tip of the cannula will usually lie in the lumen and blood will gush out of the proximal end of the cannula (**Fig. 3.6**).

Introducing the Catheter System

- Insert the wire into the cannula.
- Hold the cannula at a more acute angle so it more closely follows the course of the vessel (**Fig. 3.7**).

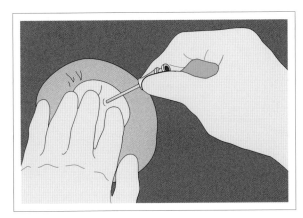

Fig. 3.3 Locating the artery by palpation.

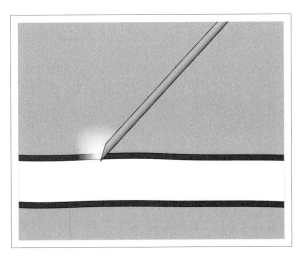

Fig. 3.5 Anesthetizing the vessel wall with the angiography cannula.

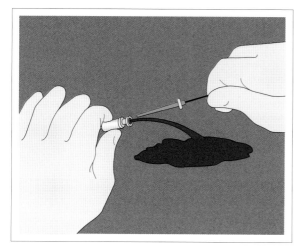

Fig. 3.6 Cannula lies within the lumen: Blood gushes out of the proximal end of the cannula. Now the wire (shown here with an introducer) can be inserted.

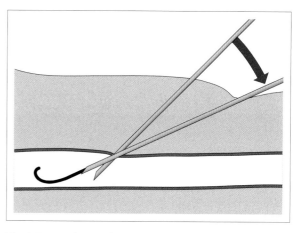

Fig. 3.7 To advance the wire, place the cannula at an acute angle (i.e., approximating the course of the vessel).

- Advance the wire into the vessel (where possible > 5 cm, yet at least far enough so that the stiff shaft of the wire lies within the vessel).
- Remove the cannula.
- Compress the puncture site (see **Figs. 3.14** and **3.16**).
- Slip the catheter or sheath over the wire (see **Figs. 3.15, 3.16,** and **3.17**).
- Advance the catheter or sheath into the vessel.

A **hard vessel wall** may require so much pressure to penetrate the proximal wall that the artery collapses, and the tip of the cannula enters the distal wall before any blood can escape through the cannula (**Fig. 3.8**). If this is suspected to be the case, withdraw the cannula slightly after it has penetrated the vessel wall. If the open lumen of the vessel cannot be reached with this maneuver, advance the cannula far enough to penetrate the distal wall as well. Then verify that the cannula is patent by injecting

a small quantity of saline solution or local anesthetic (**Fig. 3.9a**). Now carefully withdraw the cannula until blood gushes out of its lumen (**Fig. 3.9b**). This is best done while applying pressure to the adjacent skin to prevent the cannula from pulling the artery toward the skin and rapidly slipping out of both walls.

If the vessel is not penetrated, let go of the cannula and watch whether it moves with the pulsation of the artery (**Fig. 3.10a**):

- If the tip of the cannula lies lateral to the artery, the outer margin of the cannula will move medially, and vice versa. Correct the direction of the cannula accordingly (**Fig. 3.10b–c**).
- If the tip of the cannula lies short of the artery, the outer margin of the cannula will dip slightly with each pulse ("nodding," **Fig. 3.10d**).
- Another important aid: When you feel the artery but have advanced the cannula past it, press the cannula upward slightly against your palpating finger. Then you will know whether the cannula lies medial or lateral to the artery.

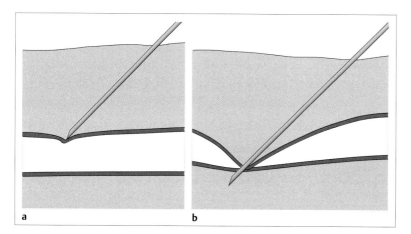

Fig. 3.8 Risk with hard or calcified vessel wall.
a The cannula compresses the vessel.
b It passes through both the anterior and posterior walls of the vessel before blood can escape from the cannula.

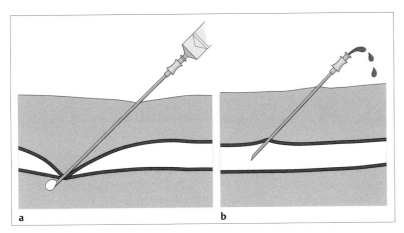

Fig. 3.9 Where perforation is suspected.
a Verify that the cannula is not obstructed.
b Blood gushes out of the cannula as it is withdrawn.

▷ **Important:** Always withdraw the cannula very slowly and watch its proximal end. It may be that the cannula has punctured or passed through an artery without any obvious signs and that blood will gush out once it is withdrawn. If you then withdraw the cannula too rapidly, it will already have left the vessel by the time you see the blood.

Very Slender Patients

In very slender patients the artery in the inguinal region occasionally lies directly beneath the skin. In such cases do not puncture the artery directly beneath the skin incision. Advance the cannula at least 1 cm farther between the skin and vessel wall. This creates a tunnel that will later provide space for a vascular closure system. Otherwise, with a system such as Angio-Seal (St. Jude Medical, St. Paul, MN, USA), part of the collagen sponge that is fixed to the outside of the vessel wall could project out of the skin incision, posing an unacceptable risk of infection.

Puncture of an Impalpable or Poorly Palpable Artery

If the puncture does not succeed, do not immediately go to the other side or the left arm. Under fluoroscopy, search for calcification along the vessel wall (see later discussion). This is best done with the cannula still in place near the artery. Then you will see in which direction you will have to correct.

When the artery is not palpable, it will almost invariably be due to one of these four reasons:
- Occlusion of the artery itself (rare)
- Occlusion or high-grade stenosis in the iliac arteries
- Severe mural calcification (attenuates pulsation)
- Severe obesity

If the contralateral artery is sufficiently palpable, catheterize the contralateral side (Crossover Catheterization, p. 60). If neither side shows a palpable pulse, then exclude occlusion of the common femoral artery with ultrasound (color Doppler ultrasound is best) before the patient is prepped and draped.

An alternate access site is the left brachial artery.

Puncture of an impalpable artery:
1. Under fluoroscopy: when there is visible vascular calcification
2. With Doppler probe
3. Using road mapping
4. Using an indwelling wire in the vascular lumen as a target (3 and 4 are options only when an endovascular catheter has been introduced at another site)

Puncture with Visible Calcification

First look for calcification. Severe calcifications make the vessel wall so rigid that it no longer pulsates. In this case the artery will usually be readily visible on the fluoroscopic image (**Fig. 3.11**) and can be punctured under fluoroscopic control.

If there is no visible calcification, have the image intensifier rotated slightly over the patient with the beam collimated. Then the vascular calcification will move relative to the bone, and calcifications of lesser density will be visible. When the image intensifier rotates to the right, the calcification will move to the left and vice versa. The same applies to a cannula that lies just short of or adjacent to an artery (see earlier discussion). Even if calcification is visible only in the external iliac artery, one can infer the further course of the vessel from that point on.

Calcification is typically seen on the medial and lateral contour of the artery, where X-ray is tangential to the vessel wall. Where there is only one visible line of calcification, it will rather be the medial contour.

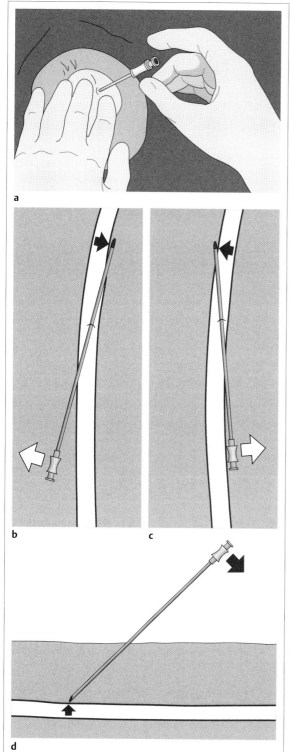

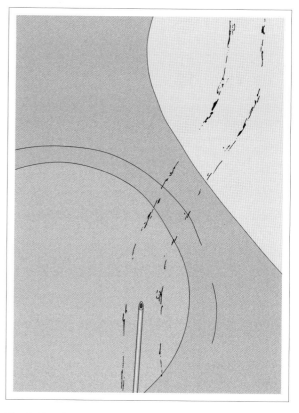

Fig. 3.11 Fluoroscopic image showing vascular calcification and tip of cannula.

Puncture with visible calcification:
- Use the lock-in function to set the fluoroscopy dose.
- Collimate the beam so that the puncture site in the vessel is well visualized but the outer end of the cannula remains outside the fluoroscopic field of view.
- To better protect the fingers against radiation attach a syringe to the cannula.
- Under fluoroscopic control, advance the tip of the cannula toward the vessel until the calcification is seen to move with the cannula.
- Turn off fluoroscopy.

◄**Fig. 3.10** Procedure where the vessel has not been punctured.
a Let go of the cannula and watch whether it moves with the pulsation of the artery.
b Tip of cannula lies lateral to the artery → End of cannula moves medially.
c Tip of cannula lies medial to the artery → End of cannula moves laterally.
d "Nodding" where the tip of the cannula lies short of the artery.

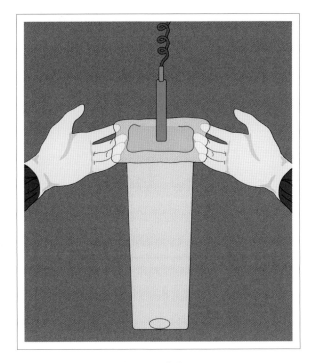

Fig. 3.12 Doppler probe in sterile bag.

- Remove the syringe from the cannula.
- Advance the cannula until blood gushes out.

Puncture with Doppler Ultrasound

In the absence of visible calcification (occluded iliac artery or severe obesity), use a Doppler probe to locate the artery. Often one can locate the artery with Doppler ultrasound and mark its course on the skin prior to administering local anesthesia and before the patient is prepped and draped. If the vessel still cannot be punctured, proceed as follows: An assistant places the Doppler probe in a sterile bag that you hold open (after first applying acoustic gel to its tip; **Fig. 3.12**). Then the device is hung by its cord in the sterile puncture area. To ensure good acoustic coupling, sprinkle a few drops of saline solution on the skin. Then grasp the probe in its sterile bag and locate the artery. The narrower the probe, the more precise the localization will be. (Very fine Doppler probes that can be advanced within the cannula to its tip are also available. One model is the SmartNeedle (Vascular Solutions, Maple Grove, MN, USA). The author has no experience with such probes.)

Puncture with Doppler ultrasound (Fig. 3.13):
- Apply the Doppler probe perpendicular to skin.
- Move it laterally, seeking maximum signal strength.
- Apply local anesthesia and make the skin incision over the course of the vessel.
- Point the cannula obliquely at the vessel in the plane of the Doppler probe.
- Advance the cannula until blood gushes out.

Possible problem: A collateral may emit a stronger signal than the artery being searched for, especially if that artery is occluded.

Puncture Using Road Mapping

Whenever a catheter is already in place proximal to an impalpable artery, the artery can be reliably visualized by road mapping and punctured. Two examples are as follows:
- Retrograde catheterization of an occluded left iliac artery is planned in the presence of an abdominal aorta catheter placed via a right arterial approach.
- Antegrade catheterization of an occluded superficial femoral artery is not feasible; catheterization is to be attempted via the popliteal artery: Contrast agent should be injected via a sheath already in place in the common femoral artery.

Procedure:
- Focus on the region of interest.
- Collimate the beam (with lock-in function as for puncture with visible calcification).
- Activate road mapping, inject contrast.
- Puncture the contrasted artery under fluoroscopy (as with visible calcification).

Instead of road mapping it is occasionally possible to advance a wire from the other catheter into the artery

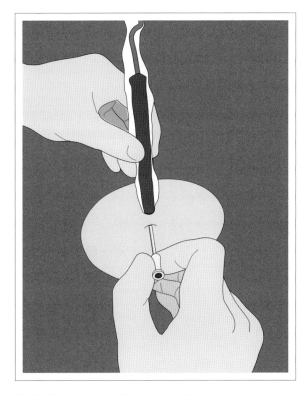

Fig. 3.13 Puncture with Doppler probe.

to be punctured. Then under fluoroscopic control one simply aims the cannula at the wire.

Whenever one is unsure whether one has punctured an artery or vein in the inguinal region, one must first answer this question before making a larger hole in the vessel wall with a catheter or sheath. A small quantity of contrast agent can be injected through the cannula and observed as to whether it flows proximally or distally. The same degree of certainty can be achieved by advancing a guidewire cranially past the iliac region. If the wire courses to the right of the spinal column, one is in the vein; if it courses to the left, one is in the artery.

Introducing a Catheter or Sheath

Once the wire has been positioned securely far enough within the artery, withdraw the cannula and compress the puncture site with the ring and middle fingers (**Fig. 3.14a**). Grasp the wire with the thumb and index finger of the same hand to prevent it from sliding out of the vessel when the cannula is withdrawn (**Fig. 3.14b**).

An assistant now slips the sheath or catheter over the proximal end of the wire after the cannula is withdrawn.

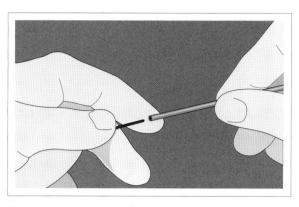

Fig. 3.15   Slipping the catheter over the wire.

This will be easier if one holds the wire with the thumb and middle finger and supports the wire and catheter tip from behind with the index finger (**Fig. 3.15**).

Without Assistance

In the absence of an assistant, it is best to use a sheath. As one slips the sheath over the wire, one presses the short outer end of the wire against the drape with the thumb of the hand that is compressing the puncture site. This will prevent the wire from whipping through the air at random (**Fig. 3.16**). Then the wire can be more easily placed on the index finger of the other hand and directed into the tip of the sheath.

If you are working alone and want to introduce the catheter without a sheath for angiography, proceed as follows: Place the wire on the drape in a wide loop (**Fig. 3.17a**) so that you can compress the puncture site while holding the end of the wire so it can be inserted into the tip of the catheter. Then push the wire through the catheter, grasp the catheter tip with the left hand, and with the right hand pull the wire out of the back of the catheter (**Fig. 3.17b**) until the loop disappears and the catheter tip has been drawn up to the puncture site (**Fig. 3.17c, d**).

Resistance at the Vessel Wall

As one introduces the tip of the catheter or sheath, the external pressure one applies helps to guide it through the subcutaneous tissue (**Fig. 3.18**). This prevents the catheter or sheath from glancing off the vessel into the soft subcutaneous tissue when it encounters the resistance of the vessel wall (**Fig. 3.19**).

Not only may the inguinal artery be difficult to locate precisely; there may also be strong mechanical resistance to introducing a cannula, catheter, or sheath. Often hard subcutaneous scar tissue from previous surgery will be encountered. Large chronic hematomas can also lead to scarring and induration. The vessel wall itself may be indurated, calcified, and very hard as a result of

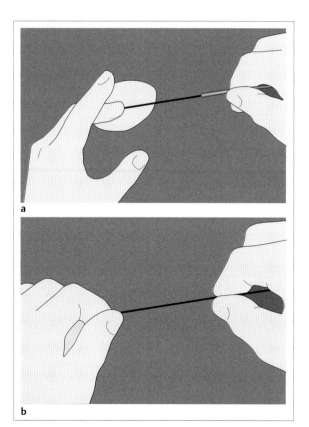

Fig. 3.14   First steps in introducing a catheter or sheath.
a Pulling out the cannula and compressing the puncture site.
b Holding the wire while maintaining compression.

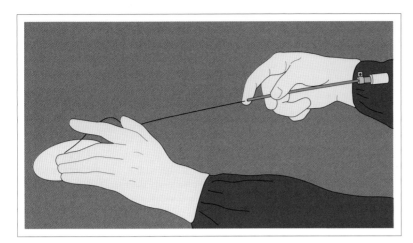

Fig. 3.16 Slipping a sheath over a short wire without assistance.

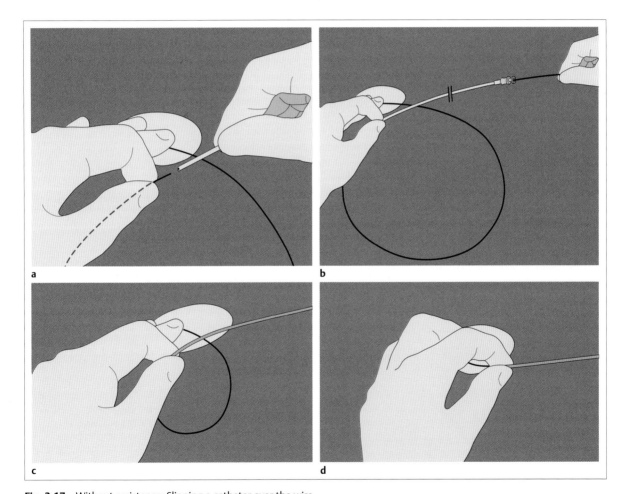

Fig. 3.17 Without assistance: Slipping a catheter over the wire.

a Place the wire on the drape in a wide loop. Compress the puncture site with your left hand while simultaneously holding the end of the wire. Slip the tip of the catheter over it with your right hand.

b Push the wire through the catheter, grasp the catheter tip with your left hand and with your right hand pull the wire out of the back of the catheter.

c Keep pulling the wire until the loop disappears.

d Advancing the catheter tip to the puncture site.

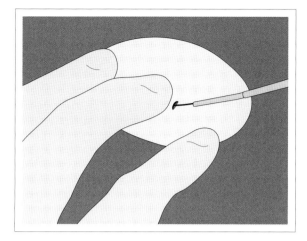

Fig. 3.18 Apply finger pressure to guide the wire and sheath through the subcutaneous tissue.

arteriosclerosis. The scar tissue at an older anastomosis is almost always very firm. Finally, very firm scar tissue usually forms around a plastic bypass.

As one **punctures** the artery, the lumen can collapse before the cannula has passed through the proximal wall (see **Fig. 3.8,** p. 44). When that happens, one will have punctured the distal wall as well without the tip of the cannula having been within the open lumen. Solution:

- During the puncture procedure, one slightly withdraws the cannula several times to allow the arterial lumen to reopen.
- One withdraws the needle very slowly while maintaining pressure on the surface of the skin.
- As soon as blood gushes out of the cannula, it is best to introduce a short **Amplatz wire** (Boston Scientific, Natick, MA, USA). Inserted far enough, this will almost always provide a secure track suitable for introducing a sheath through indurated tissue (**Fig. 3.19**).

After initially using a normal guidewire, one may occasionally find that it is not possible to introduce a sheath over the wire without kinking it. This is especially true of a hard vessel wall with soft overlying tissue (**Fig. 3.19**). In this case, one first introduces the catheter of a long 18 gauge catheter cannula or a 4 French dilator over the normal wire and then replaces it with an Amplatz wire.

In this situation the **sheath** must meet certain special requirements: It must be made of very sturdy plastic, it must be in close contact with the guidewire, and the transitions between guidewire and dilator and between dilator and sheath must be smooth transitions without a pronounced step-off (see Chapter 2, Sheaths, p. 13). There must also be a firm connection between dilator and sheath. Otherwise only the sheath will move forward, and the dilator will be pushed out of the back of the sheath.

Acute Occlusion of the Common Femoral Artery Induced by Catheter or Sheath

Rarely a patient will complain of severe pain in the ipsilateral leg shortly after catheterization of the inguinal artery. The most common cause of this is that the catheter or sheath has completely blocked a high-grade stenosis, usually due to posteromedial plaque (**Fig. 3.20**). This results in ischemia of the entire leg. The pain can be so severe and so difficult to control that an anesthesiologist will have to be called in to help.

However, it is essential to perform angiography of the inguinal region and of the entire leg if possible to visualize the causative stenosis and to exclude acute embolism. A vascular surgeon must be alerted immediately.

Catheterization Via a Plastic Bypass

Even a plastic bypass can be punctured and catheterized (an aortofemoral, femoropopliteal, or axillofemoral bypass or a dialysis shunt). Especially in the vicinity of an anastomosis, a plastic bypass is often enveloped in very

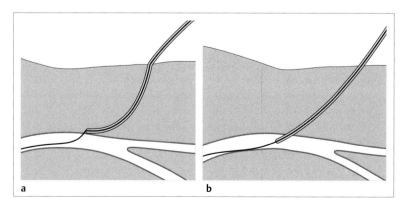

Fig. 3.19 Two examples of advancing a wire into a hard vessel wall.
a Advancing over a soft wire.
b Advancing over a very stiff wire.

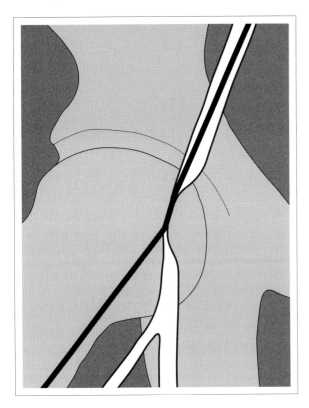

Fig. 3.20 Rare complication: A catheter or sheath occludes a stenosis of the common femoral artery.

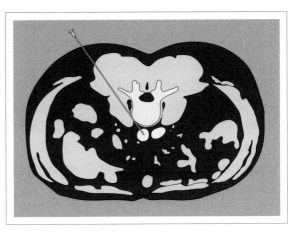

Fig. 3.21 Translumbar approach.

Translumbar Approach

During the 1970s the technique of percutaneous catheterization with guidewire and catheter introduced by Seldinger only gradually supplanted the previously predominant techniques of direct puncture of major arteries (common carotid artery, abdominal aorta, and femoral artery) with rigid cannulas. Up to that time translumbar aortography had been the standard procedure used in the diagnostic workup of peripheral arterial occlusive disease.

The patient (usually under general anesthesia) was positioned prone. A steel cannula ~ 2 mm wide was advanced toward the aorta from the left side, one hand width from the midline at the level of the L2–3 vertebra. At the time there was no tomographic imaging modality such as computed tomography (CT), magnetic resonance imaging (MRI), or ultrasonography. At best one could recognize the calcification of the aortic wall on the fluoroscopic image. And of course the aorta was not always punctured on the first attempt.

Today it is hard to imagine a situation that would require this approach. Nonetheless it would be less risky today than it used to be. CT, MRI, or ultrasound images could be used to plan the approach with a high degree of precision (**Fig. 3.21**). Local anesthesia of the cannula track would suffice. The puncture would be performed with an 18 gauge catheter cannula (1.2 mm in diameter). Then the catheter could be pointed cranially or caudally over a guidewire, or an angiography catheter of the appropriate size could be introduced.

hard scar tissue that renders catheterization difficult. Then an **extra stiff wire** (Amplatz) is often required to introduce a catheter or sheath.

> **Caution:** The following is the most important difference between this puncture and the puncture of an artery or vein: A **bacterial infection of a bypass** cannot be controlled by medication alone. Therefore the procedure should always be performed under strict aseptic conditions. To be on the safe side, the patient should also be given a broad-spectrum antibiotic prior to any puncture and catheterization of a plastic bypass.

Successful catheterization of arteries of the lower leg via the posterior tibial artery at the level of the ankle or the dorsalis pedis artery has recently been described as well (Huppert et al 2010, Schmidt and Montero-Baker 2008).

Antegrade Catheterization of the Femoral Artery

Endovascular interventions involve many complex tasks. Some of them are rarely required, whereas others represent a daily challenge. Antegrade catheterization of the common femoral artery is undoubtedly the most common of these. Performed correctly, antegrade catheterization has several **advantages** over the crossover technique:

- It is quicker.
- It requires less material.
- The decisive advantage is that without the long tortuous approach through the iliac arteries it is easier to steer the wire and catheter in the arteries of the leg (for details see Chapter 5, Superficial Femoral Artery, p. 159).

In antegrade catheterization, all of the instruments such as the guidewire and catheter lie somewhere close to the patient's face. Because it is not possible to cover the entire face with sterile drapes, this could pose problems with respect to sterility (the same applies to uncontrolled arm movements by the patient).

This does not mean that it would be better to lay the wire and catheter over the patient's legs and then conduct them to the inguinal region in a 180° curve. The operator's arms would be unnecessarily close to the fluoroscopic field. This would also reduce the immediacy of every manipulation (even in the radiologist's imagination), and a curved catheter and wire cannot be rotated as freely as straight ones. Deformations in the catheter wall create resistance to torsion (Schröder 1992).

Yet it is a very good idea to use an oblique bracket to keep the sterile drape off the patient's face (**Fig. 3.22**). Another proven solution is to attach a small extension platform alongside the table on the operator's side. This provides a tray for the guidewire, catheter, manometer syringe, and other materials (**Fig. 3.23**). Radiation shields attached to the side of the table are also helpful. The covering drape can be positioned so it forms a trough behind the shields which can be used to hold instruments.

Antegrade Puncture of the Common Femoral Artery

Everything that has been said about retrograde puncture also applies to antegrade puncture. However, the procedure involves a few additional difficulties:

- An obese abdomen often makes it very difficult to perform the puncture at the proper site and at the desired angle.
- The path through the subcutaneous fatty tissue to the vessel is significantly longer in many cases.
- The deep femoral artery will often be accessible to the wire as the direct continuation of the line of puncture (**Fig. 3.27**).
- In contrast, the superficial femoral artery courses horizontally and not in a favorable posterior direction like the external iliac artery in the retrograde puncture.
- And if the deep femoral artery is punctured instead of the common femoral artery, there will be no way to get from there to the superficial femoral artery.

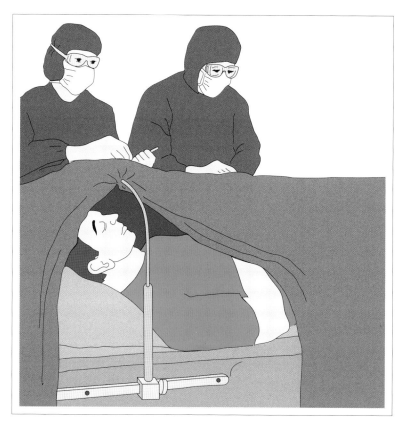

Fig. 3.22 A bracket keeps the sterile drape off the patient's face.

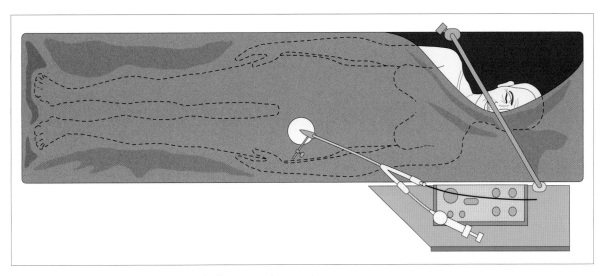

Fig. 3.23 Tray for catheters, syringes, and other required materials.

A soft, mobile abdomen can be pulled in an obliquely cranial and contralateral direction and immobilized there with long strips of bandage. These strips should not be fastened to the contralateral abdomen but to the rail on the table instead. Otherwise one will merely draw the abdomen together slightly and it will slide back into its original position (**Fig. 3.24**).

In a patient with a firm potbelly, there is little you can achieve with bandages. An assistant must push the abdomen upward when vascular access is established, or one opts for crossover catheterization (p. 60).

A long path through the subcutaneous fatty tissue also means that the skin incision must be made farther cranial in order for an oblique cannula to puncture the common femoral artery at the proper location. This requires particularly **careful planning** of the puncture level and then advancing the cannula under **fluoroscopic control**. These imaging findings may reveal that a change in the puncture angle or an incision at a different site is indicated.

In antegrade catheterization, it will not always be possible to avoid a puncture angle steeper than 45°. However, such an angle has significant disadvantages:

- The guidewire can travel cranially into the iliac arteries (**Fig. 3.25**).
- The sheath can easily kink, making it very difficult to introduce a catheter and especially a vascular closure system into the sheath (**Fig. 3.26**).

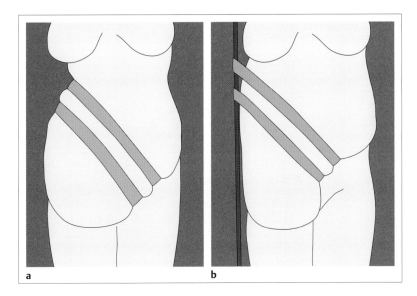

Fig. 3.24 Immobilizing a soft, mobile abdomen with strips of bandage.
a Fastening strips to the contralateral abdomen is of little use.
b Fastening strips to the rail on the table produces a better result.

a   b

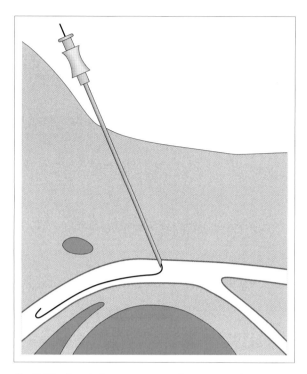

Fig. 3.25 Puncturing at a steep angle can cause the guidewire to travel cranially into the iliac arteries.

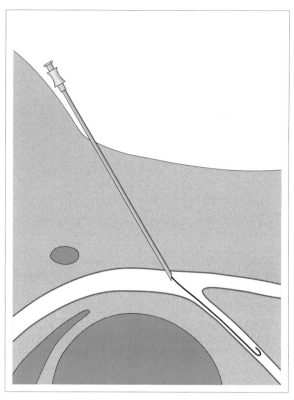

Fig. 3.27 The deep femoral artery is often the direct continuation of the cannula track.

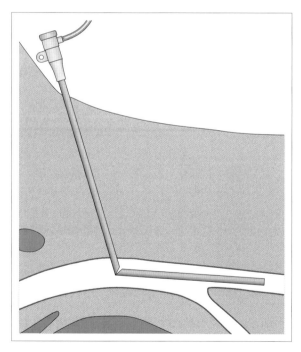

Fig. 3.26 A kink in the sheath can make it difficult to introduce a catheter or vascular closure system.

As soon as blood gushes out of the cannula, introduce the wire and try to hold the cannula at an acute angle to the skin, if necessary by turning it slightly medially, before you advance the wire into the vessel.

From the Deep Femoral Artery to the Superficial Femoral Artery

The deep femoral artery will often be accessible to the wire as the direct continuation of the line of puncture (**Fig. 3.27**). Brief fluoroscopy will usually show whether the wire has entered the superficial femoral or deep femoral artery (**Fig. 3.28**).

Into the Superficial Femoral Artery with the Aid of the Cannula

The difference is more obvious on lateral oblique fluoroscopy: If the wire is in the deep femoral artery, it will often be possible to bring it into the superficial femoral artery by withdrawing it and advancing it again with the cannula at a more acute angle to the skin and at a slightly medial angle (**Fig. 3.29**).

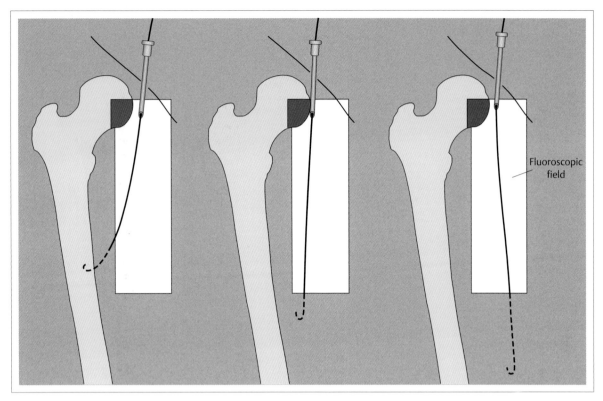

Fig. 3.28 Fluoroscopy verifies whether the catheter lies within the deep femoral artery (left) or in superficial femoral artery (right). Center: Findings are equivocal; the wire must be advanced further.

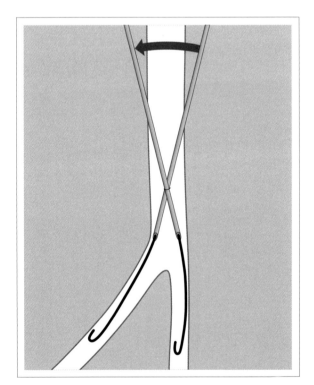

Fig. 3.29 From the deep femoral artery into the superficial femoral artery by changing the direction of the cannula.

Into the Superficial Femoral Artery with an 18 G Catheter Cannula (or 4F Dilator) and a Curved Glide Wire

The previous method may be unsuccessful and it may be doubtful that one has entered the common femoral artery far enough proximal to its bifurcation. In this case one must determine the precise location of the puncture before creating a larger hole in the vessel wall with a sheath.

The author cannot recommend withdrawing the wire and injecting contrast through the cannula for this purpose. Doing so may cause the cannula to slip out of its correct position. With the wire in place, replace the rigid cannula with a long 18 gauge catheter cannula or a 4 French dilator. This can be placed in a secure position within the vessel without greatly expanding the hole in the vessel wall. Then do the following:

- Use oblique projection (30% ipsilateral).
- Collimate the beam, focusing on the femoral artery bifurcation (lock-in function).
- Use road mapping over the catheter cannula.
- Fill the catheter with concentrated contrast agent so that its tip is clearly visualized.
- Withdraw it until proximal to the femoral artery bifurcation.
- Introduce a short curved, torqueable glide wire.
- Steer the wire into the superficial femoral artery under fluoroscopic control (**Fig. 3.30**).

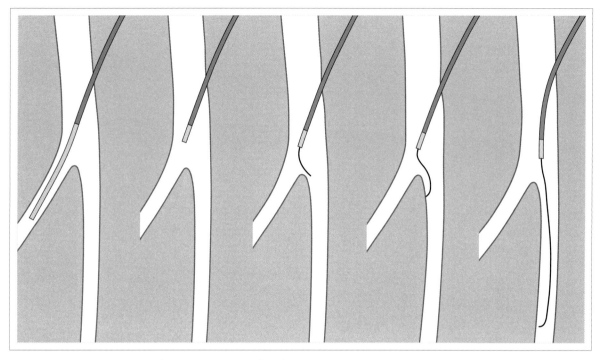

Fig. 3.30 From the deep femoral artery into the superficial femoral artery with an 18 gauge catheter cannula and curved glide wire (fluoroscopy with 30° ipsilateral oblique projection and road mapping).

It can be helpful to rotate the wire 180° as soon as its tip has reached the origin of the superficial femoral artery. The wire will hook into that artery instead of sliding back into the superficial femoral artery. Only when the wire has been positioned securely far enough within the superficial femoral artery the catheter cannula may be withdrawn and the sheath introduced.

Often the bend in the tip of the glide wire is too slight. Then the tip will fail to reach the origin of the superficial femoral artery (**Fig. 3.31**). In this case the wire should be given a more pronounced bend (see Chapter 2, Guidewires, p. 8).

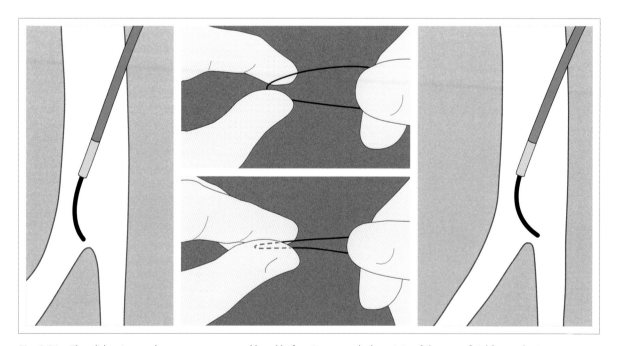

Fig. 3.31 The glide wire needs a more pronounced bend before it can reach the origin of the superficial femoral artery.

Into the Superficial Femoral Artery with a Curved Catheter (Simplest Method)

The alternative to a curved wire is a curved catheter. This has a straight shaft but must have a 90° bend immediately behind its tip (ACN 1 from Cook Medical [Bloomington, IN, USA] or BERN from various suppliers). If one rotates the tip of this catheter anteromedially within the deep femoral artery, withdrawing the catheter will cause the tip to drop back medially as soon as one leaves the deep femoral artery (**Fig. 3.32**). "Road mapping" or continuous injection of small amounts of contrast as the catheter is withdrawn will verify proper positioning. This maneuver with the curved catheter will probably work more reliably than the one with the curved wire, and the distance to the femoral artery bifurcation is not as critical in this case. In a wide vessel one may not succeed in guiding the tip of the catheter along the medial wall of the deep femoral artery. In that case, road mapping will reliably show how far to withdraw the catheter.

Shortening the catheter to a length of ~ 30 cm will greatly facilitate this manipulation.

If the catheter is smaller than the sheath (e.g., 4 French as opposed to 6 French), then one should advance only the wire into the superficial femoral artery and then replace the catheter with a dilator. Otherwise the unprotected tip of the sheath could injure the vessel wall at the carina (**Fig. 3.33**).

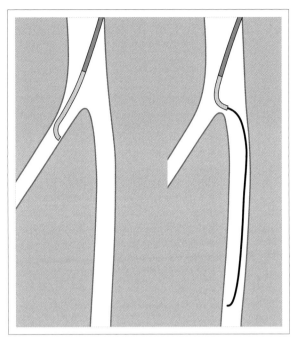

Fig. 3.32 From the deep femoral artery into the superficial femoral artery with a sharply curved catheter (such as ACN1 from Cook Medical or BERN).

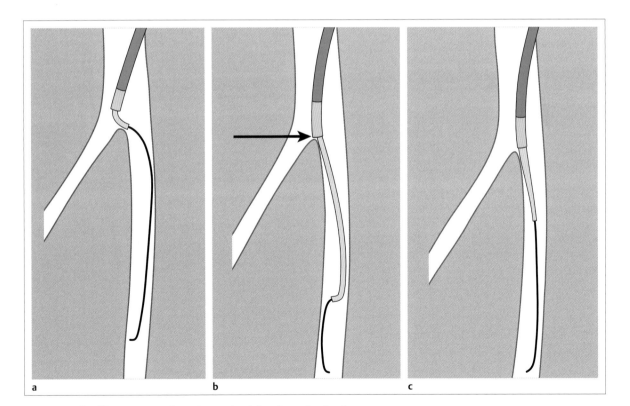

a

b

c

Fig. 3.33 The dilator protects the carina against injury from the sheath.
a 6 French sheath.
b With a 4 French catheter: The unprotected tip of the sheath (arrow) could injure the vessel wall.
c With 6 French dilator: First advance only the wire into the superficial femoral artery and then replace the catheter with a dilator.

The sheath must be long enough so that it extends at least 1 to 2 cm into the superficial femoral artery. Otherwise it can easily slip back into the deep femoral artery when one changes catheters.

Into the Superficial Femoral Artery Using the Cope Technique

Cope et al (1990) suggested introducing into the deep femoral artery a short catheter or dilator that has a side hole on the outside of a bend. Road mapping is used to place this catheter at the femoral artery bifurcation in such a manner that one can steer a 0.018 in. wire through the side hole into the superficial femoral artery (**Fig. 3.34**). Then the catheter is removed and the sheath is introduced into the superficial femoral artery over the wire. Unfortunately, the author has yet to find any company on the German market that supplies this catheter with a side hole.

When the road mapping shows that the puncture site is very close to the femoral artery bifurcation, it will often be impossible to introduce a curved wire or curved catheter into the superficial femoral artery. In that case one must withdraw the catheter cannula, compress the site for 2 to 3 minutes, and repeat the puncture.

Kink in the Sheath

Certain anatomical situations (such as a steep puncture through a thick layer of subcutaneous fatty tissue) are conducive to kinking of the sheath that could prevent insertion of a wire or catheter. Wherever there is a risk of kinking, always leave a stiff wire or catheter in the sheath. And with every new catheterization, have an assistant pull the abdomen upward!

The attempt to catheterize a kinked sheath will probably have the best chance of success if one uses a wire splinted by a dilator to within a short distance of its tip. (Use of a stopcock on the dilator ensures a firm connection between the dilator and the wire.) A fixed kink is best overcome by withdrawing the sheath slightly, advancing the wire and dilator up to the kink, and then advancing sheath, dilator, and wire together (**Fig. 3.35**).

High Bifurcation of the Common Femoral Artery

A high bifurcation of the common femoral artery or a prominent abdomen will occasionally preclude antegrade catheterization of the common femoral artery. In such

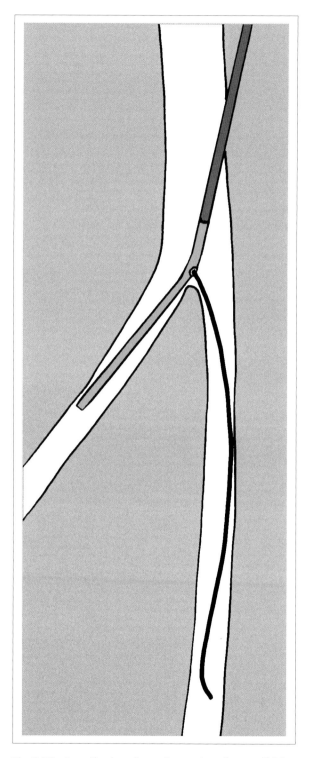

Fig. 3.34 From the deep femoral artery into the superficial femoral artery using the Cope technique.

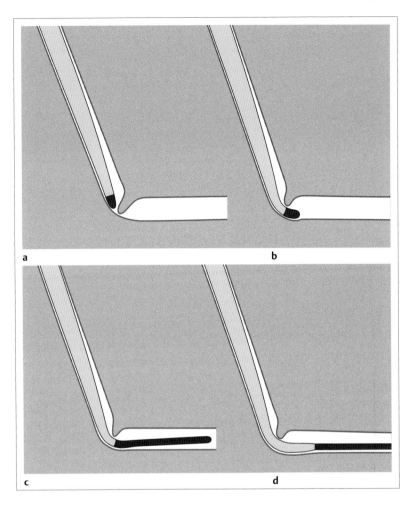

Fig. 3.35 Introducing a wire and dilator into a kink in the sheath.
a The wire is splinted by the dilator to within a short distance of its tip.
b The kink is more easily overcome by withdrawing the sheath slightly; advancing the wire and dilator up to the kink; and then advancing sheath, dilator, and wire together.
c Tip of the dilator is within the kink; wire is advanced.
d Dilator passes through the kink.

cases one may consider crossover catheterization (see later discussion) or, rarely, a superficial femoral artery puncture. For a **puncture of the superficial femoral artery** (not palpable, use a Doppler probe!) its lumen should not be less than 5 mm so that a vascular closure system can be placed to seal the puncture after the intervention. This is particularly important because there is no solid structure deep to the superficial femoral artery that could be used as a buttress to achieve compression.

In extremely **obese patients** it is possible that the inguinal regions of both sides are unsuitable for catheterization, regardless of whether antegrade or retrograde. One possible access site in such cases is the **left brachial artery**. This artery usually lies just beneath the skin even in severe obesity (see Access via the Brachial Artery, p. 65).

Retrograde catheterization of the superficial femoral artery via the **popliteal artery** is an option primarily where occlusion of the superficial femoral artery precludes proximal access. Usually this is preceded by antegrade placement of a sheath via the common femoral artery (see Chapter 5, Superficial Femoral Artery, p. 159). In the rare case of chronic occlusion of the superficial femoral artery over a long segment, one may consider **antegrade catheterization** of the popliteal artery to treat the arteries of the lower leg (Schroeder 1989).

Especially in diabetic patients with trophic lesions in one foot and possibly renal insufficiency as well, it will occasionally be necessary to determine whether intervention is indicated using a slight amount of contrast. If indicated, intervention would then be performed immediately. (CO_2 should be used for contrast in the presence of renal insufficiency—see Chapter 2, CO_2 as a Contrast Agent, p. 36.)

It is recommended to begin with angiography via an 18 gauge catheter cannula (or 4 French dilator) immediately after puncture. This cannula need only be replaced with a sheath where angiography demonstrates findings requiring treatment.

Crossover Catheterization

The term "crossover" has come to be used for catheterization and treatment of the contralateral arteries of the pelvis and legs beyond the aortic bifurcation. The technique of crossover catheterization is a crucial element in the repertoire of every interventional radiologist. For example, after retrograde catheterization it can be used to treat not only the iliac arteries of one side but also the arteries of the contralateral pelvis and leg.

The crossover maneuver is performed in several steps:
- A catheter with a suitable bend is advanced past the aortic bifurcation and hooked into the contralateral common iliac artery.
- A guidewire is advanced through the catheter far into the contralateral iliac arteries.
- The first catheter is removed and replaced with a suitable sheath.
- The sheath is advanced over the wire into a stable position in the contralateral iliac arteries.

Catheters for Contralateral Access

Various catheters with a bend of < 180° are suitable for this purpose. The segment distal to the bend should not be longer than 15–20 mm to allow the catheter to be easily directed caudally within the aorta (**Fig. 3.36**). The UF catheters from Cordis (Miami, FL, USA); the Omni Flush, Sos Omni 0, 1, 2, or 3 from AngioDynamics (Latham, NY, USA); and the Contra from Boston Scientific are all very suitable designs. Several other catheters are also recommended in the literature for initial catheterization of the contralateral iliac arteries beyond the aortic bifurcation. These include a simple hook, a Judkins catheter for the right coronary artery, and even Cobra or pigtail catheters. This latter design is not really suitable (see Chapter 2, Angiography Catheters, p. 16); the Cobra catheter is useful only with an obtuse bifurcation angle. The other

catheters mentioned have too wide a bend or insufficient strength to rotate the wire caudally nearly 180°.

The tighter bends recommended here (see **Fig. 3.36**) occasionally tend to slip back into the ipsilateral iliac artery. It is usually fairly easy to spread open the bend a little with the wire and then to guide the bend in the catheter across the bifurcation.

If one cannot find the bifurcation right away, road mapping with a small quantity of contrast will help.

The Wire's Role in Crossover Catheterization

The wire must be soft near its tip to allow it to follow the bend in the catheter (**Fig. 3.37**). Gradually increasing stiffness (over a transition of at least 5 cm) is required to allow a relatively stiff segment to pass through the bifurcation last. This is needed to extend the distal bend in the catheter so that it can be advanced across the bifurcation. An abrupt transition will cause the wire to push the catheter cranially into the aorta (**Fig. 3.38**).

Pulling the catheter downward onto the bifurcation to spread open the bend makes it a lot easier to advance the catheter into the contralateral iliac arteries (**Fig. 3.37d**). In difficult cases one can also apply external compression to try to hold the wire in its position within the common femoral artery. Then one can advance the catheter over the immobilized wire (**Fig. 3.39**). A spring wire with a very long soft tip (Bentson) is best suited for this purpose, not a "glide" wire.

If one does not succeed in introducing a normal J wire into the contralateral iliac arteries due to plaque or stenosis, a glide wire with a curved tip will almost always help. If this wire becomes caught on plaque, one can turn it and steer it past the plaque.

▷ The instructions up to this point also apply to selective angiography of the vessels of the legs.

In patients with an acute-angle bifurcation and elongated iliac arteries, a normal wire will often be insufficient to guide the relatively stiff sheath. One will then need a stiffer wire (Amplatz or similar wire). However, it will only be possible to advance this wire across the bifurcation when the catheter lies far within the contralateral iliac arteries. This case requires one to do the following:
- Advance a normal wire far into the contralateral iliac arteries.
- Advance a catheter over the wire.
- Replace the first wire with a stiffer wire (**Fig. 3.40**).

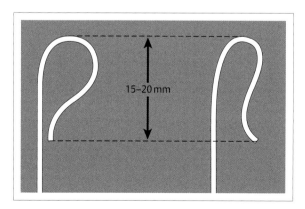

15–20 mm

Fig. 3.36 Catheter for crossover procedures.

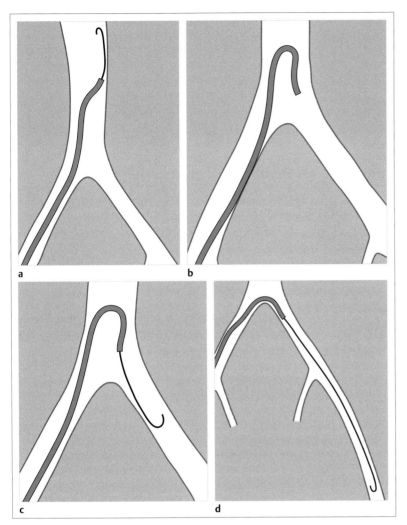

Fig. 3.37 The wire is maneuvered to the contralateral side with the proper catheter.
a Wire and catheter superior to the aortic bifurcation.
b Withdraw wire and hook catheter into the bifurcation.
c Advance wire to the contralateral side.
d To facilitate the maneuver pull the catheter downward onto the bifurcation to spread open the bend.

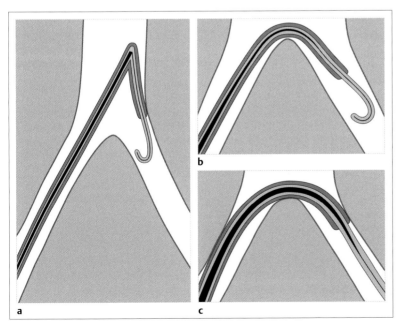

Fig. 3.38 Crossover catheterization using wire with gradual transition to stiff segment.
a A wire with abrupt transition to stiff segment pushes the catheter into the aorta.
b A wire with gradual transition to stiff segment is required for crossover catheterization.
c The stiff part of the wire expands the curve.

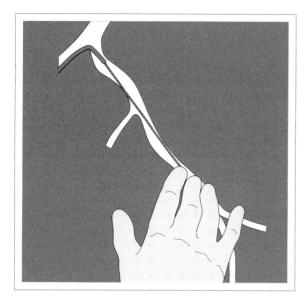

Fig. 3.39 Applying external compression traps the wire in the groin, allowing one to advance the catheter over the immobilized wire.

An acute-angle bifurcation immediately followed by a medial curve in the common iliac artery may make it impossible to advance even a curved glide wire across the bifurcation. In such cases a long taper glide wire may be helpful. This wire with its long, increasingly stiff tip will only begin to spread open the bend in the catheter once it has reached a fairly stable position in the contralateral iliac arteries. Once it has been advanced far enough it is usually stiff enough to splint the bifurcation to allow passage of the catheter.

The bend in the catheter must be spread open as the catheter passes into the contralateral iliac artery. The force required to do this acts against the passage. Therefore, if the bend in the catheter prevents it from being guided around the curve (**Fig. 3.41**), it should be replaced

with a straight 4 French catheter. This catheter will more easily follow the wire across the bifurcation. First the segment near the tip is softened with the fingers, and then the catheter is rotated as it is slowly advanced across the bifurcation. When this catheter has been advanced into the contralateral inguinal region, a stiff wire (stiff glide wire, Amplatz wire, or similar wire) is carefully inserted to spread open all the curves to allow passage of the sheath (**Fig. 3.42**).

Sheaths for Crossover Catheterization

The sheath must have the following characteristics to be advanced across an acute-angle bifurcation:
- Either the dilator and the sheath have a suitable bend (e.g., from Cook Medical, **Figs. 3.43** and **3.44**),
- or a flexible dilator projects a few centimeters beyond the tip of the sheath (e.g., Arrow International [Reading, PA, USA], **Figs. 3.43** and **3.45**).

The dilator is first advanced across the bifurcation. It splints the bifurcation so the stiffer sheath can be advanced. (This is the principle of gradually increasing stiffness.)

An acute-angle bifurcation can cause the sheath to kink, which may even make it impossible to withdraw the sheath. For this reason crossover catheterization should only be attempted using sheaths with spiral metal reinforcement in their wall.

Interventions in the arteries of the pelvis and legs may also be performed without introducing a long sheath into the contralateral vessels. However, this long sheath has two decisive advantages:
- It allows injection of contrast agent during the intervention (road mapping and evaluation of results with the guidewire still in place).
- Equally important: Without the sheath you will be unable to negotiate many stenoses and occlusions because it will not be possible to apply sufficient axial force with guidewire and catheter alone. Guidewire

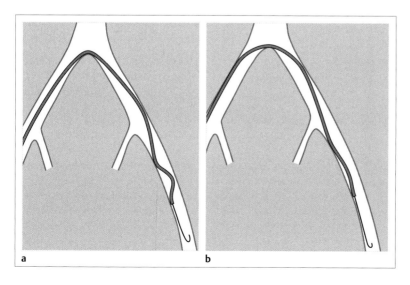

Fig. 3.40 A stiff wire is often helpful in patients with an acute-angle bifurcation.
a A soft wire will not always provide sufficient support to guide the sheath.
b A stiff wire expands the curve at the bifurcation.

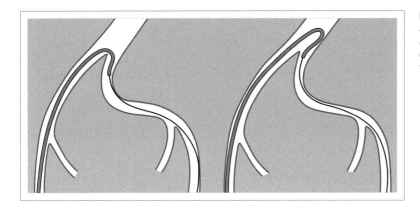

Fig. 3.41 Catheter wanders into the aorta when advanced. Trap the wire as shown in **Fig. 3.39.** Or replace the curved catheter with a straight model that will more likely follow the wire.

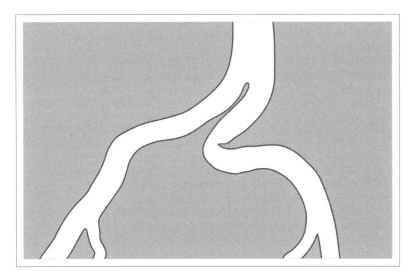

Fig. 3.42 In a case like this crossover catheterization from right to left is very difficult. It is best performed using a wire with a very long soft tip (Bentson) than one that can be immobilized in the groin as shown in **Fig. 3.39**.

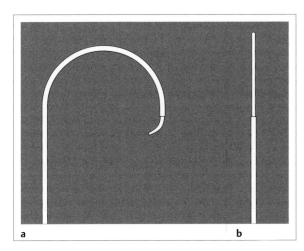

a   b

Fig. 3.43 Sheaths for crossover catheterization.
a Cook sheath.
b Arrow sheath or OptiMed Epsylar.

and catheter alone will be diverted into the abdominal aorta as soon as they encounter any significant resistance. A sheath will reliably prevent this.

▷ **Caution:** In crossover catheterizations the guidewire and catheter often spontaneously seek the internal iliac artery. This will not always be obvious from the course of the artery on a posteroanterior (PA) view. When in doubt, and especially before any intervention, rotate the C-arm to obtain a medial oblique view: The internal iliac artery courses posteriorly, the external iliac artery anteriorly.

The goal of crossover catheterization is typically an intervention. However, a balloon catheter does not allow one to choose between the deep and superficial femoral arteries. However, a curved diagnostic catheter is not

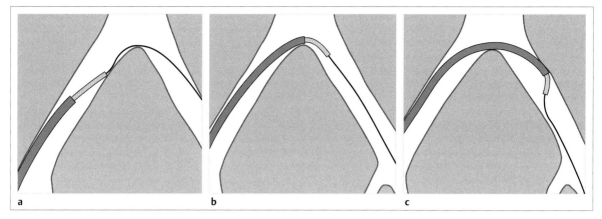

Fig. 3.44 Crossover catheterization with Cook-Balkin sheath.
a Wire within the contralateral iliac arteries.
b The curved dilator follows the wire.

c The bend in the sheath facilitates passage across the bifurcation.

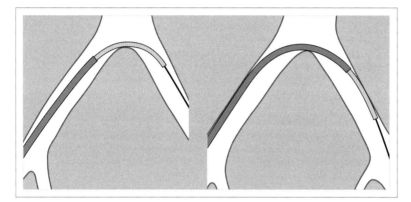

Fig. 3.45 Crossover catheterization with Arrow sheath.

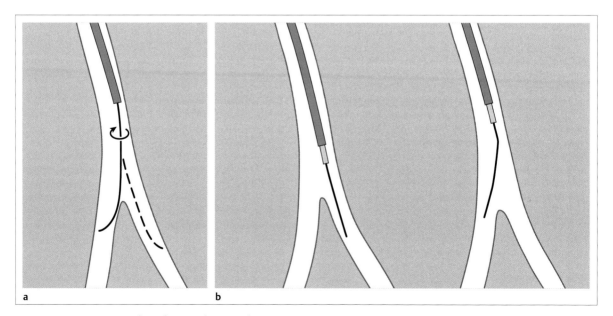

Fig. 3.46 Steering a straight catheter with a curved wire.
a The catheter often passes into the contralateral deep femoral artery instead of the superficial femoral artery.
b Solution: Steer the catheter with a torqueable, curved glide wire. If necessary, increase the bend by putting a kink ~ 3 cm behind the tip.

required if the wire and catheter pass into the contralateral deep femoral artery instead of the superficial femoral artery. Use a torqueable curved glide wire to steer the catheter under fluoroscopic control. Use an ~ 30° lateral oblique projection and road mapping (**Fig. 3.46b**). If the bend is not sufficient, withdraw the wire and increase the bend (put a kink in it ~ 3 cm behind the tip). The wire can be used like a straight wire for negotiating the artery if one then withdraws the kink into the catheter (see **Fig. 5.48**, p. 188).

Access via the Brachial Artery

Special Considerations with the Arm Approach

The left brachial artery is the most important alternative to the inguinal arteries as an approach to the arterial system. The left side has the advantage of shorter distance. The risk of cerebral complications due to embolism or vasospasm is also significantly lower because a catheter introduced on the left side only passes the origin of the vertebral artery on its way into the descending aorta. However, one must also consider the possibility of stenosis or occlusion of the subclavian artery. Both are encountered significantly more often on the left side than on the right. Therefore one should measure the blood pressure in both arms before performing the puncture.

The axillary artery was once favored for vascular access due to its size. However, it is significantly more difficult to puncture, and the difficulty in achieving effective compression significantly increases the risk of local complications.

Some cardiologists prefer the radial artery because of the availability of the ulnar artery in the event of occlusion. Note, however, that the probability of vascular occlusion is higher than in the brachial artery due to the radial artery's relatively small caliber.

If one chooses the approach via the radial artery, the **Allen test** must be performed first to verify the function of the ulnar artery as a collateral: Simultaneously compress the radial and ulnar arteries while the patient makes a fist. Then release the ulnar artery as the patient opens the fist. A sufficiently functional ulnar artery will cause the hand to turn pink within 5 to 10 seconds.

Puncture and Catheterization

The brachial artery is punctured where it is best palpated. It occasionally exhibits a tendency to avoid the cannula. Therefore, it is essential to use a sharp cannula. At least in difficult cases, it is advisable to supplement the normal puncture cannula with a puncture set (**Fig. 3.47**) that includes a thin cannula (21 gauge) and a fine guidewire such as those supplied for radial artery puncture.

Yet, if arterial blood pressure is very low, such as can occur in a proximal brachial or subclavian artery occlusion, the thin cannula can pose too much resistance for the escaping blood, particularly in a long cannula. Filling a cannula 8 cm long requires twice the pressure needed to fill one 4 cm long!

An 18 gauge plastic cannula is also a viable alternative.

Where the brachial artery is poorly palpable it is often helpful to use a Doppler probe (see p. 47). The probe should be as narrow as possible. The weak pulse can of course be due to a subclavian artery stenosis. Compare the blood pressure with the right side. In this case, one may consider dilating the subclavian artery in the same intervention. Even an impalpable brachial artery can be punctured with the aid of a Doppler probe, for example, where a proximal brachial artery stenosis or occlusion is to be treated. However, in such a case the artery would no longer provide a suitable approach for intervention in other vessels.

The standard J wire may not be used for catheterizing the brachial artery because the curve at its tip is 6 mm in diameter, which is far too wide for the narrow vessel. The wire will cause vasospasms. A 0.035 in. glide wire with a slightly curved tip is recommended.

> **Caution:** If the wire cannot be easily advanced, then it probably lies within the wall or outside the vessel! In this case, do the following:
> - Remove the cannula.
> - Apply light compression for 2 to 3 minutes.
> - Repeat the puncture.

Especially in the axillary artery, a curved wire will often enter a **branch**. At the slightest resistance, the region should be examined under fluoroscopy, and the wire should be withdrawn and then rotated to advance it beyond the branch.

The guidewire will often spontaneously enter the left **vertebral artery**. This, too, must be immediately corrected or,

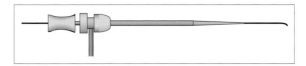

Fig. 3.47   Sheath of 5, 6, or 7 French diameter with a dilator for an 0.018 in. nitinol wire that fits a 4 cm long 21 gauge cannula (Cook).

better, avoided from the outset (use fluoroscopy!) because the catheter can trigger a vasospasm at that location.

The arm approach for interventions in abdominal, iliac, or leg arteries is thus associated with an increased risk and remains the exception. The risks include thromboembolic complications in the arteries supplying the brain and vascular occlusions in the arm. Thrombus deposition can occur on long catheters and sheaths. Withdrawing the instruments can then strip this material off and release it into the bloodstream where it can form emboli in the basilar artery or the arteries of the fingers. For this reason **heparin must be administered immediately at the beginning of any intervention**.

Approach to the Descending Aorta

Usually one must negotiate a sharp curve at the junction of the left subclavian artery and descending aorta. Often this is attempted with a pigtail catheter, which is rather poorly suited for this purpose (**Fig. 3.48a**). Instead, use a **catheter with a short distal bend** of 180° maximum (**Fig. 3.48b**), and perform this maneuver under fluoroscopic control using the 30° left anterior oblique (LAO) projection.

Long sheaths that can be introduced as needed into the vessel requiring treatment are very helpful for interventions via a brachial approach. The following maneuver is recommended to guide these sheaths into the descending aorta:
- The sheath is advanced as far as the origin of the subclavian artery.
- The dilator of the sheath is replaced with a catheter having a distal bend of 150 to 180°. (In the absence of the proper sort of catheter, one can take a long pigtail catheter and cut off the superfluous part of the bend.)
- This catheter is used to direct the guidewire into the descending aorta (**Fig. 3.49**).

- The wire is pushed far enough into the catheter to extend its distal bend (or one can withdraw the bend in the catheter into the sheath).
- Finally, the sheath is advanced with the wire and catheter into the abdominal aorta (**Fig. 3.49**).

For most interventions (those in the renal or iliac arteries), a slight bend close to the tip of the sheath is helpful. Because of the small caliber of the arteries of the arm, the diameter of the sheath becomes a critical dimension (6 French is maximum, 5 French is better). This makes it essential to work with slender systems.

Treatment of the Access Site

Requirements, Alternatives

Most complications in angiography and endovascular intervention are sequelae of insufficient or unsuccessful treatment of the arterial access site.

Since the introduction of Seldinger's percutaneous catheterization technique in 1953, the opening in the vessel wall has been closed by external compression. Even after the introduction of systems such as Angio-Seal or StarClose (Abbott Vascular, Temecula, CA, USA) that close the opening immediately at the vessel wall, compression treatment has continued to dominate to this day and accounts for 70 to 90% of all cases (Turi 2008). The ongoing trend to smaller systems (4 French rather than 6 French) will presumably help compression treatment maintain its dominance in the future as well.

Common Femoral Artery

The first step toward correct treatment of the access site at the end of the intervention is at its very beginning: the **careful choice of puncture site**. In the inguinal region, this

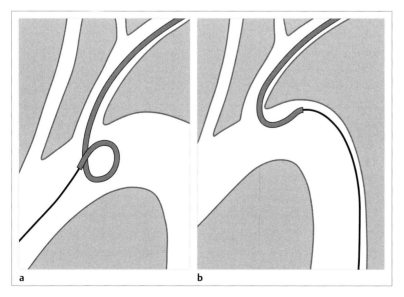

Fig. 3.48 Approach to the descending aorta from the left subclavian artery.
a A pigtail catheter tends to guide the wire into the ascending aorta.
b A catheter with a short distal bend works.

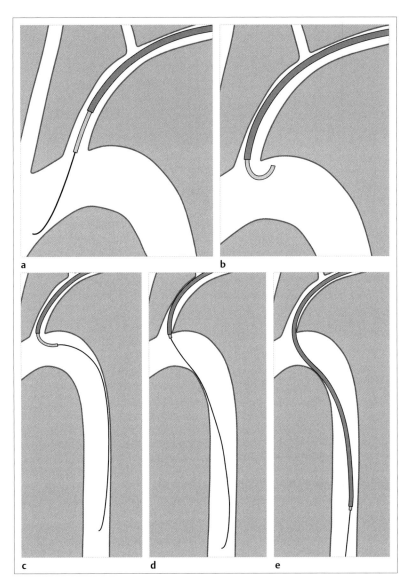

Fig. 3.49 Catheterization of the descending aorta with a long sheath via the brachial artery.
a Advance the sheath as far as the origin of the subclavian artery.
b Replace the dilator with a catheter with a bend of 150 to 180°.
c Direct the guidewire into the descending aorta with this catheter.
d Draw the curve of the catheter into the sheath.
e Advance the sheath with the wire and catheter into the abdominal aorta.

is at the level of the middle third of the femoral head, although the distal third is also acceptable. Here one has a solid structure that can be used as a buttress to achieve compression, and for a vascular closure system one will not normally have a problem with the origin of the deep femoral artery in this segment.

Closure by External Compression

If the catheter track is to be closed by compression, then the pressure applied to the skin must be high enough to press the sides of the oblique wound together and prevent any more blood from escaping. The residual blood in the cannula track will then coagulate and seal the track. On the other hand, the artery must remain patent or only collapse briefly under the pressure. If there is no palpable pulse distal to the compression site or the Doppler probe or pulse oximetry fail to demonstrate blood flow there,

then the pressure must be reduced within 2 minutes at the latest.

There are two decisive criteria for the entire aftercare phase:
- There must be no bleeding at the puncture site.
- There must be blood flow in the arteries of the legs. There must be a palpable pulse distal to the compression site (in the common or superficial femoral artery immediately distal to the compression site, in the popliteal artery, in the posterior tibial artery, or in the dorsalis pedis artery). Where there is no palpable pulse, one must look for flow signals with a Doppler probe or detect them by pulse oximetry.

The pressure exerted on the skin above the punctured vessel decreases with the depth of the tissue. One can compensate for this decrease with depth by increasing the surface on which one exerts pressure. Yet applying the same pressure over a larger area requires more exertion, which is why manual compression can be very strenuous in obese patients.

A solid **buttressing structure**, like the bones of the hip, acts as counterpressure. This force vector is added to the direct pressure to create a field of largely homogeneous compression between the compression device and the buttress (**Fig. 3.50**). A certain loss of pressure in the deeper tissue may nonetheless occur under such conditions, but this is due to the larger area of the buttress over which the force is distributed. The less the pressure decreases with depth, the more favorable will be the conditions for achieving successful compression.

With the sharp drop in pressure that typically occurs in the absence of a buttressing structure, the cannula track is often closed superficially, whereas there is insufficient pressure in the deep layer to close the puncture wound in the vessel. This can lead to a **pseudoaneurysm**: Blood continues to escape into the surrounding tissue through the puncture wound in the vessel wall. Because it moves back and forth with the alternating blood pressure, it does not coagulate (**Fig. 3.51**).

These are the typical conditions that give rise to a pseudoaneurysm when the puncture is performed too far distal, beyond the buttressing structure of the femoral head. A puncture performed proximal to the inguinal ligament will also lack this buttress for compression. The consequences can be far worse at this site because a circumscribed cavitation will fail to form in the sparse tissue. The blood tends to flow into the retroperitoneum and often forms a life-threatening retroperitoneal hematoma. (**Caution:** Ultrasound and CT studies are indicated at the slightest suspicion!) In a more favorable case it can spread out within the anterior abdominal wall, where it is less dangerous but very painful.

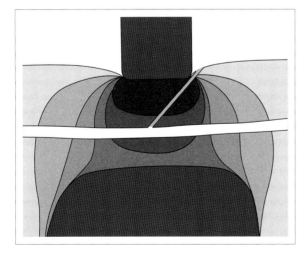

Fig. 3.50 Compression against a buttressing structure: Compression is relatively homogeneous down to the buttress.

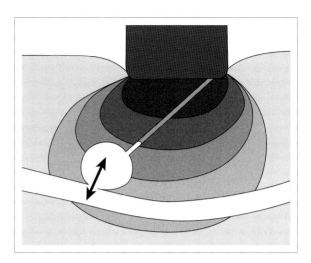

Fig. 3.51 Compression without a buttressing structure: Compression decreases greatly with depth, leading to pseudoaneurysm.

The decisive requirement for complication-free management of the arterial access site is to perform the puncture at the correct level. (Fluoroscopy is indicated to determine the puncture site.)

The compression applied during the first 2 minutes should be close to the systolic pressure. Once a thrombotic closure has formed within the cannula track, it will suffice to maintain a significantly lower pressure.

Manual Compression

External compression is still largely performed by hand these days. This is a time-consuming and often strenuous method. The time wasted is particularly great when the compression is performed on the angiography table and the next patient is kept waiting. There is another disadvantage. A patient with an indwelling catheter or sheath can be safely moved to a bed because the catheter seals the puncture site. Yet moving a patient after manual compression, with the puncture site protected only by a pressure bandage of variable efficacy, increases the risk of postprocedure bleeding. Therefore one should only perform **even manual compression after the patient has been transferred to a bed**.

Manual compression lasting 10 to 15 minutes must be immediately followed by application of a pressure bandage intended to prevent postprocedure bleeding for the next 4 to 6 hours (or up to 24 hours). The following scheme can be applied to patients treated with 4 or 5 French systems and given a single dose of 5,000 IU of heparin:

- Apply manual compression for 10 to 15 minutes, then apply a pressure bandage.
- During the first 2 hours take the peripheral pulse and check for possible bleeding every 30 minutes.
- Reduce the pressure after 4 hours.

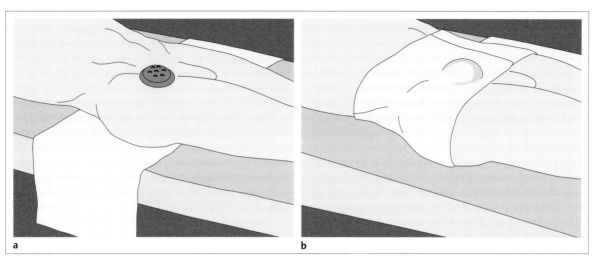

Fig. 3.52 Pressure bandage with pad of expanded polystyrene and elastic abdominal belt.
a Pad of expanded polystyrene over the puncture site, belt beneath the patient.
b Abdominal belt closed under tension.

- Remove the pressure bandage after 5 hours, slowly mobilize the patient, and allow walking after another 2 hours.

The **gauze strips** between the back and medial aspect of the thigh once commonly used as a pressure bandage are **not recommended**. They require extension in the hip to maintain their tension. A better solution is to use a **pad of expanded polystyrene** held in place and pressed onto the puncture site by an elastic abdominal belt with a Velcro closure (**Fig. 3.52**, available from Ernst Tischler, Roth, Germany). The Velcro closure allows a certain measure of subsequent correction of the compression. Another option is to use an **elastic foam rubber roll** held in place and pressed into the wound by an elastic bandage (**Fig. 3.53**). Applying

the elastic bandage requires the patient to get up several times and fixing it later is very difficult.

All of these bandages have the disadvantage that the compression applied is not measurable and cannot be gradually decreased during the course of treatment. One can only measure the peripheral pulse at various sites for orientation. Bleeding is only detectable when the bandage has turned red or blood is observed running down the medial aspect of the thigh.

Most of the complications in endovascular interventions occur at the access site, and the majority of these develop during the poorly controllable phase of those first few hours following manual compression. This situation can only be improved by mechanical compression systems that cover the entire phase of compression, are

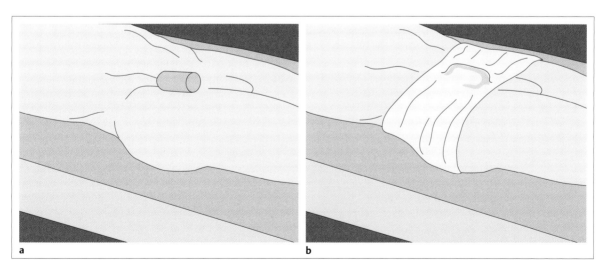

Fig. 3.53 Pressure bandage with foam rubber roll and elastic bandage.
a Foam rubber roll over the puncture site.
b Fixation with elastic bandage.

applied and adjusted before the sheath is removed, allow inspection of the puncture site, and permit gradual and preferably measurable reduction of pressure.

Internal Compression with a Percutaneous Transluminal Angioplasty Balloon

Occasionally the proximal popliteal or posterior tibial artery is punctured using road mapping to provide vascular access for retrograde catheterization of an occlusion. Postprocedure management of this access site is difficult because there is no structure to provide a buttress for external compression. An elegant alternative to external compression has recently been described for this situation (Huppert et al 2010). In these cases, percutaneous transluminal angioplasty (PTA) is usually performed via a sheath introduced into the inguinal arteries in antegrade fashion. When the vessel is again patent, one can easily advance a balloon catheter of the appropriate size to the peripheral access site and usually achieve thrombotic closure of the narrow cannula track by maintaining slight pressure for 2 to 3 minutes (**Fig. 3.54**).

Mechanical Compression Systems

Various mechanical systems are available as substitutes for manual compression. Such systems should fulfill the following criteria:

- Exact placement of compression
- Reliable pressure control
- Good fit on the surface of the body with uniform pressure distribution
- Sterility at and around the skin incision
- Good visibility of the puncture site to allow prompt detection of bleeding
- Definitive treatment that does not require subsequent application of a pressure bandage
- Minimal impairment of the patient while ensuring compression for a period of several hours
- Low material costs

The compression devices that have been available to date leave much to be desired.

The **Compressar** (Advanced Vascular Dynamics, Portland, OR, USA) is simple and inexpensive. However, it has the disadvantage of being unsuitable for prolonged use over a period of hours. The patient is constrained and confined to bed for the duration of treatment (**Fig. 3.55**) and is unable to use a bed pan. This means that the Compressar is only a substitute for manual compression. A pressure bandage must be applied for the next few hours after that.

The **FemoStop II Plus** (St. Jude Medical) is suitable for treatment over a period of several hours. A plastic frame placed across the inguinal region holds a transparent inflatable pad. The frame is held by a belt that lies beneath the patient, having been placed on the bed before the patient with an indwelling catheter gets into bed (**Fig. 3.56a**). The patient raises the buttocks to allow the belt to be positioned at the level of the puncture site.

The folded pad and frame are placed over the access site so that the center line of the dome of the pad lies directly over the site of the arterial puncture. Then the frame is connected on both sides to the belt with a clamping device, and the belt is drawn tight (**Fig. 3.56b**). Now a hand pump with a pressure gauge is used to unfold the pad and inflate it to a pressure approximately corresponding to the systolic pressure.

Note: The pressure measurements performed with this device are reproducible in the individual patient. Yet they are in no way measurements of the absolute pressure at the interface between the pad and the skin. The pad has the shape of a rigid hemisphere. Its center presses deeper into the tissue than its periphery, which is why the pressure in the center must be significantly higher. Assuming, in a slender patient, the contact interface between pad and skin is only half as large as the area of the base of the pad, then the average pressure on the skin must be twice as high as the air pressure measured in the pad.

Inflating the pad places tension on both sides of the belt. If the belt is not aligned exactly along the axis of the frame, it can change the position of the pad. In such cases it is crucial to deflate the pad and reposition the belt and frame, several times if necessary. Only when an optimal,

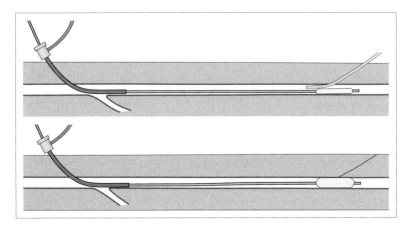

Fig. 3.54 Internal compression with a percutaneous transluminal angioplasty balloon.

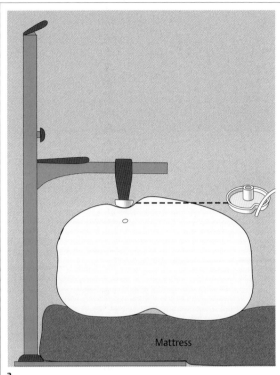

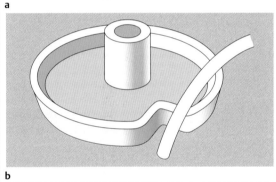

Fig. 3.55 The Compressar compression device (Advanced Vascular Dynamics).
a The Compressar system confines the patient to mattress.
b Detailed view of the pad with a notch for the sheath.

stable pad position has been achieved may the sheath or catheter be withdrawn.

If blood continues to escape, the pressure is increased. This is first done by applying manual pressure to the frame, then by further inflating the pad. Then one will have time to check the peripheral pulse, in applicable cases with Doppler ultrasound or pulse oximetry. If there is no detectable flow, then after 2 minutes the pressure must be reduced until a clear flow signal is detected. After another 5 minutes the pressure is reduced further and the pulse is checked. Now the patient can return to the ward. There the compression device remains in place for 4 hours (with a 4 French catheter; 5 hours with a

5 French catheter or 4 French sheath). Then the pressure device is removed, the puncture site cleaned, and a sterile dressing applied. At this point the patient may move again and after another 1 to 2 hours may carefully leave the bed.

The FemoStop system involves **relatively high costs**. It is not always possible to optimally position the inflatable pad with this device because it is difficult to judge the belt's influence on the pad's position once the pad is inflated. In obese patients the inguinal region rises toward the abdomen, and relatively high pressure is required due to the depth of the artery. This often causes the system to tilt distally. In rare cases, an undetected leak in the pneumatic system can lead to loss of compression.

Vascular Closure Systems

External compression is a suitable method of obtaining closure with systems 3 through 5 French in diameter. This is because the smallest available vascular closure systems initially expand the puncture site to 6 French. (Exoseal from Cordis is an exception; it is available in 5 French). However, after the intervention it may become apparent that the puncture was inadvertently performed superior to the inguinal ligament (in the external iliac artery) or distally to the femoral artery bifurcation (in the superficial or deep femoral artery). This will more likely occur in obese patients. There may be no available buttressing structure to aid in compression and there may even be a risk of life-threatening retroperitoneal hematoma. In such cases, a vascular closure system may represent the best solution, even where a small catheter size was used for the intervention.

▷ **Advantage:** Vascular closure systems work even without compression and a buttressing structure.

The option of closing the access site directly at the vessel wall is of interest for every system more than 2 mm in diameter (i.e., from 6 to 9 [-24] French). These systems may require greater care and practice with their application. Of course closure systems are also more expensive than simple external compression. However, they offer certain advantages for patients and physicians:

- The patient is no longer confined to bed for hours with an uncomfortable compression bandage or device.
- This type of treatment is the quickest for the physician.

All systems require a minimum vascular caliber for application (> 4 mm diameter for Angio-Seal). Applying such a device immediately adjacent to the origin of the deep femoral artery is thought to be risky. The presence of plaque on the anterior wall of the common femoral artery at the puncture site may compromise the system's efficacy. Therefore a vascular closure system is contraindicated in such a situation.

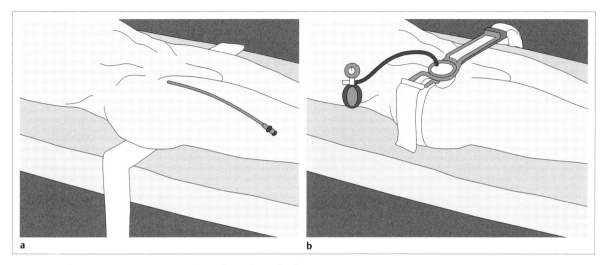

Fig. 3.56 The FemoStop compression device (St. Jude Medical).
a Belt beneath the patient, catheter still in situ in the vessel. **b** Pneumatic compression.

Unfortunately, the highest frequency of complications is observed precisely in patients in whom compression treatment is most difficult, namely obese patients with severe vascular changes in the vicinity of the access site (Fraedrich et al 2010).

The following section describes a few important examples of vascular closure systems.

Angio-Seal

The Angio-Seal system seems to be well suited for daily practice. Its simplicity also makes it a good choice for less experienced operators. It has proven effective in prospective studies of large series.

The Angio-Seal system introduces a small plastic "anchor" through the puncture into the lumen. A collagen sponge is introduced from outside along a filament that holds the anchor in place. The sponge is pressed tightly against the vessel wall and held in place with a knot. The manufacturer states that all foreign material is absorbed within 2 to 3 months. (Note the expiration date. The filament tends to lose its strength after a long period of storage.)

Before a vascular closure system is placed, the access site is first visualized on a lateral oblique view (**Fig. 3.57**). This is done after the intervention if it was not done right at the beginning. (In an antegrade procedure, you will need a short forceful injection and high

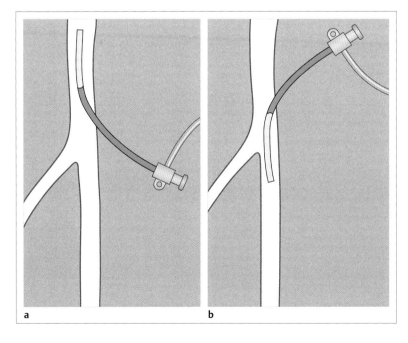

Fig. 3.57 Angiogram of the access site prior to placing a vascular closure system.
a In retrograde catheterization.
b In antegrade catheterization.

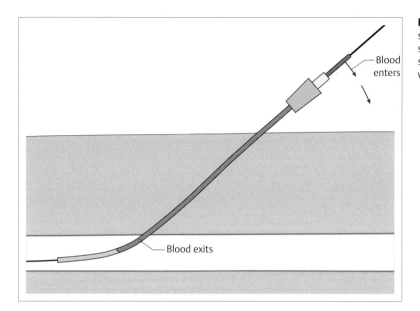

Fig. 3.58 Angio-Seal: Replacing the sheath with the sheath of the closure system. Blood escaping through this sheath indicates it is at the correct depth within the vessel.

Blood enters

Blood exits

image frequency.) Evaluate the following findings on this image:

- Diameter of the common femoral artery
- Quality of the anterior wall (possible signs of calcified plaque)
- Sufficient distance to the deep femoral artery

If none of these criteria contraindicate the use of a vascular closure system, then proceed as follows:

- Replace the sheath with the sheath of the closure system.
- Advance this sheath until pulsating blood escapes from the outer end of the sheath. This means the inner end

has entered the vascular lumen (**Fig. 3.58**). The sheath is maintained in this position.

- Now removed the wire and dilator.
- Next, introduce the applicator for the closure system into the sheath.
- When the applicator snaps into place at the head of the sheath, an anchor folds out of the sheath with a soft click (parallel to the longitudinal axis of the vessel; **Fig. 3.59a**).
- The sheath and applicator tube are now withdrawn together, maintaining continuous tension on the filament inside. This secures the anchor in position on the vessel wall (**Fig. 3.59b**).

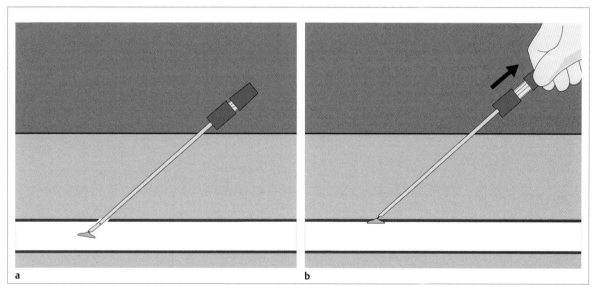

a b

Fig. 3.59 Angio-Seal: Positioning the "anchor."
a The anchor unfolds after the applicator snaps into place at the head of the sheath.

b Sheath and applicator are withdrawn together until the anchor lies against the vessel wall.

- A black tube now appears. This tube is used to press the collagen sponge and a knot against the vessel wall, where they are fixed in place by tamping them a few times with the tube (**Fig. 3.60a**). The tension on the filament must always be greater than the pressure on the tube. Otherwise one possibly pushes the sponge into the vessel lumen, a relatively common error.

When the collagen sponge has been correctly seated against the vessel wall, a black mark on the filament should come into view.

Now let go of the tube and filament and observe whether the bleeding stops. Once the bleeding has stopped, cut through the filament at its proximal end, remove the tube, and then cut off the filament beneath the skin (**Fig. 3.60b**). Apply a sterile dressing to the skin incision and you are finished. If a little blood continues to seep from the cannula track, place a few compresses on the dressing and ask the patient to press on them for a while.

Tamping the collagen sponge into place against the vessel wall can be very painful. Therefore careful anesthesia of the vessel wall is highly recommended when one is performing a puncture. If one is not sure whether the anesthesia will be sufficient, try to anesthetize the vessel wall again immediately before placing the vascular closure system, but this is more difficult.

According to the manufacturer's specifications, patients who have undergone diagnostic interventions (without anticoagulants) and been treated with Angio-Seal can get out of bed after 20 minutes and be released after 60 minutes. It is certainly no mistake to extend these times a bit.

After an intervention, the patient should remain in bed until the effect of the anticoagulant therapy has subsided (heparin has a half-life of 30 minutes; that of recombinant tissue plasminogen activators (TPAs) is 4 to 6 minutes).

Important complications. Instead of remaining on the vessel wall, the collagen sponge can be pushed into the artery. This is best prevented by pulling on the filament with greater force than one uses to push in the tube (the author has never seen a filament break).

Infections often leading to mycotic pseudoaneurysm are said to occur in up to 0.3% of all cases. The infection manifests itself on average after 8 days but in extreme cases can take more than a month to appear (Turi 2008).

After antegrade catheterization, the wire can kink at the arterial access site. This can make it impossible to introduce the relatively stiff dilator of the Angio-Seal system (see Antegrade Catheterization of the Femoral Artery, p. 51). If one anticipates this happening, one can use a stiff Amplatz wire when introducing the sheath instead of the wire supplied with the system. This will almost always make it possible to introduce the sheath. One can also switch to an Amplatz wire when the standard wire already has a kink. A long 18 gauge plastic cannula can always be inserted over the wire, and this cannula will allow one to advance an Amplatz wire into the vessel. If not, an assistant can pull the patient's abdomen upward. Even then, a kink can still develop in the system sheath that will prevent one from introducing the closure system (although this is rare). In this case, one will have to treat the access site with external compression.

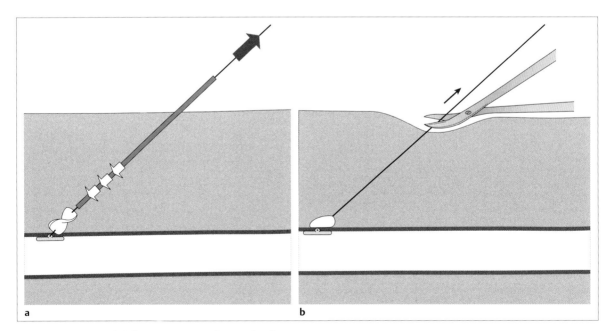

Fig. 3.60 Angio-Seal: Collagen sponge on the vessel wall.
a The collagen sponge is pressed against the vessel wall while tension is applied to the anchor filament.

b The filament is cut beneath the skin.

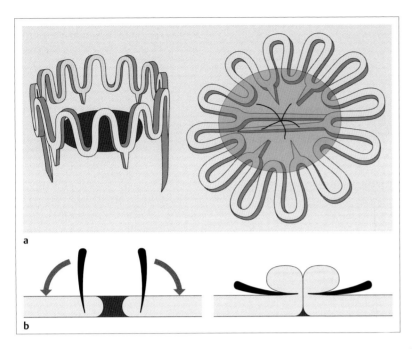

Fig. 3.61 StarClose system.
a Six hooks around the access wound are pressed into the vessel wall.
b When released, the system draws the edges of the wound together.

StarClose

The StarClose system closes the vessel wall with a ring of six interlinked metal (nitinol) hooks. These hook into the vessel wall from outside and are then drawn together toward the center (**Fig. 3.61**). The author has not had experience with this system.

Perclose ProGlide

The Perclose system (Abbott Vascular) employs the most convincing technique. It actually closes the puncture with a perfect vascular suture. The long tip of this system contains a suture two tails of which are held in the two arms of a lever mechanism. This mechanism is unfolded within the vessel and then drawn against its inner wall (**Fig. 3.62**). The outer section of the system contains two long needles that penetrate the vessel wall

exactly opposite the two suture tails. These needles then connect with the suture tails within the vascular lumen (**Fig. 3.62**). Each of the suture tails is fitted with a tiny metal sleeve no thicker than the shaft of the needle. The tip of the needle hooks into this sleeve. When the needles are then withdrawn, they pull the suture tails back out through the vessel wall, one proximal to the puncture site and one distal to it (**Fig. 3.63**). Outside the vessel the two suture tails are tied together in a knot, which is pushed against the vessel wall and then pulled tight (**Fig. 3.64**).

A larger version (Prostar XL) includes two sutures with four needles. This allows percutaneous closure of punctures up to 24 French in diameter. Unfortunately these systems are a bit more complex and may be more liable to malfunction. For this reason they are not recommended for a less experienced operator.

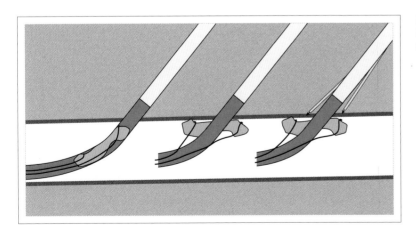

Fig. 3.62 Perclose: System introduced, lever with suture tail unfolded, needles at vessel wall.

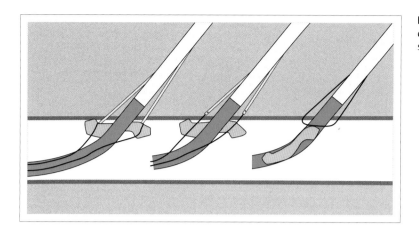

Fig. 3.63 Perclose: Needles have penetrated vessel wall, now connected with suture tails, suture loop at puncture site.

Mynx

The Mynx system (AccessClosure, Mountain View, CA, USA) closes the cannula track with a plug that absorbs fluid and expands. The precise position over the vessel wall is reached by inflating a small balloon in the vascular lumen and pulling it against the inner wall of the vessel as the plug is inserted (**Fig. 3.65**). The manufacturer states that the closure material is absorbed by the surrounding tissue within a month. (**Note:** This system is relatively new. The author has not yet had any experience with it.)

Summary and Evaluation of Vascular Closure Systems

The advantages and disadvantages of vascular closure systems are currently the subject of much discussion. Some of the study results are contradictory. Vascular closure systems indisputably save a lot of time for the physician. On the other hand, they involve higher costs. A recently published compilation of statistics on the management of a total of 2,373 inguinal artery punctures (Das et al 2011) revealed the following complication rates: manual compression

4.1%, Angio-Seal 3.1%, StarClose 8.3%, and Perclose 9.7%. The complications requiring surgery that occur as a result of vascular closure systems are more complex, and the surgical interventions are more extensive (Fraedrich et al 2010).

Treatment of the Brachial and Radial Artery Access Sites

In recent years, the arteries of the arm have increasingly been used as an approach for angiography and endovascular interventions. Although the radial artery is occluded after catheterization in 5 to 10% of all cases, cardiologists in particular prefer it to the brachial artery because its occlusion does not endanger the hand if the ulnar artery is patent. The **Allen test** (see Access via the Brachial Artery, p. 65) is used to evaluate the function of the ulnar artery.

Manual Compression

The access site in the arteries of the arm is usually treated with manual compression. To avoid injury to the

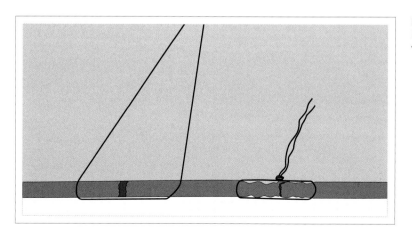

Fig. 3.64 Perclose: Knot is made between suture tails, pushed against the vessel wall, and pulled tight.

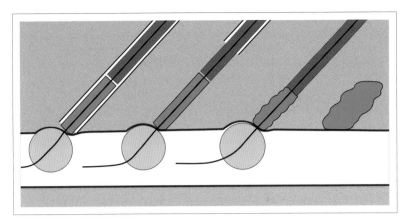

Fig. 3.65 Mynx system: An expanding plug closes the cannula track.

endothelium from shear forces, the sheath should not be withdrawn under external pressure. Because of their superficial location the brachial and radial arteries will collapse even under slight pressure. Here it is particularly important to ensure that only the cannula track collapses and not the artery itself.

When compressing the brachial artery with three fingertips of one hand for 10 to 15 minutes, one can easily check the pulse in the radial artery with the other hand. Then apply a short splint to the extensor side of the arm and wrap it with an elastic bandage. This is done primarily to prevent the patient from flexing the arm. Beneath the bandage, place a long cushion of gauze over the artery. This gently compresses the cannula track. Before sending the patient back to the ward to lie in bed for 3 to 4 hours, check the pulse in the radial artery and have the patient repeat this at brief intervals.

Mechanical Compression

The arteries of the arm are more conducive to mechanical compression than the femoral artery: The arteries' immediate subcutaneous location makes it easier to identify their course precisely. It is also a lot easier to

apply a tourniquet around the arm, which provides a reliable buttress for compression without causing the patient excessive discomfort. However, the arteries' immediate subcutaneous location also makes them more susceptible to the pressure peaks that can occur when the compression system is not entirely congruent with the surface of the arm. The subcutaneous fatty tissue in the inguinal region usually compensates for such irregularities.

Compression Systems for the Radial Artery

Various compression systems for the radial artery are available. These include RadiStop (St. Jude Medical), Adapty (Medikit, Tokyo, Japan), D Stat Radial (Vascular Solutions), and TR Band (Terumo Medical, Southaven, MS, USA). Three of these four compression devices are designed so that a narrow nontransparent block of plastic is pressed against the artery (**Fig. 3.66**). The block is attached to a frame that is pressed against the volar aspect of the forearm with the aid of a belt. It is not possible to adjust the pressure with any precision.

The device manufactured by Terumo (**Fig. 3.67**) is an inflatable transparent compression cushion integrated into a flexible plastic cuff ~ 4 cm wide, which is placed

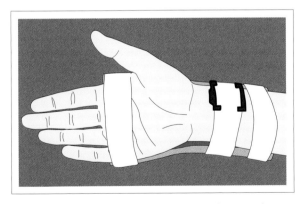

Fig. 3.66 RadiStop: A plastic block is pressed against the artery.

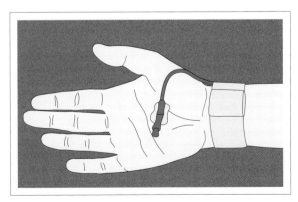

Fig. 3.67 TR Band: An inflatable compression cushion is placed over the radial artery.

on the forearm. Cubero et al (2009) demonstrated in a prospective study that this system could decrease the rate of radial artery occlusion from 12.0 to 1.1% if the compression cushion is not filled with the standard 15 mL of air but adapted to the mean arterial pressure. Thrombotic occlusion should be expected whenever arterial blood flow is interrupted by compression for several hours. An occluded radial artery can occasionally recanalize spontaneously within the next 3 months.

Vascular closure systems are very rarely used in the arteries of the arm. Angio-Seal (Belenky et al 2007) and StarClose (Puggioni et al 2008) have each been used in small series in the **brachial artery** only.

Venous Access

Catheterization of the Femoral Vein

Because the femoral vein is not palpable the artery is palpated for orientation. The vein normally lies medial and slightly posterior to the artery. It can lie partially or completely beneath the artery. If one does not hit the vein when performing the puncture medial to the artery, then one first looks behind the artery. This means advancing the cannula past the artery and then guiding it laterally.

Those who lack practice in this type of puncture can use color Doppler imaging to acquire a reliable image of the vein's location relative to the artery.

One should try to puncture the vein with the thin needle while applying local anesthesia. Because of the low pressure in the vein this does not involve any risk. If one fails to find the vein with this method, the ultrasound unit should be obtained before the patient is draped. Of course one can also use the small vascular Doppler transducer even after the patient has been draped (see Puncture of an Impalpable or Poorly Palpable Artery, p. 45).

The most important trick: Have the patient press during the puncture (**Fig. 3.68**)! Now one has a chance of puncturing only the anterior wall and not gaining access to the lumen only after partially withdrawing the cannula (one should also use this trick when looking for the vein while administering local anesthesia). Without the Valsalva maneuver, advancing the cannula will push the anterior wall of the vein against the posterior wall. One will then pass through both without noticing it. Here the Valsalva maneuver is as useful, even essential, as a tourniquet for puncturing a vein in the arm.

Some operators attach a syringe filled with saline solution to the cannula and use it to create suction while advancing the cannula. This is not necessary if the patient presses hard enough. Then blood will flow out of the cannula as soon as one penetrates the anterior wall of the vein, and one can introduce the wire without any further manipulation.

Treatment of the access site after removal of the sheath. The low venous blood pressure means there is little risk of postprocedure bleeding or hematoma. It is enough to compress the access site for 3 to 5 minutes with slight pressure and then apply a pressure bandage that is not very tight for a few hours. However, it is important for

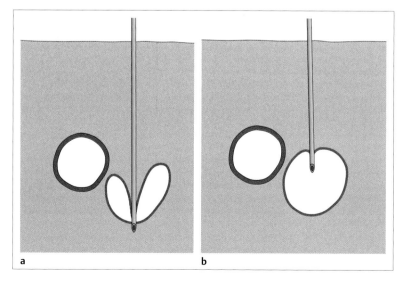

Fig. 3.68 Puncture of the femoral vein.
a Without Valsalva maneuver.
b With Valsalva maneuver.

a

b

the patient to remain in bed for the next 4 hours because venous pressure is significantly higher when the body is upright.

Catheterization of the Internal Jugular Vein

The internal jugular vein is an important access site. It must be catheterized for implanting an inferior vena cava filter, for treating superior inflow tract congestion, or for a transjugular intrahepatic portosystemic shunt (TIPS). Study the course of the vein with ultrasound prior to catheterization. Usually one will have to puncture the vein through the sternocleidomastoid muscle. To reliably exclude an air embolism, puncture the jugular vein with a syringe attached!

The approach via the right jugular vein is better than via the left side because it gives one direct access to the vena cava. The puncture is performed ~ 5 cm superior to the clavicle with the patient's head turned to the left side and the cannula angled caudally 45°. The transducer is held perpendicular to the vein 2 cm caudal to the skin incision (**Fig. 3.69**). Here too, the Valsalva maneuver is crucial! If one fails to aspirate blood while advancing the cannula, one should withdraw it slowly while aspirating.

The guidewire must not enter the right ventricle. There it would trigger extrasystoles.

The vein courses lateral to the carotid artery. If pulsating blood gushes out of the cannula, then the carotid artery has been punctured. In that case, the cannula is withdrawn and moderate pressure is applied for 5 to 10 minutes to compress the site (the carotid artery must not be sealed off by compression).

Catheterization of the Subclavian Vein

The Valsalva maneuver is of no help in a subclavian vein puncture (usually only required for placing an implantable port) because the vein lies within the chest cavity and is compressed by the maneuver. The course, depth, and patency of the vein should be evaluated with ultrasound prior to any puncture. Road mapping can also be used to facilitate a subclavian vein puncture: Contrast is injected into the cubital vein with a perfusor line connecting the venous cannula and contrast syringe. All of this is covered by a sterile drape.

It may be necessary to catheterize the subclavian vein via an arm vein, as is done when dilating a central vein in a dialysis patient. In such cases, it is far better to use the basilic vein than the cephalic vein. Not only is the approach shorter but, more importantly, one avoids the nearly right angle curve where the cephalic vein joins the subclavian vein (**Fig. 3.70**).

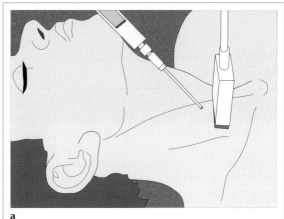

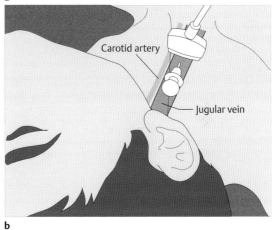

Fig. 3.69 Puncture of the internal jugular vein (using Valsalva maneuver).
a Lateral view.
b From the examiner's perspective.

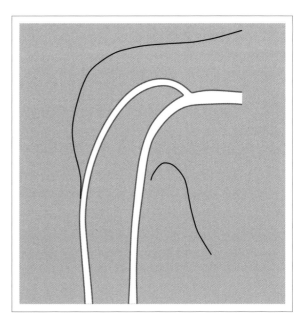

Fig. 3.70 The basilic vein is the better approach to the subclavian vein.

Angiography

General Remarks on Indication and Significance

Angiographic images can meet high aesthetic standards, and the attempt on the part of the radiologist to obtain an aesthetically appealing image is well in line with the primary purpose of the modality. However, other criteria are the crucial ones: Angiography must identify the cause of the patient's complaints, and it must visualize everything that will determine which treatment option is indicated.

This means that the radiologist must be familiar with the treatment methods of vascular surgery, interventional radiology, and angiology. Upon completion of the examination, the radiologist should know which treatment is worth considering and should clearly document its indication. The necessary knowledge and experience to make such decisions are best acquired in regular, ideally daily, discussions of findings with colleagues specializing in vascular surgery and, in applicable cases, angiology.

A previous MR or CT angiographic study significantly simplifies the planning of angiography and intervention. Even older angiographic studies regularly provide valuable information about preexisting vascular findings, the shape of the aortic bifurcation, and the position of the femoral artery bifurcation. They are helpful in planning the approach and in defining the indication and should therefore be obtained prior to any new angiography or intervention.

Digital Subtraction, Computed Tomographic, and Magnetic Resonance Angiography

Prior to any endovascular intervention precise imaging studies of the findings are required. There are three available modalities:

- Digital subtraction angiography (DSA)
- CT angiography (CTA)
- MR angiography (MRA)

CTA and MRA are generally regarded as noninvasive. At least in the case of CTA this is misleading. This is because the risk of contrast-induced nephropathy, a more severe complication than vascular trauma at the arterial access site, is greater in CTA than in carefully performed DSA. When we calculate the equivalent to contrast agent with 300 mg of iodine per mL, CTA requires between 115 and 175 mL (Sommer et al 2010) as opposed to no more than 80 to 100 mL required to perform equally precise DSA with good technique. In patients with known renal insufficiency this contrast agent can be partially or completely replaced with CO_2 in DSA. One can also limit the imaging study to a specific region, for example, one leg, and then image and treat the other after an interval of several days.

The contrast agent used in MRA also poses a specific risk for patients with impaired kidney function. Nephrogenic systemic fibrosis is an occasionally fatal disease that manifests itself primarily in the skin and for which there is no known treatment. The use of gadolinium contrast is not advisable in patients with a glomerular filtration rate (GFR) less than 60 mL/min/1.73 m² (normal value: 100 to 160 mL/min/1.73 m²; Miki et al 2009). Noncontrast MRA techniques have again become the subject of increased interest (Lanzman et al 2011).

In most cases clinical findings will determine relatively clearly whether endovascular intervention is indicated, and the ankle-brachial index (ABI; see Chapter 1, Clinical Presentation of Peripheral Arterial Occlusive Disease, p. 1) can be used to confirm the indication. Given this situation, it can be expedient to combine diagnostics and therapy in a single session. This assumes that the patient is well prepared and the examiner does not use more contrast agent than necessary. In practice it is often possible to get by with less than 100 mL of contrast for both procedures.

Important Principles for Angiography of the Extremities

Today the demands placed on angiography of the arms and legs have increased because improvements in therapeutic options have made it necessary to visualize even smaller peripheral vessels. Yet one often has the impression that this angiographic task is not taken seriously, even that the results it achieves do not really justify catheterizing an artery.

Two factors render angiography of the arteries of the arms and legs in some respects more demanding than angiography of those of any internal organ, including the coronary and cerebral arteries. These are, first, the length of the arteries and, second, the possibility of a drop in **temperature** in the hands and feet far below that of the trunk. This in turn can lead to **drastically reduced circulation**. In any patient with stage II disease according to Fontaine, it is important to warm up the patient's feet or hands prior to the angiography and keep them warm during the examination. This is not recommended in stage III and IV disease because warming increases the need for oxygen and therefore the existing oxygen deficit.

The technique of angiography of the pelvis and lower extremity must always be adapted to the equipment being used, especially the size of the image intensifier or flat panel detector. In applicable cases one must also be able to incrementally shift the image intensifier relative to the patient. This means that one should be a bit creative with the schemes suggested here until the optimum technique is found.

It is important to remember these six important principles:

- DSA systems are able to generate **a single summation angiogram from a series of sequential images**. This

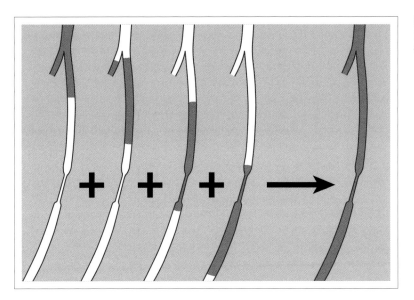

means that for one good image of a vascular segment 35 cm in length one will not need a 35 cm contrast bolus for 2 to 3 seconds. It will be enough to document a short bolus on its way through this segment in a sufficient number of images (**Fig. 3.71**). If one wants to make use of this capability, it should be noted that the **concentration of contrast agent** in the bolus is far more important than its length. The iodine content of the contrast agent and the flow rate during injection determine the concentration. One can replace a maximum of 70 to 80% of the blood with contrast agent (Schroeder 1989). Assuming 15 mL of blood flow through the lower abdominal aorta per second, one will be able to add at most maybe 12 mL per second of contrast agent to achieve the maximum possible contrast.

- On its way into the periphery the contrast bolus is thinned with blood at both ends. To ensure sufficient contrast in the periphery, one will need a longer bolus and a higher initial concentration to **visualize the arteries of the lower leg** than in the iliac arteries. It is therefore wrong to use a lower concentration (200 or even 150 mg of iodine per mL) when examining the leg arteries. Good visualization of the arteries of the lower leg and foot is the yardstick for quality in angiography of the pelvis and lower extremity.
- One will greatly improve contrast in peripheral vessels and conserve contrast agent by **injecting the contrast close to the periphery** (e.g., into the distal external iliac or distal superficial femoral artery instead of into the abdominal aorta).
- The thinning on its way into the periphery makes the contrast bolus become longer. Therefore use a **low image frequency for the lower leg**.
- A hyperosmolar contrast agent causes a sensation of heat that varies greatly between individuals and elicits reactive motion in some patients. This renders correct

subtraction more difficult. At least in sensitive patients consider using the **iso-osmolar dimeric contrast agent iodixanol**, which does not elicit this reaction even at its highest concentration (320 mg of iodine/mL).
- Most important: **Cold feet are the worst enemies of good angiography of the legs!** Cold feet lead to narrow blood vessels and drastically reduced blood flow. The result is that the contrast agent will thin to the point of invisibility and flow away via proximal branch arteries before it ever reaches the feet. Therefore it is crucial to warm up the patient's feet prior to the angiography and keep them warm during the examination. This is best done with a large plastic bag partially filled with warm water (**Fig. 3.72**). **Exception:** Patients with Fontaine stage III and IV disease (see earlier discussion).

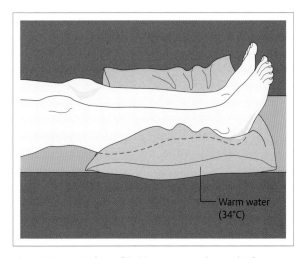

Warm water (34°C)

Fig. 3.72 A 10 L bag of 34°C warm water keeps the feet warm. It also improves image quality by optimally ensuring uniform thickness.

Intra-arterial administration of a vasodilator is no substitute for warming the patient's feet. In a patient with cold feet these agents will rarely reach the vessels they are supposed to dilate!

The dialysis ward will have suitable plastic bags for dialysis fluid and large burners for warming it to the desired temperature (34°C).

Variants of Angiography of the Pelvis and Lower Extremity

Angiography of the pelvis and lower extremity may be performed in three ways:
1. Segmental examination with selective contrast injection into the distal right and left external iliac arteries to image the arteries of the legs
2. Segmental examination with repeated contrast injection into the lower abdominal aorta
3. A single contrast injection into the lower abdominal aorta after which the image intensifier is shifted incrementally relative to the patient to follow the contrast drainage

The technique known as IV DSA was never a good method. Its major drawback was that the mediocre quality of its angiographic images hardly justified the large quantity of contrast agent it required. The capabilities of modern MRA and CTA have clearly rendered it obsolete.

Which side should be used for vascular access? Many patients are referred to the radiology department for DSA with the option of subsequent intervention in the same session. This means that one should choose the access site so as to allow the maximum number of treatment options.

Usually one should opt for arterial access on the side with less pathology because this will better allow one to treat the arteries of the pelvis and legs on the affected side in the same session.

If one catheterizes the affected side and finds that the symptoms are caused by problems in the arteries of the leg, then one may have to perform an antegrade puncture in the same inguinal region within the next few days. Then one may even have to contend with a hematoma.

Exception: One suspects the symptoms are due to iliac arterial stenosis and a sufficiently strong pulse is palpable on the affected side. In this case retrograde catheterization of the affected side will give better access to the findings requiring treatment.

Variant 1

Segmental angiography with selective contrast injection into the distal right and left external iliac arteries to image the arteries of the legs.

Distinctive features of this technique:
- It uses less contrast agent and achieves better opacification because the injection is performed close to the region of interest. (Using an end-hole catheter improves contrast.)
- Optimal collimation (with full and half aperture stops) is readily achieved without compensating devices.
- Conditions are optimal for subtraction: only a few seconds between precontrast images (mask) and contrast-filled image.
- It offers the capability of imaging abnormal findings more precisely (enlargement, second imaging plane) with just slight additional contrast agent.

Which Catheter?

The shape of the catheter must allow it to be easily hooked into the contralateral common iliac artery at the bifurcation and then advanced over a wire (see **Figs. 3.36** and **3.37**). Avoid pigtails! If the catheter then lies extended within the external iliac artery for the contrast injection into a leg, its side holes will cause the bolus to be distributed over a longer segment. Its initial concentration will be correspondingly reduced (**Fig. 3.73**). Angiography of the pelvis and lower extremity with selective injection does not require contrast flow rates over 8 mL/ per second. Therefore, it is best not to use catheters with side holes.

There is another practical disadvantage to side holes: In patients with an acute-angle bifurcation and elongated iliac arteries, one may not succeed in advancing the catheter into the contralateral arteries. In such a case, satisfactory visualization of the contralateral side will only be possible with a catheter hooked into the common iliac artery. One will then avoid losing half of the contrast agent that would flow out on the ipsilateral side through side holes (**Fig. 3.74**). Recommended catheters include appropriately shaped 4 French models without side holes (see **Fig. 3.36**) such as the Sos Omni 0 (AngioDynamics) or Contra 2 (Boston Scientific).

One will need only a sheath if the vessel wall is very hard or bleeding occurs next to the catheter. This is more likely to occur where the tip of the catheter is not in close contact with the guidewire (**Fig. 3.75**). A 4 French sheath has an outer diameter of ~ 2.1 mm, whereas a 4 French catheter measures only 1.33 mm. The area of the access opening with a sheath is ~ 2.4 times as large as without one. If one performs purely diagnostic angiography with a good catheter and dispenses with a sheath, one will do more than save money.

Performing the Procedure
- Position the patient on the angiography table.
- Check the pulse status and inspect the skin.
- Place water cushions beneath the patient's feet (10 L, 34°C) and a blanket over the legs and feet.
- Establish venous access.

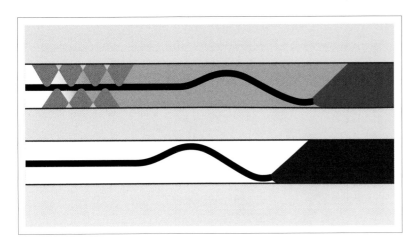

Fig. 3.73 Decreased initial concentration from a catheter with side holes (top), optimal contrast with a single end hole.

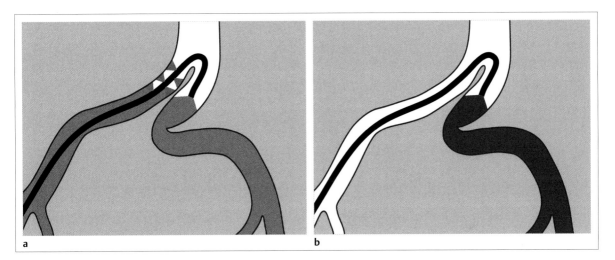

Fig. 3.74 Better contrast is obtained in the contralateral side without side holes.
a With side holes.   **b** Without side holes.

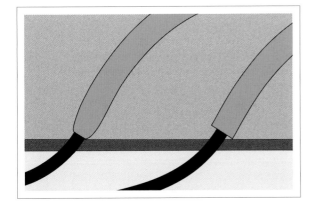

Fig. 3.75 Catheter tip is in close contact with the wire (*left*). Tip is too wide (*right*).

- Determine the level of the access site under fluoroscopy.
- Administer local anesthesia.
- Prep and drape the patient.
- Make a stab incision and puncture the proximal arterial wall with an open cannula and J wire (standard Teflon-coated steel wire).
- Advance the catheter into the distal contralateral external iliac artery (see the section on crossover catheterization, **Figs. 3.37** and **3.76**). After this maneuver the guidewire will usually no longer be needed.
- Connect the catheter to the injector (use a perfusor line instead of a high-pressure line: cheap and long instead of expensive and unnecessarily strong!)

Table 3.1 (p. 85) lists the image series obtained with variant 1. As was mentioned earlier, the specifications must always be adapted to the equipment being used, especially the size of the image intensifier.

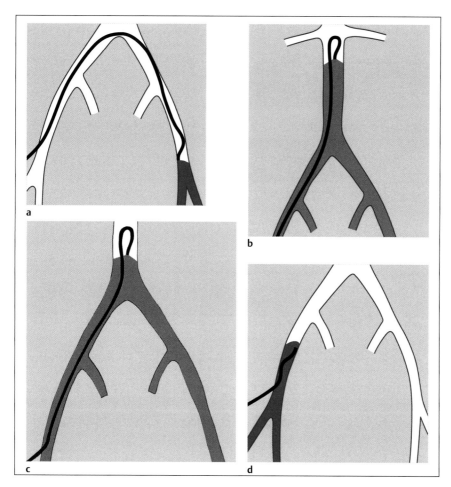

Fig. 3.76 Overview of the four positions into which the catheter is moved without using the wire (i.e., when connected to the injector).
a Distal contralateral external iliac artery.
b Infrarenal abdominal aorta.
c Distal abdominal aorta.
d Distal ipsilateral external iliac artery.

Comments about the settings. The origin and trunk of the internal iliac artery can usually be evaluated only on a contralateral (medial) oblique image. The same applies to the external iliac artery.

It is almost always the case that stenosis at the origin of the deep femoral artery is properly visualized only on a lateral oblique view. Exceptional cases may also require a medial oblique view. It is crucial to visualize the origin of the deep femoral artery because endarterectomy of this structure represents one of the most important treatment options.

Stenosis at the origin of the anterior tibial artery is easily missed where the trifurcation is visualized on a view other than a medial oblique view or the leg is in external rotation (as can occur spontaneously).

Supplements

Visualization of the **popliteal artery on a lateral view** is required for total knee arthroplasty; it may also be helpful in the presence of popliteal aneurysms or stenoses. Have the patient externally rotate the leg as far as it will go, and then rotate the image intensifier medially until it provides a lateral view of the knee. Or have the patient flex the unaffected knee. Then obtain the images using a horizontal-beam, cross-table lateral projection underneath this other knee.

A plastic femoropopliteal bypass can kink when the knee is flexed. This may be the cause of an occlusion. Similar problems can occur with stents in the distal superficial femoral artery or popliteal artery. In these cases one will need a **lateral view with the knee flexed**.

For **lateral views of a foot** (i.e., for unobscured visualization of the dorsalis pedis and plantar arteries) the same two options apply as with the knee. To obtain a plantodorsal view, tilt the unit cranially so that the imaging plane is approximately parallel to the foot.

Findings requiring treatment should also be visualized on magnified images. Measure the vessel diameter and degree of stenosis. It may be possible to treat pathology in the contralateral arteries of the pelvis and leg and in the ipsilateral iliac arteries in the same session.

Before completing the intervention check once again carefully:
- Has everything been clearly visualized?
- Has the cause of the symptoms been identified?

Table 3.1 Image series for variant 1: Segmental angiography with selective contrast injection into the distal right and left external iliac arteries to image the arteries of the legs

	Image Frequency	Contrast Volume
Injection into contralateral external iliac artery (320 mg of iodine/mL contrast at 8 mL/s)		
Common femoral artery and femoral bifurcation, 30–40° lateral	3/s	5 mL
Thigh PA	2/s	6 mL
Knee	2/s	8 mL
Lower leg, 15° medial	1/s	10 mL
Where indicated: foot, lateral, and plantodorsal	1/s	1–2 × 10 mL
Adapt the oblique projection for the lower leg series to the position of the leg. Often the legs are externally rotated. In this case, a PA projection may be appropriate. To obtain optimal opacification in the arteries of the lower leg and foot, it may be advisable to advance the catheter into the superficial femoral artery or even the popliteal artery. As long as it is not known how much the deep femoral artery contributes to the arterial supply of the lower leg, contrast must be injected superior to the femoral artery bifurcation.		
Withdraw catheter and advance it into the infrarenal aorta (320 mg of iodine/mL contrast at 8 mL/s)		
Aorta and iliac arteries PA	4/s	10 mL
Only where clinical findings might justify renal PTA (i.e., in arterial hypertension or impaired kidney function) then: **Advance catheter to the level of the renal arteries:**		
Abdominal aorta 20° LAO	4/s	10 mL
Injection into lower abdominal aorta (320 mg of iodine/mL contrast at 8 mL/s)		
Iliac arteries 30° RAO	4/s	8 mL
Iliac arteries 30° LAO	4/s	8 mL
Withdraw catheter into the ipsilateral external iliac artery (320 mg of iodine/mL contrast at 8 mL/s)		
Common femoral artery and femoral bifurcation, 30° lateral	3/s	5 mL
Thigh PA	2/s	6 mL
Knee	2/s	8 mL
Lower leg, 15° medial	1/s	10 mL
Where indicated: foot, lateral, and plantodorsal	1/s	1–2 × 10 mL
Total contrast required (without kidneys and feet): 84 mL		

Note: obese patients can require up to 50% more contrast.
Abbreviations: LAO, left anterior oblique; PA, posteroanterior; PTA, percutaneous transluminal angioplasty; RAO, right anterior oblique.

CO_2 angiography in renal insufficiency, hyperthyroidism, or adverse reaction to contrast agent. CO_2 is the best alternative to iodine-containing contrast agents in patients with hyperthyroidism, patients who have experienced a previous adverse reaction, and especially patients with impaired kidney function (see Chapter 2, CO_2 as a Contrast Agent, p. 36). Good results are most easily achieved with selective injection of CO_2. Variant 1 described earlier is the most suitable technique.

Notes on Imaging Technique

When planning angiography of an extremity, remember that the actual size of the part of the body imaged is normally smaller than the entrance field size specified by the manufacturer of the image intensifier. The data for rectangular flat panel detectors are particularly misleading. The data monitor may display, say, 48 cm as the entrance field size. This number refers to the diagonal of this rectangle. One is actually imaging 32 to 35 cm along the patient's longitudinal axis.

If the contrast agent only reaches the vascular segment of interest 10 or 20 seconds after the start of the injection, then there is invariably some uncertainty as to when exactly to begin the image series. Because the study always requires an initial precontrast image, examiners tend to begin the series too early. The result is that too many precontrast images are obtained. This leads to unnecessary radiation exposure for the patient and equally unnecessary wear and tear on the X-ray tube.

This problem is easily solved whenever there is an opportunity to obtain a precontrast image separately from the actual series itself. The first pulse, triggered about where we now begin the entire series, would only trigger the precontrast image. The image series would then be triggered with a second pulse as soon the fluoroscopic image shows good opacification.

Systems manufactured by GE and Toshiba currently provide this capability; the ones from Siemens and Philips do not.

Variant 2

Segmental angiography with repeated contrast injection into the lower abdominal aorta.

Distinctive features of this technique:

- Favorable conditions for subtraction: only a few seconds between precontrast images (mask) and contrast-filled image.
- This technique requires more contrast agent than variant 1. This is because in every series for the legs, contrast agent also flows into the iliac arteries and because the longer flow distances lead to greater thinning.
- Restless patients will often require separate manual correction of the subtraction for the left and right sides.

Which Catheter?

To avoid unnecessary thinning of the contrast agent, the catheter should release it within a very short segment of the aorta. The contrast agent should therefore be released from the end hole at the level of the few, closely spaced side holes (see **Fig. 2.21b**). Many pigtail catheters release

part of the contrast against the flow and are therefore unsuitable (see **Fig. 2.21a**). One should also be able to advance the catheter easily into the contralateral vessels (see **Figs. 3.36** and **3.37**). This makes it easier to visualize details and initiate treatment during the same session where indicated. Therefore, use a catheter such as the UF (Cordis), OmniFlush (AngioDynamics), or Contralateral Flush (Boston Scientific) instead of a pigtail design.

One will only need a sheath if the vessel wall is very hard or bleeding occurs next to the catheter. This is more likely to occur where the tip of the catheter is not in close contact with the guidewire (see **Fig. 3.75**).

Performing the Procedure

The procedure is identical to variant 1 with one exception: The catheter is immediately advanced into the infrarenal abdominal aorta and pulled down to the lower aorta after the first series (**Table 3.2**).

Variant 3

A single contrast injection into the lower abdominal aorta after which the image intensifier is shifted incrementally relative to the patient to follow the contrast drainage.

Distinctive features of this technique:

- The subtraction is particularly susceptible to error because there is a relatively long time between the precontrast images and the contrast-filled images.
- Collimation settings and other thickness compensation must be adjusted beforehand, and it is best to fix the patient to the table.

Table 3.2 Image series for variant 2: Segmental angiography with repeated contrast injection into the lower abdominal aorta

	Image Frequency	Contrast Volume
Catheter in the infrarenal aorta (320 mg of iodine/mL contrast at 12 mL/s)		
Aorta and iliac arteries PA	4/s	10 mL
Only where clinical findings might justify renal PTA (i.e., in arterial hypertension or impaired kidney function) then: **Advance catheter to the level of the renal arteries:**		
Abdominal aorta 20° LAO	4/s	10 mL
Injection into lower abdominal aorta (320 mg of iodine/mL contrast at 12 mL/s)		
Iliac arteries 30° RAO	4/s	10 mL
Iliac arteries 30° LAO	4/s	10 mL
The oblique images must extend sufficiently distally to allow reliable evaluation of the femoral artery bifurcations.		
Thigh PA	2/s	20 mL
Knee	1/s	20 mL
Lower leg (slightly externally rotated)	1/s	25 mL
Total contrast required (without kidneys and feet):		**85 mL**
Note: obese patients can require up to 50% more contrast. Abbreviations: LAO, left anterior oblique; PA, posteroanterior; PTA, percutaneous transluminal angioplasty; RAO, right anterior oblique.		

Table 3.3 A single contrast injection into the lower abdominal aorta after which the image intensifier is shifted incrementally relative to the patient to follow the contrast drainage

	Image frequency	Contrast Volume
Catheter in the infrarenal aorta (320 mg of iodine/mL contrast at 12 mL/s)		
The contrast syringe is connected when adjustments for thickness compensation have been made and the patient has been immobilized. Further steps: • Precontrast images from distal to proximal • Start contrast injection: 40–50 mL at 12 mL/s • Shift from proximal to distal controlled by fluoroscopy; images of every segment are obtained. • The incremental shift is triggered manually at each segment as soon as the arteries in the segment currently visualized have filled as far as the distal edge of the image. Next: **contrast injection into lower abdominal aorta (320 mg of iodine/mL contrast at 12 mL/s)**		
Iliac arteries 30° RAO	4/s	10 mL
Iliac arteries 30° LAO	4/s	10 mL
The oblique images must extend sufficiently distally to allow reliable evaluation of the femoral artery bifurcations.		
Total contrast required is approx.		**70 mL**

Note: obese patients can require up to 50% more contrast.
Abbreviations: LAO, left anterior oblique; RAO, right anterior oblique.

- Theoretically, 25 mL of contrast should be sufficient for the entire distance from the aorta to the lower legs. In practice one will need significantly more to have sufficient tolerance for incrementally shifting the image intensifier relative to the patient to follow the contrast drainage.
- Incomplete visualization can be a problem if there is a difference in the flow rates on the right and left sides.

Catheter
As in variant 2 (see earlier discussion).

Performing the Procedure
The procedure is identical to that for variant 2: The catheter is immediately advanced into the infrarenal abdominal aorta (**Table 3.3**).

Restrictions
- Incomplete visualization can be a problem if there is a difference in the flow rates on the right and left sides.
- Incomplete visualization will also occur where there is retrograde filling of one superficial femoral artery due to pathology such as a short proximal occlusion (**Fig. 3.77**).
- Even an artery that is occluded distally by an acute thrombus fills very slowly. This means that in the presence of embolic occlusion one will have to obtain a long stationary series for the correct diagnosis.
- Not every patient lies still enough to allow flawless subtraction using the precontrast images obtained on the first attempt. It is possible to make manual corrections. However, they will often have to be done separately for the left and right sides.

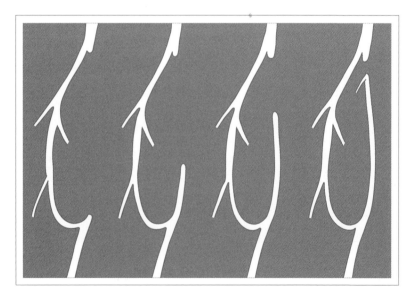

Fig. 3.77 These findings are typically overestimated when shifting the image intensifier incrementally relative to the patient: A short proximal occlusion of the superficial femoral artery fills only slowly in retrograde fashion. By the time the superficial femoral artery has filled completely, the unit is already over the lower legs.

Angiography of a Leg

Retrograde catheterization is recommended for **purely diagnostic angiography** because the technique is simpler. A long 18 French plastic cannula or a 4 French dilator is used for the angiography itself. The deep femoral artery is reliably visualized only by retrograde injection. The puncture is performed with the normal steel cannula. This is then replaced over a short wire with the plastic cannula, which lies more securely within the lumen. The image series are identical to angiography of the pelvis and lower extremity as described under variant 1 (see earlier discussion).

Angiography and Percutaneous Transluminal Angioplasty in a Leg

When a patient has trophic changes in one or both feet (Fontaine stage IV disease), it is important to determine whether stenoses or occlusions of the arteries of the leg are present and require treatment. Two thirds of these patients are diabetics; therefore many of them have impaired kidney function as well. When the inguinal pulses are strong and there is no ultrasound evidence of iliac arterial stenosis, then one can limit the examination to angiography of the leg using an antegrade approach in anticipation of possible intervention:

- Perform the puncture with the normal steel cannula. Then switch to the longer plastic cannula over a short wire.
- Perform angiography; determine whether intervention is indicated.
- For intervention in the lower leg, replace the cannula with a sheath 40 to 50 cm long.

Limit yourself to one leg per session. It is often possible to perform the diagnostic examination and PTA with no more than 30 or 40 mL of contrast. Remember, too, that CO_2 can be used as a contrast agent. If the other leg requires treatment as well, this should be done 2 or more days later to minimize the burden on the kidneys (**Table 3.4**).

Angiography of the Abdominal Aorta

The principles of contrast administration already discussed also apply to angiography of the abdominal aorta.

Diagnostic evaluation of the most important disorder of the aorta, aortic aneurysm, is the domain of CT. However, endovascular treatment is performed under angiographic control. The most important problems that require aortography are **stenoses at the origins of the major branches of the aorta**: The celiac trunk and superior mesenteric artery arise close to each other on the anterior aspect of the upper abdominal aorta. Because their origins are visible on a lateral projection, they are best visualized using a horizontal-beam, cross-table lateral projection with the patient positioned supine.

The great depth of the object being imaged leads to a relatively high amount of scattered radiation. Therefore one should use a very narrow collimation setting. The patient's arms will not be visible in the image if the arms lie flat on the table. To achieve a sufficient imaging frequency of two or three images per second in spite of the great depth of the object being imaged, one must keep a short distance between the X-ray tube and the image intensifier. Push the patient close to the image intensifier. The contrast bolus need only be short but must be sufficiently concentrated. Inject, say, 20 mL at a flow rate of 14 mL per second.

Angiography of the renal arteries is discussed in Chapter 4, Intervention Technique (p. 125).

Angiography of the Upper Extremities

To a certain extent the predominant lines of inquiry in angiography of the upper extremities differ from those that are important in the lower extremities.

Arteriosclerotic stenoses and occlusions occur at the origins of all the supra-aortic branch arteries. Stenosis or occlusion of the subclavian artery typically occurs between the artery's origin on the aortic arch and the origin of the vertebral artery. These lesions are significantly more common on the left side than on the right. Typical

Table 3.4 Image series for diagnostic angiography of a leg

	Image frequency	Contrast Volume
Common femoral artery and femoral bifurcation, 30° lateral	3/s	5 mL
Thigh PA	2/s	6 mL
Knee PA	2/s	8 mL
Lower leg, 15° medial	1/s	10 mL
Total contrast required		**29 mL**
Additional views where indicated:		
Foot, lateral, and plantodorsal	1/s	2, 3, 10 mL
Note: obese patients can require up to 50% more contrast.		

clinical symptoms include loss of strength in the arm and unilaterally decreased blood pressure. A subclavian steal syndrome may also be present (see also Chapter 6).

Often one will be asked to document a **thoracic outlet syndrome** caused by the adjacent anatomy. Some authors maintain that this can be diagnosed by color Doppler imaging alone without the need of angiography.

In elderly patients (primarily women) there are occasionally stenoses or occlusions in the axilla and upper arm as a result of **giant cell arteritis**. In the forearm, it will sometimes be necessary to evaluate conditions for placing or replacing a **dialysis shunt**.

Yet the most challenging task is **imaging the arteries of the hands and fingers**. Certain disorders of widely varying etiology (arteriosclerosis, endangiitis obliterans, Raynaud disease, scleroderma, aneurysms of the arteries of the hand with emboli in digital arteries) can present more or less characteristic pictures in hands and fingers.

Examination Technique

The line of inquiry largely determines the examination technique.

Stenoses or occlusions of the subclavian artery close to its origin. A thoracic aortogram showing the aortic arch is obtained (30° LAO projection, **Fig. 3.78**). Visualizing a

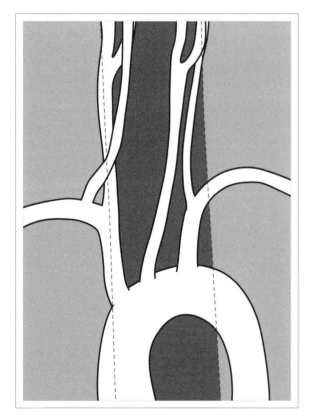

Fig. 3.78 Angiography of the supra-aortic arteries. 30° left anterior oblique projection, half aperture stops on both sides of the spine.

subclavian steal syndrome requires a long series of images (**Fig. 3.79**), possibly including supplementary views of the right side using a right anterior oblique (RAO) 30 to 45° projection.

The supra-aortic arteries should invariably be visualized in inspiration. This extends the vessels and better visualizes their origins in particular.

Thoracic outlet syndrome. It is important to image the aortic arch with the patient's arms raised and outwardly rotated.

Axillary artery and upper arm arteries. Where possible, contrast is injected selectively into the respective subclavian artery.

Forearm and hand. Where one only needs to image one side, the contrast is injected into the brachial artery at the elbow.

Positioning

Use equalization filters when imaging the supra-aortic arteries (see **Fig. 3.78**)!

When the arteries of the arm are to be imaged, the arm should be abducted 30 to 45°. The field of view is adjusted by turning rotating apertures or by rotating the flat panel detector. Imaging the forearm and hand usually requires pivoting the angiography table toward the contralateral side.

Which Catheter?

When imaging the aortic arch, do not use a pigtail catheter, but a catheter such as the Universal Flush (Cordis), OmniFlush (AngioDynamics), or Contralateral Flush (Boston Scientific). It should be 90 cm in length. Blood flow in the aorta is very fast, ~ 60 to 80 mL per second. For a series of good quality, one should select a contrast flow rate of 15 to 20 mL per second and an injection time of 1 to 1.5 seconds, and obtain four images per second. Intense pulsations often interfere with subtraction. It may be difficult to find a suitable mask for a good contrast-filled image. In such cases, it may be that the findings appear clearest without subtraction.

Catheterization of the right subclavian artery is best performed using a catheter with a short 90° distal bend and then a relatively broad curve in the opposite direction. This catheter reliably conforms to the aortic arch in such a manner that the distal bend points cranially and can be easily hooked into any branch artery arising from the aorta (JB3 or JB2, see **Fig. 2.41**, p. 24). A curved "glide" wire is advanced through this catheter into the brachiocephalic trunk, then the bend in the wire is rotated laterally into the subclavian artery. In wide vessels the distal bend may not be big enough to hook the wire into the subclavian artery. In that case, one can increase the range of this curve by adding a slight additional bend to allow visualization of the subclavian artery (see **Fig. 2.9**, p. 11).

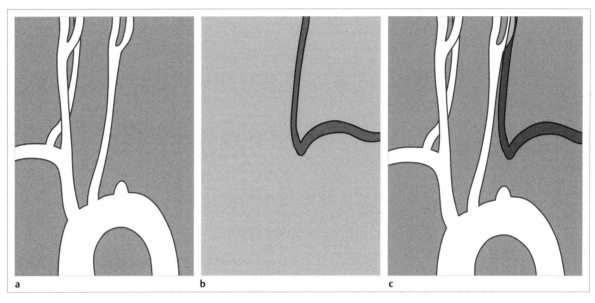

Fig. 3.79a–c Left subclavian artery occlusion with subclavian steal.
a Early phase.   **b** Late phase.   **c** Subtraction using late

With its distal bend, the wire can easily enter branches of the subclavian or axillary arteries. Care must be taken to guide it under fluoroscopy past the vertebral and internal mammary arteries in particular. Once the wire has reached the axillary or brachial artery, one can usually advance the catheter (4 French) over it without any problem. For the left side, other suitable catheters in addition to this one include straight models with a short distal bend of 20 to 30° ("vertebral artery catheters").

Contrast Agents

In addition to the face (external carotid artery), the hands are the regions of the body that react with the greatest pain to the stimulus produced by a hyperosmolar contrast agent. For this reason a less concentrated contrast agent should be used (200 or even 150 mg of iodine per mL). This results in diminished opacification and therefore image quality as well. It is much better to use the iso-osmolar dimeric contrast agent iodixanol (Visipaque, GE Healthcare, Piscataway, NJ, USA), which is tolerated at any concentration. Therefore, without hesitation, it can be used at its highest concentration of 320 mg of iodine per mL. It is recommended whenever contrast is to be injected into the subclavian or brachial arteries to image the arteries of the hand. Remember that the concentration of the contrast agent will diminish significantly on its long way to the hand.

Angiography of the Arms and Hands

Ischemic disorders of the hand and fingers can be due to a wide variety of causes. Where the clinical findings clearly involve only one hand, one can initially limit the procedure to angiography of the forearm and hand. It is usually sufficient to examine only one side when dealing with a disorder of the finger arteries that involves both hands and usually affects both sides. Proceed as follows:

- Inject the contrast into the brachial artery at the elbow via a 20 gauge plastic cannula.
- Use a perfusor line to connect the plastic cannula to a 20 mL contrast syringe with a stopcock.
- Inject manually.
- Place the hand in supination for all arm views.
- Obtain an image series of the hand (at one per second) until venous filling is seen in the fingers.

The worst enemy of angiography of the hand is a **cold hand**. Injecting a vasodilator does not help, although some books recommend it. It can only act on those arteries it can reach. Neither the contrast nor the vasodilator reaches the finger arteries in cold hands. Angiography of cold hands is usually worthless. The contrast agent is often detectable only as far distally as the wrist. Therefore do the following:

- Check the temperature of the hands prior to angiography.
- Immerse the forearm and hand in a warm bath where indicated.
- Keep the patient's arms and hands warm (under a blanket on the abdomen) until they are positioned for the examination.

When positioning the hand for the examination, place a bag filled with warm water around the hand in such

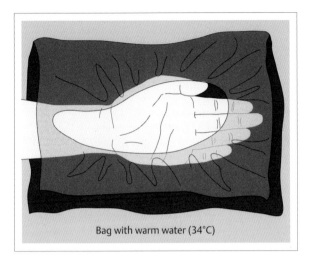

Bag with warm water (34°C)

Fig. 3.80 Bag with warm water warms and immobilizes the hand and also ensures uniform thickness.

a manner that the bag covers the dorsum and palm. Then fix the bag to the armrest with belts or adhesive strips (**Fig. 3.80**). Aside from providing effective warming this method has two additional advantages:

It eliminates motion and optimally ensures uniform thickness.

A practice that was occasionally recommended in the past was to prepare the hand for angiography by first cooling it (even in ice water) and then warming it. This is not helpful. In a cold hand, all findings appear similar; even healthy arteries are very narrow and occasionally are not visualized at all.

If angiography of the hand produces unequivocal findings consistent with arteriosclerosis, Raynaud disease, thromboangiitis obliterans (Buerger disease), or scleroderma, then the examination will have reached its objective. However, if there are signs of embolic vascular occlusion in the absence of an aneurysm in the hand, then the examination must be supplemented by transfemoral imaging of the aortic arch and the proximal segments of the respective arm. An embolism may be due to a subclavian artery aneurysm or atheromatous changes.

The other important line of inquiry for angiography of the arm is evaluating the function of a dialysis shunt. This usually requires imaging the arteries of the lower arm and the draining veins as far as the superior vena cava (see also Chapter 6, Dialysis Shunt, p. 194).

Wherever both hands are to be examined it is of course a good idea to use a transfemoral approach.

Measuring Vessel Diameter

Precise knowledge of vessel diameter is a requirement for high-quality PTA and stent implantation. More recent angiography units usually include a **measuring program** in their software. Precise measurement requires sufficient contrast in the vessel. It also helps to use a small entrance field size with the image intensifier.

A unit that is not equipped with a measuring program is no excuse for not measuring. The simplest workaround is this: Tape two small pieces of wire placed exactly 5 cm apart to the image intensifier entrance field using adhesive tape. This gives a reference guide that one can use to measure vessel diameter, allowing for the magnification.

A more elegant solution is this: Determine the magnification for certain reliably reproducible geometric constellations by obtaining a once-off measurement image.

The conditions are defined as follows:
- Set maximum possible table height (= greatest distance that can be set between focus and table surface).
- Place a lead ruler 10 cm above the table.
- Place the image intensifier entrance field 20 cm over the table.
- Set the smallest entrance field size (= maximum magnification).
- Display at maximum magnification on a specified monitor.

Then measure the magnification at which this monitor displays the lead ruler (e.g., a factor of 2.6 or 3.2).

To **measure vessel diameter** obtain an angiogram with the table at its maximum height, the image intensifier close to the patient, and both the image intensifier and the monitor set to their maximum magnification. Then divide the vessel diameter measured under these conditions by the magnification factor determined by the once-off measurement already described. This of course will be influenced by the distance between the table surface and the image intensifier entrance field (i.e., by the thickness of the patient). Increasing the distance by 2 cm will increase the magnification by ~ 1% (at a table height of 70 to 80 cm above the focus). This is relatively unimportant when choosing between balloon sizes of 5 or 6 mm, which themselves vary by 20%.

Thinking one can get by without a measurement risks dissection or rupture of the vessel by choosing too large a balloon or risks wasting time and material by starting with one that is too small.

When possible, verify the correctness of the measurement in the abdominal aorta with a sizing catheter. In the arteries of the pelvis and leg, check it against the metal markings in the balloon catheters (the package will specify the exact distance).

Percutaneous Transluminal Angioplasty

PTA involves expanding (dilating) narrow vascular segments with the aid of a balloon introduced via a percutaneous transluminal approach. Inflating the balloon creates tension in the wall of the balloon and the wall of the vessel. According to **LaPlace's law**, this tension is proportional to the product of pressure (P) and diameter (d) of the balloon or vessel (P d). On the one hand, this explains why smaller balloons can withstand far higher pressures than large balloons. On the other hand, the same applies to vessel size: The wider the vessel, the higher will be the tension in the wall that is generated by dilation at a certain pressure.

A crucial factor in the reliability of PTA is that the balloon generally reacts to the pressure far less than the vessel wall. This means that a 6 mm balloon made of a pressure-resistant material expands to a diameter of 6 mm at the recommended pressure. The pressure that the balloon exerts on the vessel wall at this diameter depends on the width and elasticity of the vessel.

The choice of balloon basically determines only the maximum diameter to which one will expand the vessel. It does not determine the pressure that will be exerted on the vessel wall.

If one wants to tear tissue, it is best done with a sharp tug. But to expand it without tearing it, one must increase the tension slowly and steadily.

Dilation should not tear the vessel wall but gently expand it. Any mural plaques should be pressed flat wherever possible. Rapidly expanding the wall increases the risk of a tear (i.e., the mechanism of vascular dissection). For this reason it is advisable to increase pressure **slowly** when dilating the vessel.

Some observations suggest that deformation and compression of the plaque material also contribute to the effect of PTA in up to 30% of all cases (Losordo et al 1992). For one thing, this would mean that moisture is being expressed. This is a process that takes time. Anyone with the patience to try to improve the results of PTA with longer and repeated dilation using the same balloon and the same pressure can observe that this does indeed lead to better results. The conclusion to be drawn from this experience is that it is best to dilate for longer than ~ 30 seconds as a matter of course. This spares all those patients requiring a second dilation unnecessary contrast administration. Moreover it spares them a second catheterization of the stenosis with the slight additional risk of dissection or thrombus mobilization (in the early days of PTA the watchword was "do not reenter!"). And cost-effectiveness is hardly the only reason why it is better to achieve a good result before having to switch to a larger balloon.

Both these things, the slow expansion and the long dilation (with repeated flushing of the catheter), are greatly facilitated by the use of a manometer syringe. The typical dilation procedure is as follows:

- Connect the manometer syringe (with contrast agent with 300 mg of iodine per mL thinned 1:1) to the lumen of the balloon.
- Slowly inflate the balloon under repeated fluoroscopic control; increase pressure over a period of 30 to 60 seconds to, say, 8 bar (**Fig. 3.81**).
- Maintain pressure for 90 seconds; flush the catheter.
- Compare the balloon diameter with the width of the vessel (road mapping); deflate the balloon.

Fig. 3.81 Dilation with manometer.

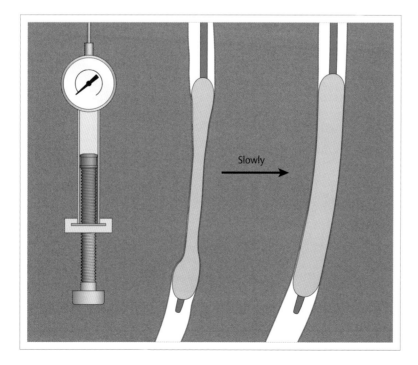

Slowly

- When reinflating, observe whether the balloon unfolds completely at low pressure (1 to 2 bar).
- Then perform a second dilation at 8 bar for over 90 seconds.

Although the recommended 3 minutes for a dilation represent at most a tenth of the time required for the entire procedure, the patience is often lacking for this brief period of what appears to be inactivity. It is easier to endure if one uses the unit's integral stopwatch or some similar timer. This allows one to concentrate on things other than time, such as chatting with the patient or with coworkers.

During dilation, care must be taken to avoid blood coagulating in the dead space in front of and behind the balloon or even within the catheter lumen. Therefore the catheter lumen should be flushed regularly and the balloon deflated at intervals of 1.5 to 2 minutes.

One can get an initial impression of the success of the dilation by initially reinflating the balloon to only 1 to 2 bar and observing whether the balloon unfolds completely at this low pressure. Upon completion of the dilation, withdraw the balloon and check the findings. For best results, use a minimum of contrast agent injected via the balloon catheter (this requires an "over the wire" balloon). Where residual stenosis is present, one can use a balloon with compliance to dilate once more with higher pressure. By increasing the pressure from, say, 8 to 14 bar one can expand the balloon's diameter by up to 10%; 5 mm will become 5.5 mm (**Fig. 3.82**). Otherwise one will probably need a larger balloon for the second dilation. A correspondingly short balloon is recommended for a short residual stenosis.

Some dissections can be tacked down by protracted dilation with slight pressure. Where that fails and especially where the dissection impairs blood flow it can be helpful to implant a stent. However, in the days before stents it was often observed how exposed plaques projecting into the lumen would disappear completely within a period of months or years.

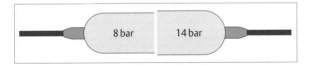

Fig. 3.82 Balloon catheter with "compliance."

Measuring vessel diameter. Good results will only be achieved when one matches the balloon to the vessel width as precisely as possible. Average values are suitable only for verifying the plausibility of values one has measured!

The measurement is performed in a segment of the vessel that appears normal but is located in close proximity to the findings requiring treatment. Comparison with the contralateral side may be helpful as well. Those who rely on average values risk having to switch catheters unnecessarily if the first one is too small or, worse, risk causing a dissection if it is too large.

Angiographic measurement of vessel diameter is an integral part of every percutaneous transluminal angioplasty or stent implantation.

Length of the balloon. Wherever possible the balloon should be a little longer than the stenosis. Otherwise the balloon could conceivably push mural deposits into adjacent vessel segments. If the available balloon is shorter than the lesion requiring treatment, one should proceed as follows: In the arteries of the leg, begin at the distal end and position the balloon so it extends a little past the lesion. Then continue the dilation proximally so that the treated segments overlap. If the balloon tends to slip out of the stenosis, advance it far enough in that it tends to slip out distally, away from the access site. Then keep tension on the catheter while the balloon is inflating.

Road mapping is extraordinarily helpful, especially for PTA of the arteries of the legs. It shows the exact position and length of the lesion in the long arteries. It shows whether the size of the selected balloon is adequate. And it can be updated at any time by injecting contrast through the sheath.

Percutaneous transluminal angioplasty with a sheath. In the early years of their use, it was common to introduce balloon catheters without a sheath. However, it has since been shown that there is significantly less trauma to the vessel wall when a sheath is used. This is because when the balloon folds up after PTA it is never as smooth as it was when first introduced. The sheath protects the vessel wall against injury when the balloon is withdrawn. Of course it is also a lot easier to change catheters with a sheath, and it eliminates bleeding next to the catheter.

Stent Placement

Balloon-Expandable Stents

Balloon-expandable stents are usually supplied attached to balloons of the appropriate size. They are introduced through sheaths and brought into the proper position with an overlay, using road mapping, under angiographic control, or according to reliable anatomical landmarks such as bone margins or mural calcifications. Once in position, they are pressed against the vessel wall by the inflated balloon.

Overlay images can be used for anatomical orientation in stent placement. Note that caution is advised if these

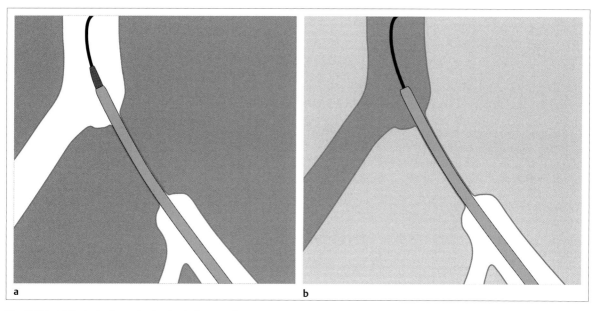

Fig. 3.83 Catheterization prior to stent placement.
a Advancing a wire and sheath through an occlusion.

b Road mapping via the sheath after removing dilator.

have not been obtained immediately before the implantation procedure. Shifting the patient even slightly can lead to improper stent placement.

The stent mounted on the balloon is an object with a relatively rough surface. It is not advisable to advance it through the vessel without protection. The stent can also be knocked off the balloon when it is advanced through a narrow, calcified stenosis. For this reason, a narrow stenosis should first be dilated. An alternative in

cases where it is technically feasible is to use a sheath of sufficient length. The sheath is first advanced into the stenosis (**Fig. 3.83**), and then the stent is brought into the desired position within the sheath. (See the section on the renal arteries for special considerations in that region.)

Once the stent has reached the proper position, the sheath is withdrawn far enough to expose the stent and balloon within the lumen (**Fig. 3.84**). The sheath must no

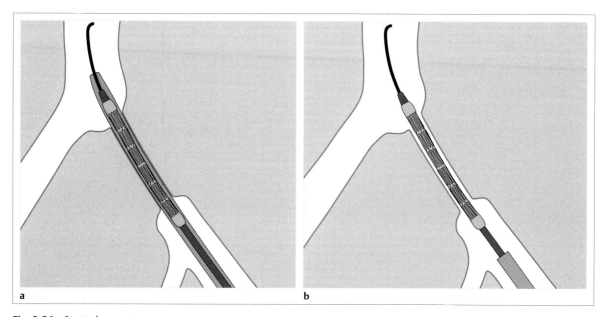

Fig. 3.84 Stent placement.
a Advance balloon catheter with stent into correct position.

b Withdraw sheath.

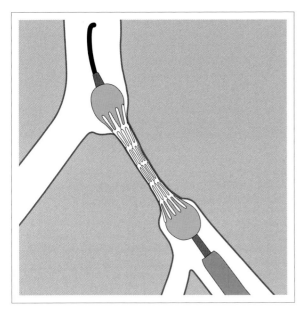

Fig. 3.85 Typical shape of balloon and stent when initially deployed. The balloon first expands at the ends outside the stent.

Now the balloon is slowly inflated with the aid of a manometer syringe to deploy the stent. The procedure is observed on fluoroscopy so that any errors can be immediately corrected (**Fig. 3.85**). Once the balloon is fully inflated, the stent will disconnect from it (**Fig. 3.86**). The balloon can then be deflated and withdrawn through the sheath. The wire remains in the stent for now. This will make it easier to introduce a larger balloon for supplementary dilation should this become necessary. Despite this precaution, a second balloon advanced to the site can still become caught on the stent. Usually it will be possible to separate the balloon from the stent by withdrawing the balloon while carefully rotating it. Under no circumstances should one advance a wire or balloon that has become caught on the stent at the back. Otherwise one will risk severely deforming the stent.

In vessels with a strong pulse the angiogram can create the impression that the stent lies slightly outside the vessel. When in doubt, obtaining an unsubtracted image will give a reliable answer.

Wherever residual stenosis is present or the stent is not in contact with the vessel wall at every point, a larger balloon may be used to further expand the stent over its entire length or only on one end (see **Fig. 2.55b** and **Fig. 3.87**).

longer cover the rear (proximal) end of the balloon either. Otherwise the balloon will only expand distally when inflated, which could push the stent off the balloon. If necessary, the position of the stent can now be verified again by injecting contrast through the sheath. The position can be corrected as long as the balloon is not inflated and stent has not been deployed.

Self-Expanding Stents

Self-expanding stents are supplied on application systems in which they lie on an inner catheter covered by a thin-walled outer catheter. Once the stent has been introduced

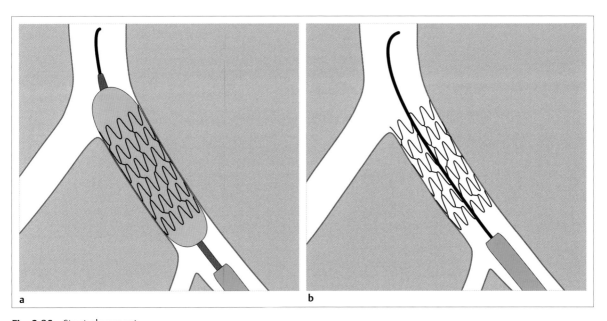

a

b

Fig. 3.86 Stent placement.
a Fully expanded stent.

b The deflated balloon is removed through the sheath, then angiography is performed.

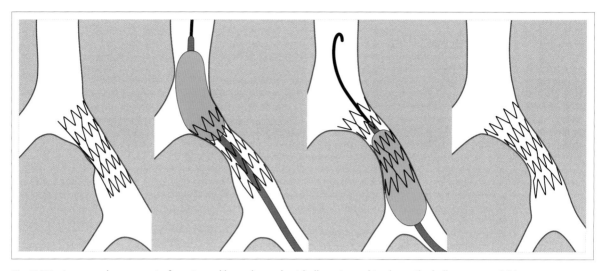

Fig. 3.87 In a vascular segment of varying caliber, a large short balloon is used to shape the balloon-expandable stent to conform to the vessel wall.

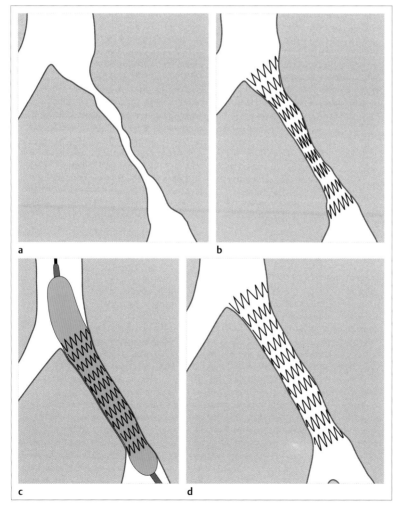

Fig. 3.88 A self-expanding stent has failed to expand the stenosis sufficiently. Subsequent dilation produces a good result.
a Initial situation.
b Unsatisfactory expansion from self-expanding stent.
c Subsequent dilation.
d Good result.

through a sheath and brought into the correct position, the outer catheter is withdrawn to deploy the stent (see **Fig. 2.57**). **Important:** In this maneuver the inner catheter must not be moved and the outer catheter must not be immobilized (see **Fig. 2.58**)!

There is a risk associated with short self-expanding stents. Their elasticity can cause them to slip out of the outer catheter and lodge in an incorrect position before the outer catheter has been fully withdrawn. This can only occur where the free end of the stent is not yet fully expanded, which fixes it to the wall. The radial force with which it presses itself into the vascular wall reaches its maximum only under the influence of body temperature; the material has a "memory effect." This occurs after a slight delay. Especially when placing a short stent one should wait for it to expand completely before withdrawing the outer catheter any further. With this in mind, some product designs include a connection between the stent and application system that separates only when the outer catheter has been completely withdrawn.

Often the strength of the stent will be insufficient to eliminate the stenosis. In most cases the residual stenosis can be eliminated by additional balloon dilation (**Fig. 3.88**). To ensure that the stent is reliably pressed against the vascular wall, one should always select the nominal stent size 1 mm larger than the vessel diameter measured. Subsequently inflating a balloon cannot expand the nitinol stent any further. For this reason it is not possible to use balloon dilation to fix in place a stent that has insufficient contact with the wall.

The essential advantage of nitinol stents lies in their flexibility (see also Chapter 2, Self-Expanding Stents, p. 31). They can better conform to vessels of varying caliber than steel stents. This assumes that one selects a sufficiently large stent.

Select a nitinol stent larger than the vessel to be treated but be careful not to select too large a size, especially in a narrow vessel. Placing, say, a 5 mm stent in a 3 mm vessel puts too much metal in the narrow vessel. For this reason special stents are available for the arteries of the lower leg.

A longer stenosis is also best treated with a single long stent. Where several stents must be placed in succession, they should overlap by at least 5 mm.

Occasionally it has been recommended to dilate a stenosis prior to planned stent implantation. This only serves a purpose where the results of PTA will determine whether additional placement of a stent is indicated. Otherwise the only plausible case would be where the stenosis is so narrow and rigid as to prevent the passage of a sheath or the application system for the stent. Where primary stent implantation is feasible, it is not only the quickest and cheapest solution. It also diminishes the risk of thrombus material from the occluded segment entering the bloodstream. As soon as it is unfolded, the stent's mesh restrains all coarse thrombus material that might otherwise be mobilized.

Local Thrombolysis

Type of Thrombolysis

The dissolving of a thrombus in blood vessels is referred to as thrombolysis. Thrombi are held together by a network of fibrin strands. Fibrin dissolves under the influence of plasmin (**Fig. 3.89**). Plasmin is produced when the precursor plasminogen reacts with a plasminogen activator (PA). Large quantities of plasminogen are present, at least in acute thrombi. This means that administering a plasminogen activator alone will suffice to dissolve the thrombus.

Streptokinase, the first thrombolytic agent available for clinical use, is hardly used today. Urokinase was very well tolerated by patients but had to be taken off the market in 1999 due to problems with production in the United States. Since then it has never regained the position it once held. Today the vast majority of medications used are recombinant TPAs produced by genetic engineering (such as alteplase). Ten milligrams of alteplase should be dissolved in 10 mL of water, 20 mg in 20 mL, and 50 mg in 50 mL. Reteplase and tenecteplase are similar substances. The recombinant TPA is bound to fibrin (**Fig. 3.89**). This increases its efficacy by a factor of 400 compared with freely circulating TPA (Roberts 2006a).

Not every thrombus can be lysed with equal ease. This **increased resistance to lysis** is presumably due more to a high thrombocyte content (white thrombus) than to a lack of plasminogen. Thrombocyte-rich components are often found at the ends of the thrombus,

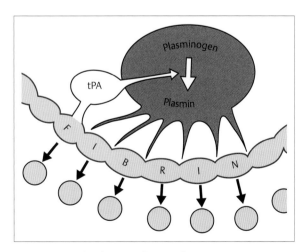

Fig. 3.89 Mode of action of tissue plasminogen activator.

especially at the proximal end. One particular advantage of local thrombolysis is that it breaks through this barrier.

The following forms of lysis are differentiated (**Fig. 3.90**):

- **Systemic lysis** is a treatment in which the thrombolytic agent acts throughout the entire cardiovascular system (arterial and venous circulation). The agent is usually administered via peripheral venous access.
- One refers to **regional lysis** where a thrombolytic agent is infused into an artery without direct infiltration of the thrombus.
- **Local lysis** is where a thrombus is dissolved by direct infiltration with a thrombolytic agent.

Indications and Contraindications

Indication for local thrombolysis:
- Acute occlusion of an artery
- Acute occlusion of a bypass or dialysis shunt
- Chronic arterial occlusions more than 3 to 5 cm in length, especially in wide arteries, if a guidewire can be easily advanced through them

Absolute contraindications:
- Cerebral stroke (hemorrhage or infarct) within the last 2 months
- Neurosurgical procedure within the last 3 months
- Craniocerebral trauma within the last 3 months
- Gastrointestinal hemorrhage within the last 10 days
- Hemorrhagic diathesis
- Thrombosis of a bypass within 4 weeks of implantation

Relative contraindications:
- Cardiopulmonary resuscitation (last 10 days)
- Major surgery, eye surgery, trauma (last 10 days)
- Intracranial tumor
- Hypertension over 180/110 mm Hg
- Puncture of incompressible vessels
- Thrombolysis will make a woven **Dacron prosthesis** permeable.
- A **venous bypass** that has been occluded for 3 days will usually be irreparably damaged.

Requirements for Successful Thrombolysis

It can be very confusing to read what various sources have to say about local lysis. The techniques described, the dose of thrombolytic agent, the duration of lysis, and the complication rates all vary greatly. Yet when one observes the **following basic principles** it soon becomes relatively clear how best to perform local lysis:

1. The actual process of thrombolysis only takes a few minutes.
2. However, the thrombolytic agent diffuses into the thrombus only very slowly (< 1 cm per hour).
3. There is very little space in the thrombus for fluid (i.e., the thrombolytic agent).
4. The half-life in thrombus of TPA, the most commonly used thrombolytic agent, is several times what it is in plasma (Fröhlich and Stump 1995).
5. Severe bleeding complications usually occur only with lysis of protracted duration.

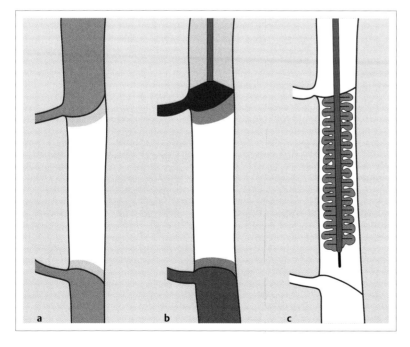

Fig. 3.90a–c Systemic (left), regional (center), and local lysis (right).

a The thrombolytic agent diffuses into the thrombus from both ends at a low concentration.

b Like **a** but with a higher concentration.

c The thrombolytic agent is distributed directly in the thrombus.

The most important requirements for successful local lysis may be deduced from conditions 1 and 2:

- We must ensure that the thrombolytic agent reaches the entire thrombus in a short time and in a high concentration.
- Long, time-consuming diffusion paths must be eliminated.
- And we must ensure that a large portion of the thrombolytic agent remains in the thrombus and does not drain into the system (condition 3).
- In summary: Inject highly concentrated thrombolytic agent into the thrombus in multiple portions of very small volumes each!

Avoid injecting contrast into the thrombus when performing the initial angiography. It will provide little information but will have the disadvantage of later displacing or diluting the thrombolytic agent.

All the thrombolytic agent that drains out is diluted in a volume of plasma that is 1,000 times greater (3,000 mL). Its local effect is therefore negligible. Moreover, the more thrombolytic agent that drains out, the greater the risk of systemic bleeding. Therefore one should inject the thrombolytic agent in the highest possible concentration and avoid injecting more active ingredient than the thrombus can accommodate. A thrombus in the superficial femoral artery with a length of 10 cm has a volume of ~ 3 mL! If one injects more than 1 mL within a short period of time, one can be sure that a large share will drain into the system. Yet there have been recommendations in the literature that a "first bolusing" be performed using doses of thrombolytic agent dissolved in 50 to 80 mL of fluid!

Another important requirement for successful therapy:
A thrombotic occlusion usually has an anatomical cause. This is best eliminated in the same procedure wherever possible. Usually this will be an arteriosclerotic stenosis in an artery or a stenosis at the bypass anastomoses. Removing residual thrombus by aspiration can also reduce the duration of treatment dramatically in certain cases. Therefore select the approach that offers the shortest route to the thrombus. In many cases this will be an antegrade approach via the groin. A 6 French sheath is recommended because it not only accommodates the 5 French lysis catheter but also allows the most important supplementary procedures such as aspiration, PTA, and stent placement.

> **Important:** When a vessel is reopened after acute occlusion, sensitivity usually returns before the ischemic pain subsides. In this situation one must expect a brief period of extremely severe pain which must be immediately relieved with a strong analgesic.

Pulse-Spray Lysis

Pulse-spray lysis allows for the following conditions:
- The volumes must be kept as small as possible. Therefore the TPA is applied in the greatest possible concentration.
- To ensure that the thrombolytic agent sprays out of all the side holes at sufficient speed, it is important not to choose excessively small injection volumes when injecting manually. This is compensated for by relatively long intervals.
- The half-life for TPA usually cited in the literature (4 to 6 minutes) refers to the concentration in plasma and reflects inactivation by metabolism in the liver. A **half-life of 30 to 40 minutes** has been measured for the clearance of TPA from tissue. The substance's thrombolytic activity within the thrombus persisted for more than 1 hour in an experimental setting (Fröhlich and Stump 1995).

The goal of distributing the thrombolytic agent throughout the entire thrombus simultaneously is best achieved using the **pulse-spray technique** (**Fig. 3.91**). This technique involves injecting the highly concentrated thrombolytic agent from a section of the catheter 5, 10, 15,

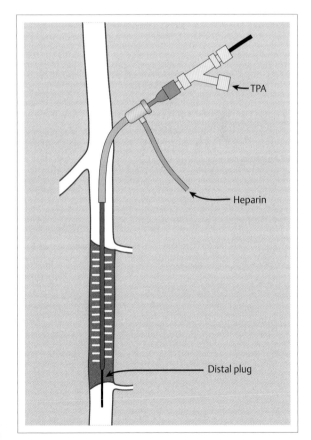

Fig. 3.91 Pulse-spray lysis.

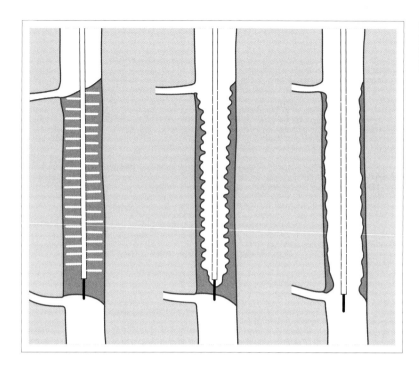

Fig. 3.92 Action of pulse-spray lysis: Infiltration of thrombus (left), advanced lysis (center), largely patent lumen (right).

or 20 cm in length in brief high-pressure spurts (at long intervals). This only works where the end hole is reliably sealed with a wire, the side holes are very fine, and the agent is injected under high pressure. At low pressure the agent seeps out of the first few side holes. High pressure also expels the thrombolytic agent from the catheter in fine, high-velocity streams that better penetrate the thrombus. It has even been suggested that this may cause mechanical fragmentation.

A plug ~ 2 cm long at the distal end of the thrombus should initially be left untreated. This prevents thrombolytic agent from draining into the periphery and concentrates it within the thrombus (**Fig. 3.92**). The plug also minimizes the risk of distal embolization from incompletely dissolved thrombus fragments.

Not all pulse-spray lysis systems supplied by the industry are of equal quality. In some models the side holes are too large. This does not allow adequate pressure to build up within the catheter. The result is that the thrombolytic agent does not spray out of all the side holes evenly. Bard/Angiomed (Covington, GA, USA) supplies a very satisfactory complete system: The tip of the 5 French catheter is sealed by the guidewire (**Fig. 3.93**) and the outer (proximal) end by a Tuohy-Borst adapter. The thrombolytic agent is injected into the space between the catheter wall

and the guidewire via a side connection on the adapter (**Fig. 3.94**). It can only escape through numerous fine side holes in a segment 5, 10, or 15 cm long close to the catheter tip. This segment is marked by metal rings.

The ev3 company (Plymouth, MN, USA) supplies a catheter with a valve on the tip under the trade name Cragg-McNamara. This valve eliminates the need to seal the tip with the guidewire. This design achieves sufficiently high flow rates even in 4 French catheters, which is particularly interesting for the arteries of the lower leg. Even smaller lumens are accessible using a 0.035 in. wire that carries the thrombolytic agent between its core and a plastic sleeve. The agent is expelled through side holes close to the tip. This system is also supplied by ev3. The injection is performed with a 1 mL syringe. After each injection the syringe is refilled with thrombolytic agent from a 10 or 20 mL syringe connected via a three-way stopcock.

Where the side holes are arranged in a helical pattern, each offset 90° and 2.5 mm from the previous one, every fifth hole will face in the same direction as the first and will be 10 mm away from it. The thrombolytic agent would have to diffuse 5 mm through the thrombus until it reaches the diffusion area of the next hole facing in the same direction. This distance can be halved by withdrawing the catheter 5 mm after the first injection and

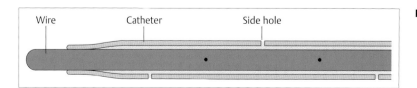

Fig. 3.93 Pulse-spray catheter.

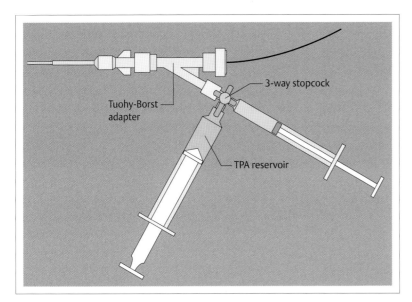

Fig. 3.94 Injection system for pulse-spray lysis.

creating a depot between the first two with a second injection (**Fig. 3.95**).

Tissue Plasminogen Activator Dosage

The recommendations in the literature usually do not allow for the size of the thrombus requiring treatment or, respectively, the distance over which the thrombolytic agent is expelled from the catheter. The following suggestions for pulse-spray lysis follow the dosage specified in a consensus document published in 2003. They have proven effective in the author's practice. In light of the broad range of recommendations made in the literature,

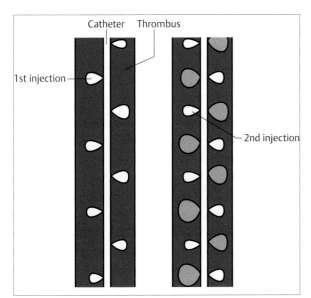

Fig. 3.95 Better infiltration is achieved by withdrawing the catheter 5 mm before second injection.

the suggestions made here are necessarily of a tentative nature. However, specific schemes are necessary for a smooth procedure. Moreover, only a largely standardized process will allow the experience required for subsequent optimization.

The following data apply to the size relationships in the superficial femoral artery or a femoropopliteal bypass. Vessels with larger diameters (such as iliac arteries) will require appropriate corrections. The injection volumes and the shifting of the catheter 5 mm between two consecutive injections apply to the Bard/Angiomed system: The catheter has four side holes per centimeter, each offset 90° from the previous hole. Each hole has a diameter of 0.15 mm. (Lysis catheters with a diameter of 4 French such as those supplied by ev3 are recommended for local lysis in the arteries of the lower leg.)

The individual doses specified in the following section can only serve as an approximate guide, especially in the case of manual injection. Moderately exceeding these values is presumably safe. A total dose of no more than 10 mg of TPA administered within 4 hours hardly involves a risk of systemic bleeding.

Lysis Distance of 5 Centimeters

- Prepare a solution of 10 mg of alteplase dissolved in 10 mL of water.
- Inject 0.2 mL, withdraw the catheter 5 mm, again inject 0.2 mL.
- Return the catheter to the original position.
- Wait 30 minutes.

Repeat this four times, then (after a total of 2 hours) measure partial thromboplastin time (PTT) and perform angiography via the sheath (TPA dose up to this point is 1.6 mg). If contrast agent does not yet flow through the treated segment, continue treatment according to the same scheme for another 2 hours (total TPA dose is now 3.2 mg). Then (after 4 hours) measure PTT and again perform angiography, this time injecting contrast via the lysis catheter after withdrawing the wire as far as the Tuohy-Borst adapter.

Lysis Distance of 10 Centimeters
- Prepare a solution of 10 mg of alteplase dissolved in 10 mL of water.
- Inject 0.2 mL, withdraw the catheter 5 mm, again inject 0.2 mL.
- Return the catheter to the original position.
- Wait 20 minutes.

Repeat this six times, then (after a total of 2 hours) measure PTT and perform angiography via the sheath (TPA dose up to this point is 2.4 mg). If contrast agent does not yet flow through the treated segment, continue treatment according to the same scheme for another 2 hours. (Total TPA dose is now 4.8 mg.) Then (after 4 hours) measure PTT and again perform angiography, this time injecting contrast via the lysis catheter after withdrawing the wire as far as the Tuohy-Borst adapter.

Lysis Distance of 15 Centimeters
- Prepare a solution of 10 mg of alteplase dissolved in 10 mL of water.
- Inject 0.3 mL, withdraw the catheter 5 mm, again inject 0.3 mL.
- Return the catheter to the original position.
- Wait 20 minutes.

Repeat this six times, then (after a total of 2 hours) measure PTT and perform angiography via the sheath (TPA dose up to this point is 3.6 mg). If contrast agent does not yet flow through the treated segment, continue treatment according to the same scheme for another 2 hours (total TPA dose is now 7.2 mg). Then (after 4 hours) measure PTT and again perform angiography, this time injecting contrast via the lysis catheter after withdrawing the wire as far as the Tuohy-Borst adapter.

Thrombus More Than 15 Centimeters Long
Such a thrombus can occur in a femoropopliteal bypass.
- Prepare solution of 10 mg of alteplase dissolved in 10 mL of water.
- Inject 0.3 mL, withdraw the catheter 5 mm, again inject 0.3 mL.
- Withdraw the catheter 15 cm.
- Inject 0.3 mL, withdraw the catheter 5 mm, again inject 0.3 mL.
- Withdraw the catheter 15 cm.

Repeat this until the entire length of the thrombus has been infiltrated.
- Return the catheter to the original position.
- Wait 20 minutes.

Repeat this six times, then (after a total of 2 hours) measure PTT and perform angiography via the sheath. If contrast agent does not yet flow through the treated segment, continue treatment according to the same scheme for another 2 hours. Then (after 4 hours) measure PTT and again perform angiography, this time injecting contrast via the lysis catheter after withdrawing the wire as far as the Tuohy-Borst adapter.

Heparin and Aspirin

Thrombolysis involves a dynamic balance between lysis and new formation of thrombi. Thrombin released from its bond with fibrin contributes to the formation of new thrombi; thrombin is also a potent thrombocyte activator. Therefore the patient should receive a **platelet aggregation inhibitor** (usually aspirin) prior to thrombolysis; during and after thrombolysis treatment with **heparin** (initial dose 5,000 IU, later 500 to 1,000 IU per hour, according to PTT) is indicated.

Heparin can be mixed with urokinase. This has the advantage of reaching the thrombus in a high concentration. One should not mix TPA with heparin because this could cause TPA to precipitate. In this case the heparin is infused through a sheath (Roberts 2006b).

Organizing the Thrombolysis

For each of the 2-hour periods between angiographic controls one can return the patient to rest in bed. There the patient will be more comfortable and the angiography table will be free for another patient. Prior to moving the patient, fix the sheath to the skin with a suture and apply a sterile bandage to mark the place on the catheter where it enters the sheath.

The more acute the occlusion, the more quickly thrombolysis will lead to success. Methodical application of the pulse-spray technique can be expected to produce successful results after ~ 2 to 4 hours of treatment (Bürkle and Bürkle 1991, Tran 1998). By then patency will usually have been largely restored to the occluded vessel. Then a precise **angiographic examination** is indicated to evaluate residual thrombi, possible peripheral emboli, and causative stenoses. Residual thrombi and peripheral emboli can often be removed by aspiration. One possible alternative is to continue treatment in the form of regional thrombolysis under intensive monitoring (typical dose is 20 mg of alteplase over 24 hours). If no significant residual thrombi are detectable then the causative stenoses are treated with PTA and, where indicated, with stent placement.

The local anesthesia must again be administered before replacing the sheath in the event it becomes necessary, and before introducing a vascular closure system. The sheath should be removed 30 minutes after completion of the thrombolysis at the earliest. This corresponds to

~ 6 half-lives of TPA. However, cleavage products with thrombolytic activity (fragment X) remain within the circulatory system for up to 24 hours.

Closure of the access site is then obtained with Angio-Seal or a similar system.

Aftercare:
- Heparin perfusor for 3 days
- Aspirin, 100 mg daily for an indefinite period
- After stent placement: clopidogrel for 6 weeks

Intensive Care Unit

Pulse-spray lysis according to the criteria defined here does not usually last more than 4 hours. Such treatment would be nearly impossible to perform in the intensive care unit (ICU). As long as one can be relatively certain that the lysis will remain local there is no need for the patient to be there. Only systemic lysis is associated with major risks, and such treatment is rarely performed under the conditions discussed earlier.

Regional lysis (infusion of a thrombolytic agent without direct infiltration of the thrombus) is indicated to treat residual thrombi after local lysis and to treat occlusions in minor peripheral arteries (or cerebral arteries).

Regional lysis has an advantage over systemic lysis only during the first passage through the affected region. The more often the agent recirculates, the more all other arteries become involved and the less the difference in concentration. Therefore regional lysis should always be performed using a thrombolytic agent with a very short half-life (such as recombinant TPA).

At least when treating acute thrombosis, it is not recommended to restore patency by mechanically removing part of the thrombi and then continuing with regional lysis to eliminate the residual thrombi. Then one would no longer have the opportunity to eliminate thrombi by direct infiltration with concentrated thrombolytic agent. Moreover, the costs would be higher, the risks of systemic complication greater, and the arterial puncture larger.

Special Indications for Thrombolysis

Thrombolysis in Chronic Occlusion

Where an occluded segment of an artery resists the passage of a wire or catheter, there is an alternative to simple mechanical restoration of patency and subintimal recanalization (see superficial femoral artery occlusions). The occluding material can be infiltrated proximally with thrombolytic agent. To do this, a catheter with only one end hole is used. Wherever possible, the catheter is advanced slightly into the occluding material. A perfusor then introduces a trickle of concentrated thrombolytic agent via the catheter. After 1 to 2 hours it may be possible to pass a wire or catheter.

Treating an Occluded Synthetic Femoropopliteal Bypass or Dialysis Graft

A dialysis graft frequently offers no opportunity for establishing access outside of the thrombosed segment. To treat the graft as a whole, it is necessary to work with two crisscrossed catheters introduced in opposite directions (see **Fig. 6.11**). A similar technique can be used with a synthetic femoropopliteal bypass if neither antegrade nor crossover catheterization appears feasible (**Fig. 3.96**).

> **Important:** A bacterial infection of a plastic bypass cannot be controlled by medication alone and may necessitate surgical removal of the implant. Therefore, in addition to painstaking attention to sterility, a single dose of a broad-spectrum antibiotic is indicated prior to any puncture or catheterization of a plastic bypass.

Once the sheath lies securely within the beginning of the bypass, advance the assembled system (lysis catheter with Tuohy-Borst adapter and guidewire; side connection completely filled with thrombolytic agent) to within 2 cm of the distal anastomosis. If the bypass can only be reached with a guidewire, first introduce the lysis catheter and Tuohy-Borst adapter over the guidewire. Then replace the guidewire with the wire included in the lysis system. This is important because that wire reliably seals the tip of the catheter.

If one has not introduced the system complete with guidewire and filled with thrombolytic agent, then one will first need 1.5 mL to fill the catheter. As soon as blood flows through the bypass again, the occluding wire is removed and the Tuohy-Borst adapter is replaced with a normal stopcock. Then a precise angiogram of the entire bypass is obtained to determine whether any residual thrombosis is present. If there are slight quantities of residual thrombus, it is best to try to remove them by aspiration (see the following section). On the other hand one may find that many residual thrombi are present, possibly distributed over longer segments of the bypass. In this case, the thrombolysis is continued in the ICU using a perfusor (20 mg of recombinant TPA over 24 hours). The perfusor is best connected directly to the sheath, which is sutured to the skin to fix it in position. If the larger part of the sheath lies outside the body, then the sheath is fixed in place with a second suture positioned immediately at the site where the sheath enters the skin.

The final step in the procedure is to identify possible causes for the occlusion. Do not neglect to do this. Most often you will find a stenosis at the distal anastomosis or, less often, at the proximal one. In many cases such stenoses can be eliminated with PTA (**Fig. 3.97**). In a synthetic bypass, the thrombosis may also be attributable to a kink that occurs when the knee is flexed. This is best evaluated by obtaining an angiogram with the patient's knee flexed. Prophylactic placement of a stent may be considered. The SUPERA stent (IDEV Technologies, Webster, TX, USA) is particularly well suited for addressing this problem and should be discussed with a vascular surgeon.

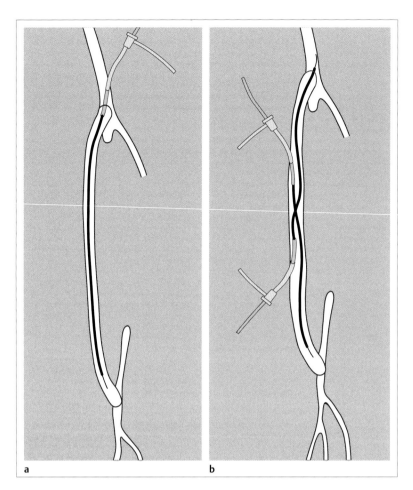

Fig. 3.96 Two options for thrombolysis in a femoropopliteal bypass to the third popliteal segment.
a Using a single catheter.
b Using two crisscrossed lysis catheters.

a

b

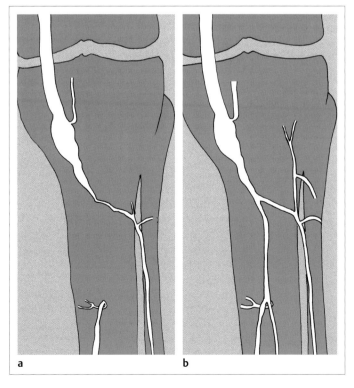

Fig. 3.97 Seventy-eight-year-old woman. Femoropopliteal bypass to the third popliteal segment reopened by pulse-spray lysis.
a Probable cause of the occlusion is a high-grade stenosis of the distal popliteal artery and occlusion of the tibiofibular tract.
b Successful treatment by percutaneous transluminal angioplasty.

a

b

Aspiration of Thrombus

Acute emboli or residual thrombi after local lysis can often be eliminated by removing them from the vessel through a large-bore catheter with suction (**aspiration thrombectomy**). The aspiration catheters supplied for this purpose are distinguished from standard catheters by their particularly large end hole. The sheath through which the aspiration catheter is introduced should be equipped with a removable valve wherever possible. Not all suppliers have such sheaths in stock. They are available from OptiMed (Ettlingen, Germany), Angiomed, or Terumo.

Before introducing the aspiration catheter, fill it and an attached 20 or 50 mL syringe with a small quantity of dilute contrast agent. This will help one localize the thrombus (with road mapping or simple fluoroscopy) after one has advanced the catheter close to the site. Then advance the tip of the catheter to the thrombus and apply powerful suction to aspirate it into the catheter. If it is too large for this, then apply continuous suction to hold it in place against the catheter tip. Then one can withdraw the thrombus and catheter through the sheath together (**Fig. 3.98**).

Where one is planning thrombus aspiration from a site such as the distal popliteal artery as a separate therapeutic procedure, one should use an aspiration catheter of the appropriate size (e.g., 8 or 9 French). This will require a relatively large puncture, which one then seals with a vascular closure system. It is also best to use a long sheath that extends to the site of the findings. Then one can introduce the aspiration catheter several times even

without protection while avoiding the risk of injury to the vessel wall.

Small thrombi will be aspirated through the catheter and directly into the syringe. To avoid missing them, filter the blood from the syringe through a gauze compress when draining it into a bowl.

Performed successfully, aspiration thrombectomy is an elegant procedure with minimal invasiveness that is unmatched. However, it can hardly be expected to succeed every time. There are several reasons for **failure**:
1. Thrombi adhering to the vessel wall cannot be mobilized.
2. The thrombi are too big for the aspiration catheter or sheath.
3. The thrombus lies eccentrically along the vessel wall and the catheter glides past it.

Causes 2 and 3 can be controlled in some cases.

Regarding cause 2: Very often the suction pulls in thrombi that are too big to be completely aspirated through the catheter. Some of these are stripped off again when the tip of the catheter is withdrawn into the sheath. Yet it often occurs that the thrombus is successfully drawn into the catheter and only lodges in front of the valve (**Fig. 3.99**). This is to be expected when there was suction in the syringe until one withdrew the catheter from the sheath yet found no thrombus at the tip of the catheter. This suspicion is confirmed when one can no longer aspirate blood through the side connection of the sheath. Then one should close off the sheath with a

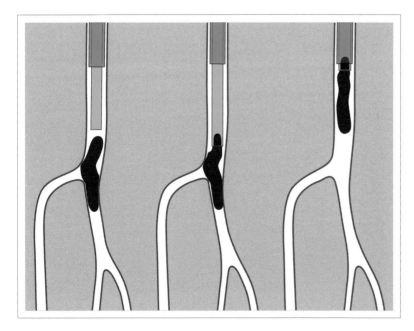

Fig. 3.98 Aspiration of an embolus from the distal popliteal artery.

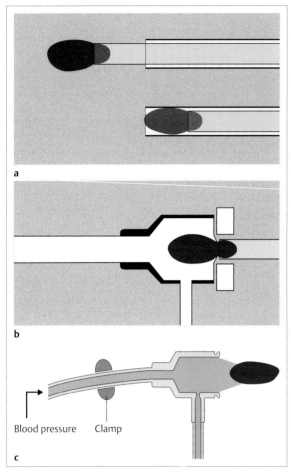

Fig. 3.99a–c Thrombus aspiration.
a A large thrombus can still be drawn into the sheath.
b But it will lodge at the valve.
c Blood flushes the thrombus out of the open sheath.

clamp, remove the valve, and open the clamp briefly to allow the blood to flush the thrombus out of the sheath (**Fig. 3.99**). Of course one must then close off the sheath with a finger or clamp once the catheter or thrombus is outside and then reattach the valve.

Fig. 3.100 As a segmental occlusion in the distal superficial femoral artery is reopened by percutaneous transluminal angioplasty (PTA), an embolus occludes the distal popliteal artery. Successful aspiration thrombectomy.
a Initial situation.
b Reopened by PTA.
c Embolic occlusion of the popliteal artery due to **b**.
d Successful aspiration thrombectomy.

Often the unforeseen necessity of aspirating a thrombus or embolus will arise during PTA (**Fig. 3.100**). When this occurs, one will usually be using a sheath with a valve one cannot remove. Here, too, it is usually possible to press out a thrombus that has lodged in front of the sheath valve. One must then seal the shaft of the sheath and forcefully inject fluid through the side connection of the sheath (**Fig. 3.101**).

> **Caution:** Turn the sheath valve so that the ejected thrombus will land on the drapes, or hold a hand or cloth in front of the opening!

Regarding cause 3: Thrombi that lie eccentrically along the vessel wall require an aspiration catheter with a slight bend close to the tip. The catheter being used can be shaped under steam (see p. 25) to give it the proper bend (**Fig. 3.102**). Alternative: Use a straight or curved guiding catheter.

There are also aspiration catheters available that are advanced over a previously introduced wire to protect the vessel wall (**Fig. 3.103**). This is a very good alternative, especially for the arteries of the lower leg. The catheter shown in **Fig. 3.104** has a diameter of 5.1 French and lumen of 1.1 mm and with a diameter of 5.7 French and lumen measuring 1.3 mm. The operating radius of such a catheter can be expanded slightly by rotating the catheter around the wire. A monorail system is available for crossover aspiration.

Fig. 3.101 Pressing out a thrombus lodged in front of a nonremovable valve.
a Seal the shaft of the sheath and forcefully inject fluid through the side connection of the sheath.
b Seal the sheath with a clamp.
c Kink the line with the hand if a clamp is not available.

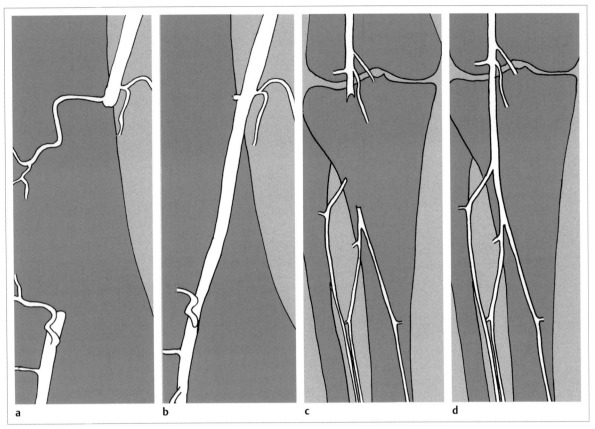

Fig. 3.100

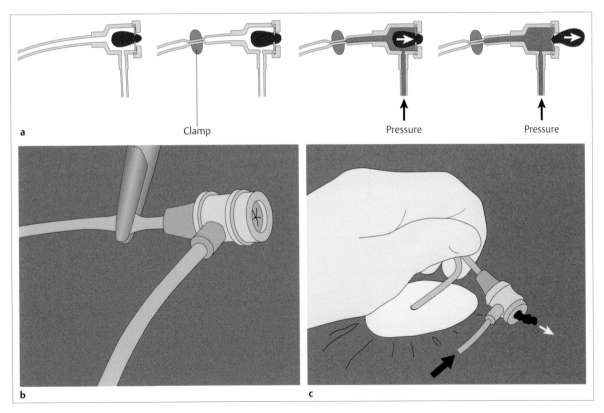

Clamp   Pressure   Pressure

Fig. 3.101

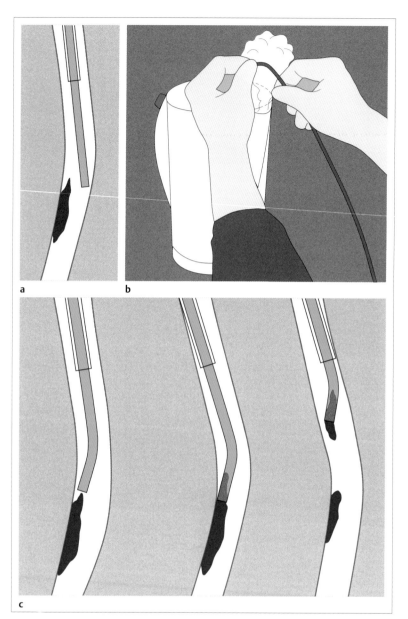

Fig. 3.102 Aspiration of thrombi that lie eccentrically along the vessel wall.
a A straight catheter is unsuitable for this purpose.
b Use steam to bend the tip of the catheter.
c A slight bend near the tip facilitates contact with the thrombus.

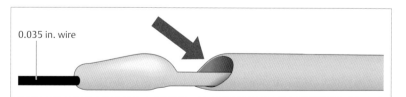

Fig. 3.103 Pronto 35 10 French catheter (Vascular Solutions).

0.035 in. wire

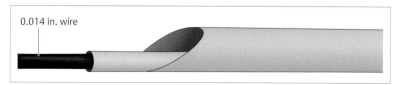

Fig. 3.104 Diver C. E. Max 5.1 French catheter (Invatec, Minneapolis, MN, USA).

0.014 in. wire

Subintimal Recanalization

In the early 1990s Bolia convincingly demonstrated in a large group of treated patients that it is possible to reopen occluded segments of the superficial femoral artery even outside the true lumen (Markose and Bolia 2008). In a manner similar to spontaneous aortic dissection, a false lumen is opened between the intima and media proximal to (or within) the occluded segment and rejoining the true lumen distal to the occlusion. According to Bolia, balloon dilation can stabilize this false lumen so well that there is usually no need for stents.

Because there are no arteriosclerotic changes in the wall of the false lumen, the chances of recurrent occlusion at this site are minimal.

It is common for the guidewire and catheter to spontaneously enter the subintimal space during an attempt to catheterize an occlusion. One can also seek to enter the subintimal space proximal to the occluded segment so as to open a new lumen completely outside the arteriosclerotic segment (**Fig. 3.105**). The important thing is to reenter the true lumen immediately distal to the

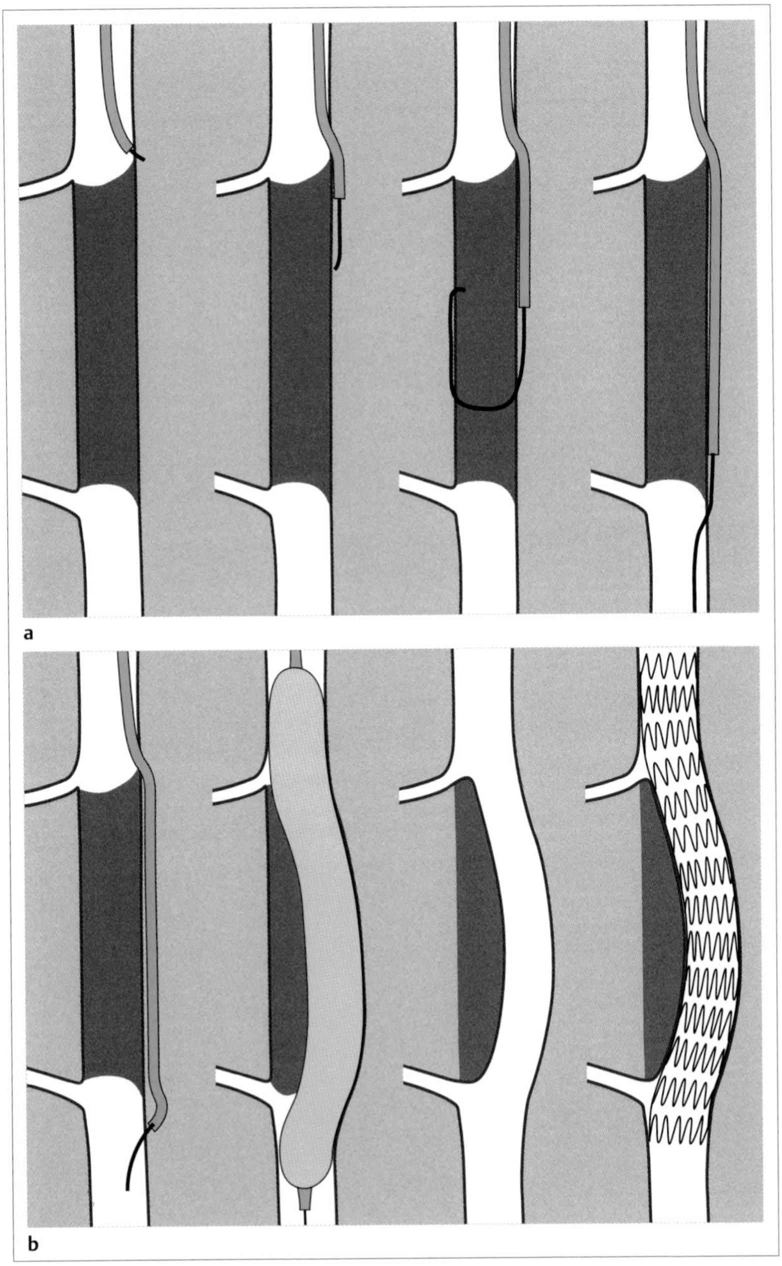

Fig. 3.105 Subintimal catheterization.
a Reentry with the wire alone.
b Reentry with the aid of a curved catheter, dilation, and stent placement.

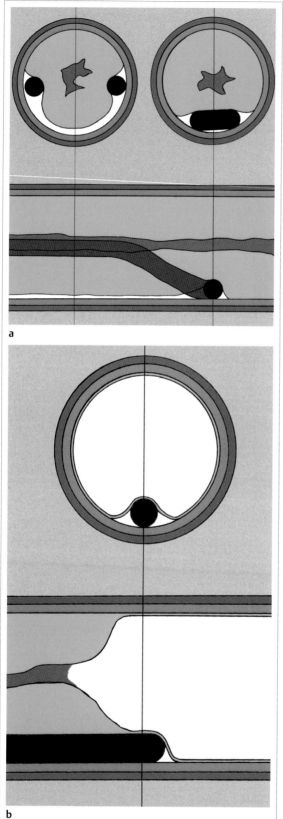

a

b

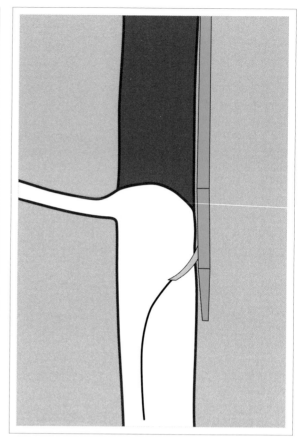

Fig. 3.107 Reentry into the physiologic lumen with the Outback catheter.

occlusion (**Fig. 3.105b**). This can prove very difficult, particularly in the presence of severe mural calcifications. Yet experienced operators can achieve this in ~ 80% of all cases.

To create the new channel in the vessel wall, a u-shaped loop is formed in a glide wire lying distal to the tip of the leading catheter. The catheter then pushes this loop to the end of the occluded segment.

One pulls back the wire and attempts to perforate the luminal aspect of the intima with the short curved tip. Then one advances the wire through the opening and follows with the catheter. This maneuver often requires curved catheters and a variety of different wires.

◀ **Fig. 3.106** Subintimal recanalization (relative sizes as in an artery 5 mm in diameter with a 0.035 in. glide wire), cross section and longitudinal section.
a The curve in the glide wire bluntly dissects the thickened intima off the media.
b Tip of the wire beneath the thin healthy intima.

It is not easy to understand how the guidewire can find its way back into even the narrow lumen of an artery in the lower leg after its subintimal passage. For this to work, the wire and catheter must not leave the vessel completely but continue to course within the media and adventitia. From here, the passage back into the lumen is the path of least resistance. Where it is not thickened by plaques, the normal physiologic intima is a fine membrane that is significantly easier to perforate than the outer layers of the vessel wall (**Fig. 3.106**). Only the subintimal passage straight ahead along the same line offers less resistance.

Several very expensive special catheters (Outback from Cordis and Pioneer from Medtronic, Minneapolis, MN, USA) have recently been introduced on the market. These catheters allow targeted intimal puncture with a curved cannula. A 0.014 in. wire is then advanced through this cannula to provide a secure track back into the true lumen (**Fig. 3.107**). This capability is particularly interesting where a subintimal passage has been successfully opened through an occluded common iliac artery but severe atheromatous calcification prevents reentry into the aortic lumen.

The final step is invariably dilation of the new lumen. Many operators also like to place a stent.

Atherectomy

The problem of reopening occluded vessels and removing stenosing plaques has driven the development of several mechanical aids, many of them very elaborate. Only a few have been able to establish themselves on the market. One important means of managing chronic stenosis and occlusion that warrants mention is atherectomy. This is a method of removing plaque material by means of a high-speed rotating cutting head shaped like a pot. The cutting head is pressed against one side of the wall. In earlier versions this was done with a balloon; in the SilverHawk system commonly used today this is achieved by a sharp bend in the system induced from outside (**Fig. 3.108**). Dispensing with the balloon has the advantage of avoiding the trauma of expanding the vessel wall (Kedhi et al 2008).

Typical indications for atherectomy include eccentric plaques that are poorly manageable by PTA in a region where it is best not to use stents (popliteal artery). Of course one can also use this method to remove material that has caused recurrent stenosis in a stent. However, in such a situation one can also usually achieve satisfactory results by patiently performing intermittent dilation over a period of 10 to 20 minutes.

Recent studies have shown that in atherectomy with the SilverHawk system, relatively large particles are mobilized and carried off into the periphery (Kaid et al 2009). Therefore it is recommended to use a protective system when performing the atherectomy (Berger 2010).

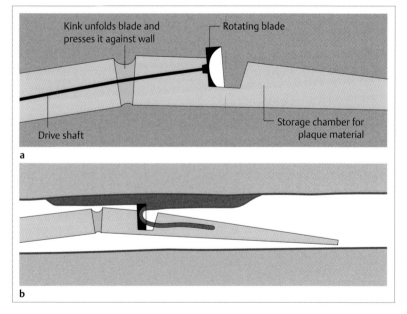

Fig. 3.108 SilverHawk system.
a Structure.
b Atherectomy.

Excimer Laser

After discouraging experience with lasers in the 1980s and early 1990s, there is now a renaissance in their use in the recanalization of occluded arteries of the legs. There were several problems with earlier systems. They developed excessively high levels of heat in continuous operation (pulse duration of up to 3 seconds), and they could not be reliably steered with the vessel. The excimer lasers now commonly used work with a pulse duration in the nanosecond range. They are invariably introduced over a wire that has been previously advanced into the vessel.

The photomechanical, photochemical, and photothermal effects of the laser energy pulverize plaque material, thrombi, and, to a lesser extent, calcifications to tiny particles. This makes it a suitable method for removing larger plaques and widening high-grade stenoses or occlusions (Kedhi et al 2008). A study of patients with critical ischemia in the extremities and involvement primarily of the arteries of the lower leg showed that technical success was achieved in 99% of all cases where it had been possible to advance a wire into the occluded segment. The long-term results were also above average (Laird et al 2006).

Embolization

General Principles

The intentional occlusion of blood vessels for therapeutic purposes achieved with the aid of a catheter is referred to as embolization. These therapeutic purposes include the following:
- Management of bleeding
- Occlusion of arteriovenous malformations
- Occlusion of aneurysms
- Occlusion of organs or parts of organs

Embolization also plays an increasingly important role in the treatment of tumors with cytostatic agents, especially in tumors of the liver. Today it has become a broad field with many highly specialized applications, for example, in neuroradiology. In some areas it is challenging in terms of technique, and it is also very risky. This section will be limited to the discussion of a few basic principles and simple indications.

Intentional vascular occlusion by means of embolization can be performed for different purposes and in very different forms. Permanent occlusion is for instance desirable in the case of arteriovenous malformations. However, when treating traumatic bleeding one usually wants to obtain a reversible occlusion of the arterial feeder. And a vascular malformation must be occluded at the level of the arteriovenous shunts wherever possible.

Material for **a potentially reversible occlusion includes the following:**
- Gelfoam particles (Pfizer, New York, NY, USA) (gelatin sponge)
- Autologous blood clots

Material for **a permanent occlusion includes the following:**
- Coils
- Polyvinyl alcohol (PVA) sponge or plastic particles
- Histoacryl (TissueSeal [Ann Arbor, MI, USA])

Proximal occlusion is best obtained with larger coils. Small coils can be placed far in the periphery with microcatheters (**Fig. 3.109**). Gelfoam particles produce a more or less proximal occlusion, depending on their size. PVA or plastic particles are supplied in various sizes. The smaller the particle, the farther peripherally it will cause occlusion (**Fig. 3.110**). Liquid embolic agents such as Histoacryl can be used to fill vessels far into the periphery (**Fig. 3.111**).

So-called occluders are supplied for occluding large vessels such as the common iliac artery. These devices lodge within the vessel and block its entire diameter. Finally, there are highly specific and very elaborate systems for occluding aneurysms in neuroradiology. This is usually done with coils.

Caution: Anyone who lacks extensive experience in interventional radiology is best advised to be very judicious in the use of embolization.

Embolic Material

Coils

Many varieties of embolic coils are available. They are designed similarly to guidewires (spring wires) but lack their solid core. They usually contain only a thin elastic wire that gives the deployed coil its shape. Textile fibers are usually incorporated into the coil to facilitate thrombosis of the vessel (**Fig. 3.112**).

Each coil is identified by three sizes: the thickness of the coil (e.g., 0.035 in.), its diameter (e.g., 8 mm), and the length of the extended spring wire (e.g., 5 cm). The diameter of the coil must be larger than the diameter of the vessel it is to occlude; angiographic measurement of the vessel's diameter and length is indicated. The thickness of the coil must fit the catheter used. Its lumen

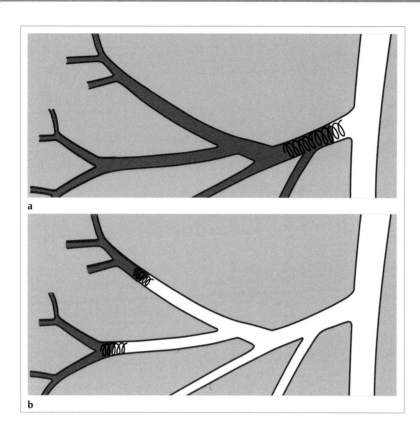

Fig. 3.109 Embolization with coils.
a Large coils.
b Small coils.

must not be significantly larger than the thickness of the coil. Otherwise the guidewire used to advance the coil could become wedged together with the coil inside the catheter.

The required or maximum possible **length** depends on the volume that the coil is intended to fill. A single 10 cm coil is equally as effective as two coils 5 cm in length. However, the longer the coil chosen, the greater the risk of misjudging the volume it is intended to fill. It then may not be possible to fit the entire length of the coil in the vessel, maybe only because its windings do not lie close together in the manner anticipated. A coil that cannot be placed completely within the target vessel must usually be removed. This can usually be done by snaring the free end of the coil and then pulling it out with the snare loop (**Fig. 3.113**).

Performing Coil Embolization. Gianturco coils (Cook Medical) are supplied in steel tubes with a plastic sleeve on their proximal end. Before a coil can be introduced, the catheter must lie securely within the vessel to be embolized. The carrier tube is then inserted into the catheter as far as the plastic sleeve permits. Then the coil is pushed out of the tube and into the catheter shaft with a guidewire. This is best done with the stiff end of the guidewire. Some companies supply for this purpose a special straight wire of the appropriate thickness and length with a grip on the proximal end. Then the guidewire is withdrawn,

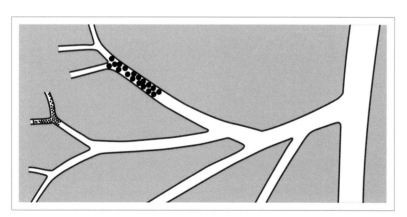

Fig. 3.110 Embolization with large and small particles.

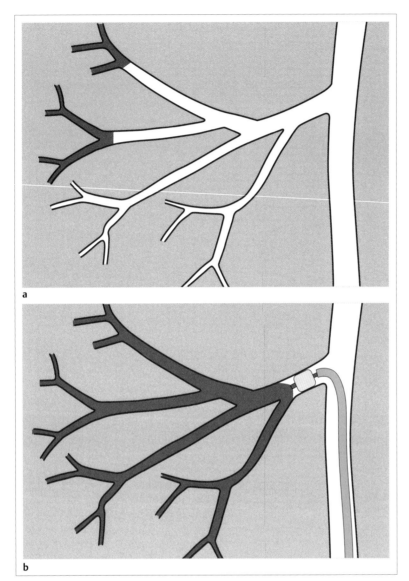

Fig. 3.111 Embolization with a liquid embolic agent.
a Peripheral.
b Central.

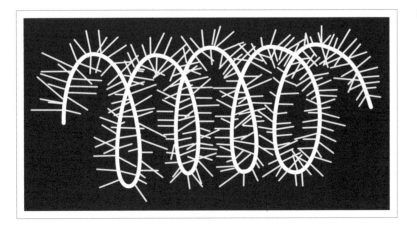

Fig. 3.112 Coil with textile fibers.

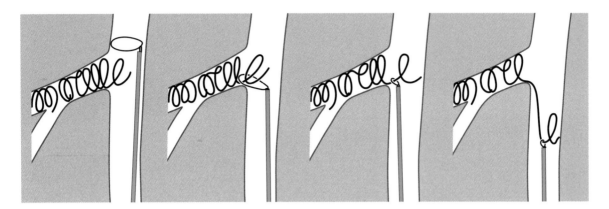

Fig. 3.113　A coil that was too long is extracted with a snare.

the sleeve is removed, and the coil, in front of the soft tip of the wire, is advanced under fluoroscopy nearly as far as the tip of the catheter. Prior to deploying the coil, the wire is slightly withdrawn to verify it has not become wedged together with the coil inside the catheter.

Then the coil is advanced under fluoroscopic control into the target vessel. When you deploy the coil, make sure that it has an opportunity to expand into shape within the vessel (i.e., that the coil is deployed slowly). Occasionally, one can use the catheter or guidewire to help push the coil windings closer together. Often several coils are required to fill the vascular lumen. A spring wire is usually better than a glide wire for maneuvering the coil.

For critical situations there are coils that are firmly connected to a special guidewire (by a threaded connection or other means). These are then deployed only when they have been securely positioned in the proper location. One interesting further development of this principle is a vascular plug: Amplatzer plug (St. Jude Medical). This consists of a mesh of fine nitinol wires arranged in a configuration resembling a fish trap. The folded system is introduced through a catheter. Once deployed, it expands to the diameter of the vessel at several planes along the segment (**Fig. 3.114**). A threaded connection firmly attaches the system to the wire with which the system is advanced through the catheter. If the system is initially positioned incorrectly, it can be withdrawn into the catheter with the wire and redeployed in the correct position. Only then is the screw connection released by rotating the wire.

This system is available in 11 different sizes for vessels 3 to 22 mm in diameter. It is particularly interesting for large vessels, which are not easily occluded by simpler means. One example of an indication would be a major artery supplying an arteriovenous malformation in the lung or kidney.

Gelfoam

Gelfoam is supplied in the form of small slabs. This is a dry brittle material that is cut up into tiny cubes before use

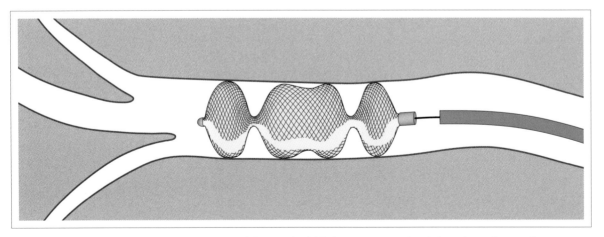

Fig. 3.114　Amplatzer II: a wire mesh resembling a fish trap. The folded system is introduced through a catheter. When deployed, it expands to the diameter of the vessel at several planes along the segment.

(**Fig. 3.115a**). The cubes are put into a syringe, contrast agent is added to a second syringe, and both are mixed back and forth between the syringes until they form an injectable sludge (**Fig. 3.115b**). This sludge consists primarily of contrast agent and is therefore easily monitored when injected.

Embolization should always be performed with a sheath. This will allow removal of the catheter with excess embolic material without loss of vascular access.

Particles

Particle suspensions have been used since the 1970s to occlude minor peripheral vessels (i.e., small arteries and arterioles just proximal to the capillary network). These particles are made of PVA and are available in various different size classes. Within the last few years PVA particles have largely been supplanted by small plastic spheres, usually with a hydrophilic coating. These are easier to handle and can be placed more reliably because they do not tend to clump. The particles can be placed via microcatheters that can be introduced coaxially through catheters of 4 or 5 French diameter far into small vascular branches. Today the main area of application is the embolization of uterine myoma.

Cyanoacrylates

The most interesting liquid embolic agents are the cyanoacrylates. These are fast-hardening tissue adhesives (Histoacryl or Bukrylat). The liquid substance is mixed with lipiodol, an oily iodine-containing contrast agent, at a ratio of 1:2 or 1:3. Its low viscosity makes it suitable for embolizing even very narrow vascular branches. The hardening process begins upon contact with an electrolyte-containing liquid (i.e., blood). For this reason the catheter and the vessels to be embolized must first be flushed with 40% glucose solution before Histoacryl is injected. Where embolization is to be performed in several steps, it is best to use a new catheter each time rather than flushing the old one with glucose solution. This is because it is not possible to reliably determine the amount of residue injected while flushing the catheter. In larger vessels, a balloon occlusion catheter (catheter with a latex balloon at its tip, see also p. 31) should be used for the injection. This will reliably prevent retrograde flow into adjacent vessels. After the injection the catheter must be withdrawn immediately to prevent its tip from adhering to the embolic material.

Microcatheters

Embolization of small vascular branches with minicoils or particles is performed with microcatheters introduced coaxially through catheters of 4 or 5 French diameter. These

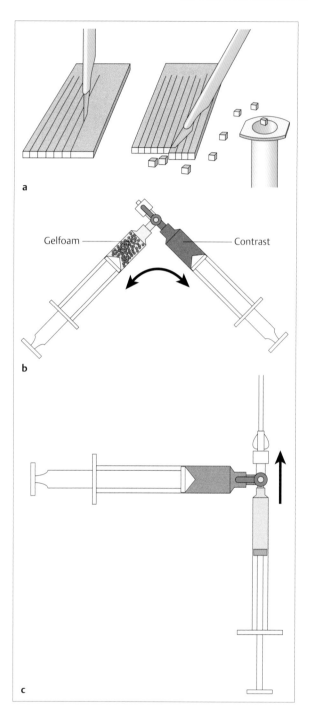

a

Gelfoam   Contrast

b

c

Fig. 3.115   Gelfoam.
a Cutting Gelfoam into cubes.
b Impregnating the Gelfoam with contrast agent. Both are mixed back and forth between the syringes to form an injectable sludge.
c Injection. (The cytostatic is mixed with lipiodol in the same manner for chemoembolization of the liver.)

microcatheters are very flexible and can be steered with a very fine wire (0.010 to 0.018 in.). The outer diameter of the microcatheters ranges between 1.5 and 2.8 French; the proximal end is usually thicker to facilitate steering.

The target vessel is first catheterized with an angiography catheter, which is advanced as far as possible. Before it is advanced to the site, the microcatheter is first fed through a hemostatic valve or a Tuohy-Borst adapter that seals the space between the two catheters and allows

flushing and injection of contrast agent. The guidewire used with the microcatheter usually requires a slightly curved tip. A twist grip is attached to the proximal end of the wire to steer it. The actual catheterization procedure involves introducing the wire into the desired branch and then, once the wire has achieved a sufficiently stable position, advancing the microcatheter over it. If necessary this process is repeated several times until the catheter tip has reached the desired position.

Extracting Foreign Bodies and Pull-Through Technique

Since the very beginning of interventional radiology, instruments have been described for removing foreign bodies from the circulatory system. The most important ones include snares (**Fig. 3.116**), baskets (**Fig. 3.117**), small forceps (**Fig. 3.118**), and pigtail catheters.

Extracting Foreign Bodies

Intravascular foreign bodies are almost invariably iatrogenic in origin. They may be catheter fragments, guidewires, electrodes, embolic coils, displaced stents, or inferior vena cava filters. The instruments used to remove them are primarily snares that expand due to their own elasticity when they are advanced out of a catheter. The operator attempts to maneuver the snare loop around the free end of the foreign body and pull it tight, thus

trapping the foreign body. A different device is required only where no free end is accessible on the foreign body. One example of this is a catheter fragment that has lodged transversely or obliquely in the right atrium, with one end at the wall and the other in the right ventricle. In such a case one advances a strong hook or a pigtail catheter past the fragment, hooks it, and dislodges it from its position. Another method is to advance a wire and a snare past either side of the foreign body and then grasp the wire with the snare distal to the foreign body. This creates a loop around the foreign body that can then be tightened and withdrawn to dislodge it.

Not every foreign body can be drawn into a sheath and then removed from the body. However, a lot is gained if the surgeon only has to open a vein or artery in the inguinal region instead of a major vessel within the chest or retroperitoneal space.

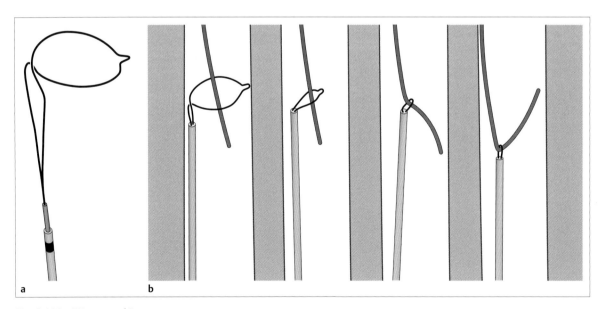

Fig. 3.116   "Goose-neck" snare.
a Structure.   **b** Capturing a wire with a goose-neck snare.

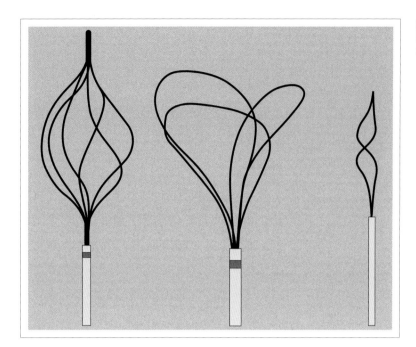

Fig. 3.117 Other snares: Dormia basket (left), snare for small vessels up to 2 mm in diameter (right).

Now that there are nitinol snares, most other instruments are no longer required. When advanced out of the catheter, these loops reliably expand to a certain size and assume a position perpendicular to the longitudinal axis of the vessel (like the head of a goose on its neck, hence the term "goose-neck" snare, **Fig. 3.116**). The goose-neck snares are available in 5, 10, 15, 20, 25, and 30 mm diameters. They are rarely needed, but there may always be unforeseen situations in which they are indispensable.

Pull-Through Technique

The most common use of snares today is to grasp a guidewire introduced via a separate access site (contralateral side or brachial artery) to facilitate advancing a balloon catheter or stent into position. One example of this is the occlusion of one common iliac artery, which cannot be catheterized via a distal approach. However, it is possible to advance a wire through the occlusion via a curved catheter introduced from the contralateral side. The snare to capture the wire is then introduced via a sheath on the ipsilateral side (the side of the occlusion). The end of the wire is caught and then pulled outside the body with the snare (**Fig. 3.119**). Now a balloon catheter or the application system for a stent can be advanced through the occluded segment over this wire.

Another example may be found in Chapter 5, Access via the Popliteal Artery (p. 179): An occlusion of the superficial femoral artery that cannot be catheterized via a proximal approach can in certain cases be catheterized distally via the popliteal artery. The access site in the popliteal artery need not be larger than 4 French if one captures the wire via a sheath in the common femoral artery and then performs the actual intervention itself via the inguinal region.

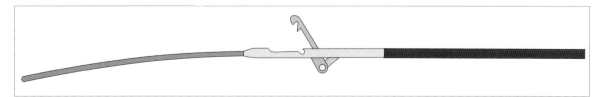

Fig. 3.118 Forceps for grasping foreign bodies (Cook Medical).

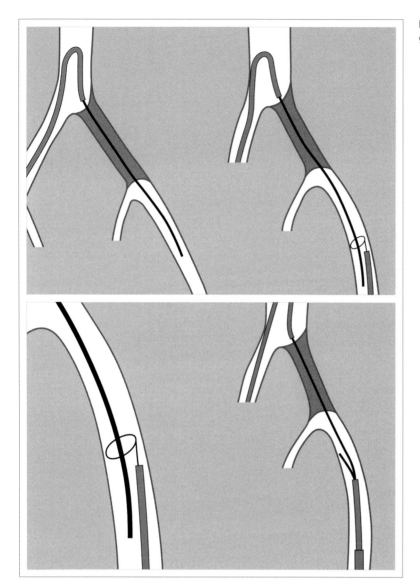

Fig. 3.119 Capturing a wire with a goose-neck snare in the iliac arteries.

References

Belenky A, Aranovich D, Greif F, Bachar G, Bartal G, Atar E. Use of a collagen-based device for closure of low brachial artery punctures. Cardiovasc Intervent Radiol 2007;30(2):273–275

Berger HJ. Einsatz von Protektionssystemen zur Vermeidung von peripheren Embolien im Bereich der femoropoplitealen und renalen PTA: Ein sinnvoller Einsatz? Berlin: Deutscher Röntgenkongress; 2010

Bürkle G, Bürkle H. The place of local, low-dose, short-duration fibrinolysis in the management concept of arterial occlusive diseases [in German]. Rofo 1991;155(5):393–404

Cope C, Burke DR, Meranze SG. Atlas of Interventional Radiology. Philadelphia, PA: Lippincott; 1990:7:18

Cubero JM, Lombardo J, Pedrosa C, et al. Radial compression guided by mean artery pressure versus standard compression with a pneumatic device (RACOMAP). Catheter Cardiovasc Interv 2009;73(4):467–472

Das R, Ahmed K, Athanasiou T, Morgan RA, Belli A-M. Arterial closure devices versus manual compression for femoral haemostasis in interventional radiological procedures: a systematic review and meta-analysis. Cardiovasc Intervent Radiol 2011;34(4):723–738

Fraedrich G, Klocker J, Gratl A, et al. Verschlusssysteme: Chirurgische Therapie sekundärer vaskulärer Komplikationen. 91. Berlin: Deutscher Röntgenkongress; 2010

Fröhlich J, Stump DL. Recombinant tissue plasminogen activator. In: Comerota AJ, ed. Thrombolytic Therapy in Peripheral Vascular Disease. Philadelphia, PA: Lippincott; 1995:103–114

Huppert P, Mueller W, Bauersachs R. Alternative Zugangswege bei der Rekanalisation von Extremitätenarterien. Berlin: Deutscher Röntgenkongress; 2010

Kaid KA, Gopinathapillai R, Qian F, Salvaji M, Wasty N, Cohen M. Analysis of particulate debris after superficial femoral artery atherectomy. J Invasive Cardiol 2009;21(1):7–10

Kedhi E, Tanguay JF, Bilodeau L. Pathophysiology of restenosis. In: Heuser RR, Henry M, eds. Textbook of Peripheral Vascular Interventions. 2nd ed. London: Informa UK; 2008:763–769

Kedhi E, Bilodeau I. Interventional therapy: new approaches. In: Heuser RR, Henry M, eds. Textbook of Peripheral Vascular Interventions. 2nd ed. London: Informa UK; 2008:772–773

Laird JR, Zeller T, Gray BH, et al; LACI Investigators. Limb salvage following laser-assisted angioplasty for critical limb ischemia: results of the LACI multicenter trial. J Endovasc Ther 2006;13(1):1–11

Lanzman RS, Schmitt P, Kröpil P, Blondin D. Nonenhanced MR angiography techniques [in German]. Rofo 2011;183(10):913–924

Losordo DW, Rosenfield K, Pieczek A, Baker K, Harding M, Isner JM. How does angioplasty work? Serial analysis of human iliac arteries using intravascular ultrasound. Circulation 1992;86(6):1845–1858

Markose G, Bolia A. Subintimal angioplasty. In: Heuser RR, Henry M, eds. Textbook of Peripheral Vascular Interventions. 2nd ed. London: Informa UK; 2008:83–91

Miki Y, Isoda H, Togashi K. Guideline to use gadolinium-based contrast agents at Kyoto University Hospital. J Magn Reson Imaging 2009;30(6):1364–1365

Puggioni A, Boesmans E, Deloose K, Peeters P, Bosiers M. Use of StarClose for brachial artery closure after percutaneous endovascular interventions. Vascular 2008;16(2):85–90

Roberts A. Principles of selective thrombolysis. In: Baum S, Pentecost MJ, eds. Abrams Angiography, Interventional Radiology. 2nd ed. Philadelphia, PA: Lippincott Williams & Wilkins; 2006a:220–232

Roberts A. Thrombolysis: clinical application. In: Baum S, Pentecost MJ, eds. Abrams Angiography, Interventional Radiology. 2nd ed. Philadelphia, PA: Lippincott Williams & Wilkins; 2006b:233–256

Schmidt A, Montero-Baker M. Below the Knee Occlusion. Leipzig: Interventional Course; 2008

Schroeder J. Catheter lysis and percutaneous transluminal angioplasty below the knee via the popliteal artery in a patient with femoral artery obstruction: technical note. Cardiovasc Intervent Radiol 1989;12(6):344–345

Schröder J. Control of catheters in coronary angiography—resistance to torsion in the aortic arch [in German]. Z Kardiol 1992;81(8):449–452

Sommer W, Reiser M, Nikolaou K. CT-Angiographie der Becken- und Beingefäbe. Berlin: Deutscher Röntgenkongress; 2010

Tran VK. Perkutane Rekanalisation bei Verschlüssen von Beinarterien. Inauguraldissertation Kiel; 1998

Turi ZG. Vascular closure devices. In: Heuser RR, Henry M, eds. Textbook of Peripheral Vascular Interventions. 2nd ed. London: Informa UK; 2008:168–184

4   Abdomen

Renal Arteries

The initial euphoria about interventional treatment of renal artery stenosis has given way to a more sober, even skeptical assessment. Good results are still being reported (Patel et al 2009), with a significant decrease in complications (Schillinger and Zeller 2007). Yet recent studies indicate that the regulation of blood pressure and restoration of kidney function achieved with stent angioplasty are on average no better than the results achieved with medical treatment alone (Lenz 2010). However, one of these studies has been criticized for flaws in its methodology. Regardless of how this dispute is likely to be resolved, the radiologist should exercise restraint in determining whether the treatment is indicated. Close consultation with specialists in allied disciplines is essential.

Renal artery stenosis is a major cause of impairment or loss of function. Yet renal artery stenosis is a probable cause of arterial hypertension in at most 5% of patients.

The kidneys have an autonomous blood pressure regulation system. When one kidney detects too low pressure (e.g., due to renal artery stenosis) it secretes renin to increase pressure throughout the system (renal hypertension). This mechanism is referred to as Goldblatt hypertension in honor of the physician who first discovered it. Eliminating the causative stenosis can improve or eliminate the hypertension in this case. About 90% of renal artery stenoses are due to arteriosclerosis. The rest are caused primarily by fibromuscular dysplasia (FMD). Restenosis rates of 14% have been observed in arteriosclerotic renal artery stenoses treated by stent placement (Sapoval et al 2005).

Indication

Suspicion of renal artery stenosis usually arises when hypertension is poorly controllable with medication, when it occurs at a particularly early age (< 30 years) or late age (> 50 years), and when it worsens under therapy with angiotensin-converting enzyme (ACE) inhibitors. Rapid deterioration of kidney function can also be a sign of renal artery stenosis.

A stenosis grade of 70% or even 80% is generally regarded as the threshold defining the indication for intervention. Today it is felt that intervention is not usually indicated in patients with well controlled hypertension and in older hypertensive patients with normal kidney function.

The reliability of magnetic resonance imaging (MRI) and computed tomography (CT) in detecting stenosis is highly dependent on the specific equipment and examination technique. Magnetic resonance angiography (MRA) in particular often produces false-positive results. Because of the toxicity of the contrast agent, both modalities are problematic in patients with impaired kidney function. Ultrasound is a relatively reliable method in a slender patient if the equipment is very good and the examiner is experienced. Sensitivity and specificity are reported to be ~ 90% (Henry et al 2008). Captopril-enhanced renal scintigraphy (too costly) and separate renin measurements for each side (too unreliable) are no longer recommended for routine clinical practice (Henry et al 2008). Angiography will occasionally fail to detect an ostial stenosis where the ostium cannot be visualized separately from the aorta.

> Renal insufficiency can be due to renal artery stenosis. Eliminating it can improve long-term function. However, in 20% of the cases with renal insufficiency it initially leads to worsening of the condition (Henry et al 2008). Therefore great care should be taken when determining whether treatment is indicated, and specialists from every discipline involved should be consulted, especially the nephrologist.

Percutaneous Transluminal Angioplasty or Stent? Ostial stenoses are now usually treated by primary placement of a stent. This is because they are usually very rigid and because the balloon only temporarily presses the occluding material into the aortic lumen. From there it falls back into the ostium after dilation (**Fig. 4.1**). Because they have higher radial strength and can be placed with greater precision, balloon-expandable stents are used almost exclusively in the renal artery (average length 15 mm).

Good results can often be achieved with dilation alone in stenoses distal to the ostium. FMD should only be treated with a stent in exceptional cases.

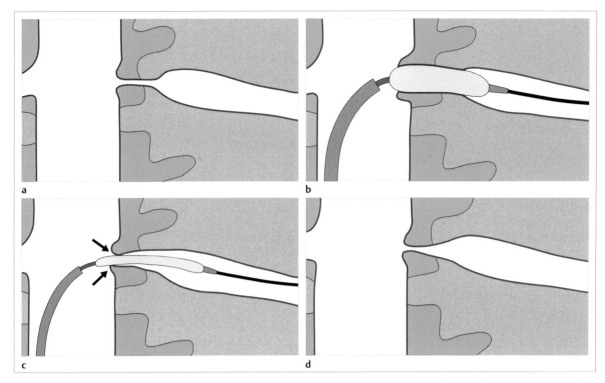

Fig. 4.1 Percutaneous transluminal angioplasty (PTA) in ostial stenoses. In an ostial stenosis, the PTA balloon often only pushes the plaque material into the aorta. It then falls back into the ostium.

a Ostial stenosis.

b Dilation. The balloon pushes plaque material into the aorta.

c Then it falls back into the ostium.

d No improvement in findings.

Risks and Complications

Renal Insufficiency

Deterioration of kidney function is the most important risk to be anticipated in an intervention in the renal arteries. The main reason for this is the nephrotoxicity of the contrast agent. Therefore the decisive prophylactic measure is to use contrast agent extremely sparingly. Note that a normal serum creatinine level does not exclude renal functional impairment. Serum creatinine increases over the normal value of 1 to 1.1 mg/dL only when the glomerular filtration rate (GFR) drops to 50%.

Renal insufficiency can be the decisive indication for elimination of renal artery stenosis. Because the condition is usually progressive, even stabilization of renal function may be regarded as a successful outcome. The more severe the insufficiency, the more likely it will improve with treatment. Yet at the same time the risk to residual function posed by the contrast agent increases with the severity of the functional impairment. The average rate of worsening of renal function secondary to intervention ranges from 15% (Schillinger and Zeller 2007) to 21%

(Henry et al). It can probably be reduced to less than 5% (Sos and Trost 2008) by good preparation and very sparing use of contrast agent, possibly substituting CO_2 (see also Chapter 2, CO_2 as a Contrast Agent, p. 36).

> ▷ Kidney function should invariably be evaluated before the patient is discharged!

Aside from contrast toxicity, the embolization of cholesterol particles within the kidney is also an important causative factor in possible deterioration of kidney function. This is triggered by mechanical action on plaques. Therefore there is an increased risk of cholesterol embolization in an aorta with severe changes in the form of unstable plaques. Cholesterol emboli can occur up to 3 days after the intervention (frequency up to 3%, Schillinger and Zeller 2007). Protection systems such as those used in the interventional treatment of carotid stenosis are currently being tested. There have not yet been any definitive recommendations for their use.

Mechanical Risks

The mechanical risks associated with the treatment of renal artery stenosis include incorrect placement of the stent, dissection, perforation of the kidney with a guidewire, rupture, and avulsion of the renal artery. The most important measures for avoiding mechanical complications include the following:

- Slender catheter systems
- Correctly matching the balloon and stent size to the vessel diameter, which requires precise angiographic measurement
- Slowly inflating the balloon while closely observing the patient: Is there a sensation of pressure? Pain?
- Correct placement of the stent
- Angiographic monitoring prior to deploying the stent
- Avoiding any uncontrolled movement of the wire (a monorail system should be preferred)

Incorrect placement of the stent. A stent placed in the ostium should project 1 to 2 mm into the aortic lumen. This prevents plaque material from falling back into the ostium after dilation. The most important step in avoiding incorrect placement of the stent is to visualize the ostium in an optimal projection (**Fig. 4.2**). This is best achieved by using cross-sectional MR or CT images as the basis for planning the procedure.

A stent that projects too far into the aorta (> 2 mm) will render any reintervention difficult. The guidewire will tend to enter the mesh of the stent rather than its lumen (**Figs. 4.3** and **4.4**).

A renal artery dissection occurs significantly more often than a rupture. The dissection most commonly occurs during dilation in the vicinity of a rigid plaque, although it can also be caused by a guidewire. It can usually be managed by placing a stent.

Perforation of the kidney with a guidewire (usually a glide wire). One must have the guidewire in view during any manipulation. Should one have neglected to do so and the patient complains of a stabbing pain in the kidney region, then one must check the wire immediately. It may be that it has entered the parenchyma or even perforated it. If that is the case, do not immediately withdraw the wire. First administer protamine to neutralize the heparin. Then advance a 4 French catheter over the wire to the end of the vessel. Remove the wire, and inject contrast agent through the catheter to demonstrate any bleeding. In the event there is bleeding, a 2 mm coil is placed in the wound canal. A CT image is later obtained to exclude a hematoma.

Rupture of a renal artery. This will most likely occur where the balloon is too large for the renal artery and where the stenosis is severely calcified. The best prophylaxis is to precisely measure vessel diameter and avoid excessive dilation. When in doubt, use a smaller balloon or stent. If this proves to be too small, one can always dilate again with a larger balloon. If the patient complains of intense pain during dilation, deflate the balloon and perform angiography via the sheath. If any extravasation is detected, inform the vascular surgeon immediately.

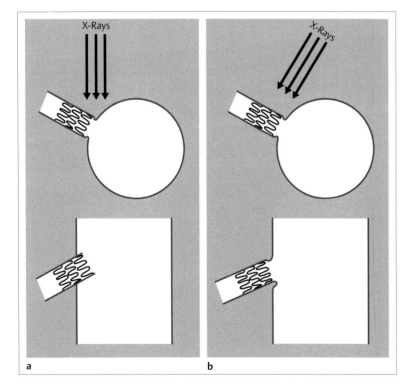

Fig. 4.2 If the ostium is not correctly visualized perpendicular to the beam, a stent that lies too far distal (shown here in cross section) will be projected onto the aortic lumen on the angiographic image.
a Incorrect projection.
b Correct projection.

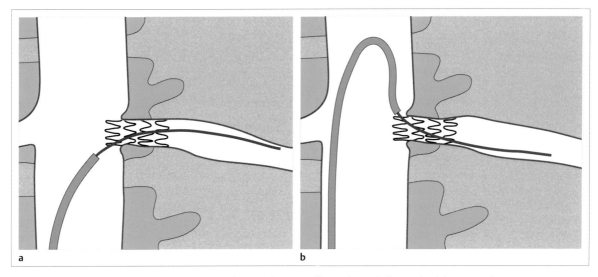

Fig. 4.3 If the stent lies too far within the aortic lumen, the wire will pass through the mesh of the stent when reintervention is attempted.
a Caudal approach.   **b** Cranial approach.

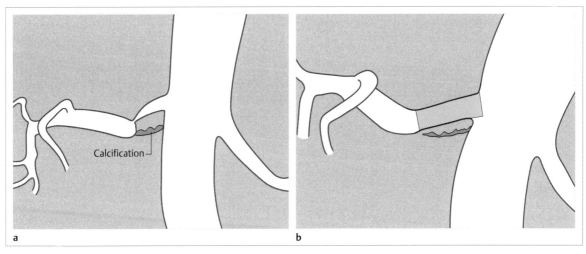

Fig. 4.4 Where the renal artery arises at an acute angle, the caudal aspect of the stent must project farther into the aortic lumen.
a Eccentric calcifications in a stenosis near the ostium.   **b** The caudal aspect of the stent projects farther into the aortic lumen than its cranial aspect.

Then one can attempt to tampon the bleeding with the balloon (at low pressure). At the same time, neutralize the heparin with protamine. (Caution: There is a risk of anaphylactic reaction, especially in patients who are allergic to fish protein.) If this does not succeed, place a covered stent. This can be difficult because the covered stent is less flexible than a regular stent.

Avulsion of a renal artery is a very rare event and is thought to occur more often in the presence of a severely calcified ostium. In this case one must occlude the aorta proximal to the renal artery with a large occlusion balloon and prepare for immediate vascular surgery.

Material for emergency treatment (according to Schillinger and Zeller 2007) includes the following:
- Covered stents 4 to 7 mm in diameter, 15 to 20 mm long
- Large balloons to seal off the aorta
- Embolization coils 2 to 6 mm
- Aspiration catheter that fits a 0.014 in. wire
- Thrombolytic agent
- Protamine ampoules containing 1,000 or 5,000 IU for intravenous (IV) administration: 1,000 IU of protamine; deactivate 1,000 IU of heparin (risk of anaphylactic reaction; see earlier mention)

Table 4.1 Complications of intervention in the renal arteries

Complication	Avoidance	Treatment
Contrast-induced nephropathy	Hydration Preparation using cross-sectional images of the aorta Catheterize renal artery without contrast Small doses of contrast with high image frequency CO_2 as contrast agent where feasible	
Incorrect placement of stent	Correct projection (cross-sectional images!) Angiographic monitoring Stiff wire: bend	
Perforation	Do not use glide wire Monorail system	Embolization (surgery)
Dissection		Stent
Rupture	Precisely measure vessel diameter Caution where calcification is present Be alert to pain sensation!	Balloon tamponade Covered stent (surgery)
Cholesterol embolization	Atraumatic technique Slender systems	
Thrombosis, embolus Spasm	Aspirin, clopidogrel, heparin Verapamil, nitroglycerin	

The complication rate in large series used to be ~ 10 to 14%. Since the introduction of long guiding sheaths and smaller systems (0.014 or 0.018 in. wires, monorail) it has decreased to less than 3% (Schillinger and Zeller 2007, **Table 4.1**).

Preparation for Intervention

- Measure urea and creatinine serum levels, creatinine clearance, wherever possible GFR.
- Measure blood pressure over 24 hours.
- Determine medication.
- Perform duplex ultrasound scan.

Any error or omission in renal percutaneous transluminal angioplasty (PTA) can have serious consequences for the patient, including dependence on dialysis, loss of a kidney, and death. This justifies any additional expense that improves safety.

Whatever can be resolved beforehand or would require additional contrast agent to resolve during the intervention should be resolved beforehand. This includes the anatomy of the abdominal aorta and the iliac arteries (MRI or CT) and, particularly important, the direction of the origins of the renal arteries (where feasible, without contrast agent). If this has not been resolved beforehand, one will end up groping toward a halfway decent projection of the renal artery on the basis of two or three aortograms. Cross-sectional CT or MR images usually show this with perfect clarity. Therefore make an effort to obtain previous imaging studies (CT, MRI, angiography). Where no such studies are available, obtain at least a noncontrasted CT scan of the kidney region prior to the intervention. Aside from the direction of the origin, these images will also show major calcifications.

If the angular adjustment is off by only a few degrees, then the ostial stenosis will be obscured by the contrasted aortic lumen. Where the renal arteries arise at different angles (**Fig. 4.5**), two separate image series are needed for the left and right renal arteries.

Preparing the Patient

On the day of the intervention begin with hydration of the patient: Administer 1 to 1.5 mL per kg body weight per hour of a normal or half normal saline solution 12 hours before and 12 hours after the intervention. In patients with heart failure, the fluid must be balanced with the volume of urine.

Also begin therapy with acetylsalicylic acid and clopidogrel on the day before the procedure (300 mg on the first day, thereafter 75 mg daily). Oral acetylcysteine, a strong antioxidant, is often administered as prophylaxis against kidney damage (600 mg each the day before and on the day of the intervention).

Intervention Technique

Fundamentals

Before the advent of stent treatment it was customary to work with only one catheter via a short sheath. The

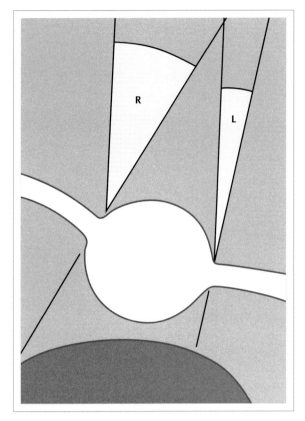

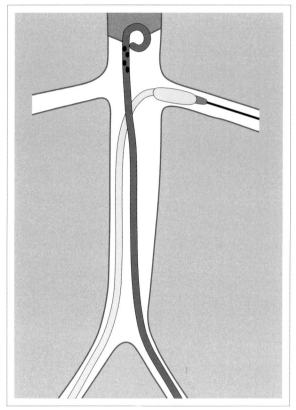

Fig. 4.5 Differences in the direction of the origins of the left and right renal arteries.

Fig. 4.6 Once a common procedure with two catheters, now no longer recommended.

balloon catheter had to be withdrawn and replaced by a diagnostic catheter to verify the results of treatment. The development of the stent gave rise to the need to verify the stent's precise position angiographically during the procedure. This was initially done by introducing a pigtail catheter via the contralateral inguinal artery and advancing it into the aorta parallel to the first one (**Fig. 4.6**). This can no longer be recommended. The quantity of contrast agent required is significantly higher than when injected via a long guiding sheath. Additionally, catheterization of the contralateral groin increases the risk of complications.

The decisive advance came with the introduction of long guiding sheaths (**Fig. 4.7**). These devices provided a significantly more reliable means of advancing the stent up to and into the renal artery. They allowed angiographic control with very small volumes of contrast, and they are also required for the use of monorail systems. A long sheath without a bend (**Fig. 4.8**) allows the use of a monorail system. However, it does not aid in advancing the wire or catheter and requires equally large volumes of contrast as the pigtail catheter technique described earlier. In addition, the spread of contrast along the aorta is even more pronounced than in the use of a pigtail, resulting in bad image quality. This means it cannot be recommended at all.

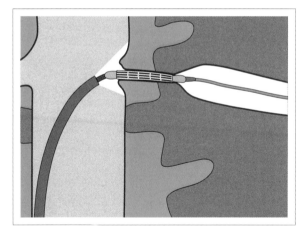

Fig. 4.7 Intervention via a long sheath. Angiographic monitoring prior to deploying the stent.

Intervention Technique in Detail

Guiding Sheaths and Guiding Catheters

Guiding sheaths and guiding catheters are supplied with various curvatures (**Fig. 4.9**). The width and curvature of the aorta and the angle of the renal artery origin are the decisive criteria for selecting the sheath. For a renal artery that arises nearly horizontally it is best to choose a sheath

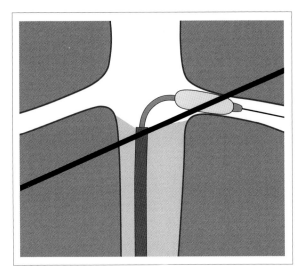

Fig. 4.8 Long sheath without a bend. The quantity of contrast agent required is higher than with a pigtail catheter. Image quality is poor due to superimposition!

the tip of which is angled perpendicular to the aortic wall. Where the renal artery courses caudally from its origin, it is best if the sheath has a more pronounced bend.

Where the sheath is to be advanced into the renal artery, a model with a less pronounced bend is recommended. A sheath with a sharp bend can be required to compensate for a bend in the infrarenal aorta (**Fig. 4.10**, left). For the contralateral side one will need for the same constellation a straight sheath with a short bend at its tip (**Fig. 4.10**, right). The popular Renal Double Curve (RDC) model is not recommended. The RDC sheath has a sharp bend near its tip that can prevent the passage of a stent. This risk is significantly reduced where the sharp bend is replaced by a harmonious curve (**Fig. 4.11**).

Catheters are specified by their outer diameter but sheaths by their inner diameter (see Chapter 2, Size Specifications for Cannulas, Guidewires, Catheters, and Sheaths, p. 7) (i.e., according to the catheter that fits in the sheath). This explains why a 6 French guiding sheath has the same inner and outer dimensions as an 8 French guiding catheter. When an 8 French guiding catheter is used, the 8 French sheath that is also required will naturally create a larger puncture wound in the wall of the femoral artery. Transbrachial catheterization (**Fig. 4.12**) may be the better approach in the presence of a slender aorta, acute-angle renal artery origin, or greatly elongated (tortuous) iliac arteries. However, this approach is associated with a higher risk, especially where placing a larger stent requires the use of a 6 French sheath that can occlude the lumen of the brachial artery. Thrombi mobilized by the sheath can cause a cerebellar insult.

Aortography

The intervention begins with abdominal aortography with a high degree of collination (obtained in the optimal projection determined on the basis of prior CT or MRI studies). This image serves to verify the indication and determine the position of the ostia. Where no cross-sectional images are available, an initial attempt with a 20° left anterior oblique (LAO) projection is recommended.

Using the smallest possible volumes of contrast to optimal effect for the aortography requires that the contrast agent be deposited over a very short segment of the aorta. The pigtail catheters commonly used distribute the contrast over a long segment of the aorta through too many side holes. Another problem is that the end of the pigtail points cranially and therefore separates up to 50% of the contrast agent from the bolus. For this reason it is better to use a catheter whose tip points caudally and has only a few side holes close to it (**Fig. 4.13**). (The most elegant solution would be a catheter without an end hole and with side holes that expel contrast agent only in the direction of the renal arteries.) If the level of

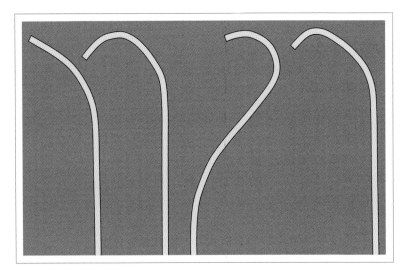

Fig. 4.9 Guiding sheaths of various shapes.

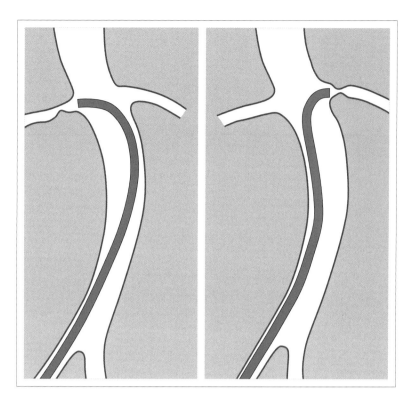

Fig. 4.10 Adapting the shape of the sheath to a curved aorta.

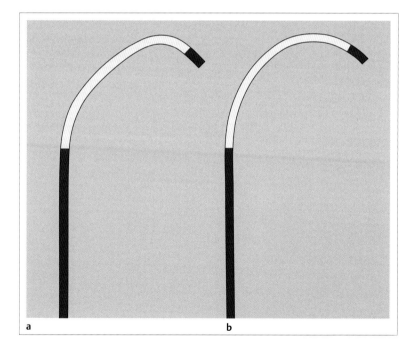

Fig. 4.11 The unnecessarily sharp bends in the Renal Double Curve (RDC) sheath (left) can interfere with the passage of a stent. The sheath on the right exhibits the same angle between shaft and tip but with a harmonious curve.
a RDC sheath.
b Harmonious curve.

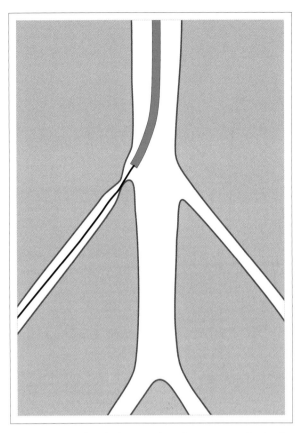

Fig. 4.12 Transbrachial approach in the presence of a slender aorta and acute-angle renal artery origin.

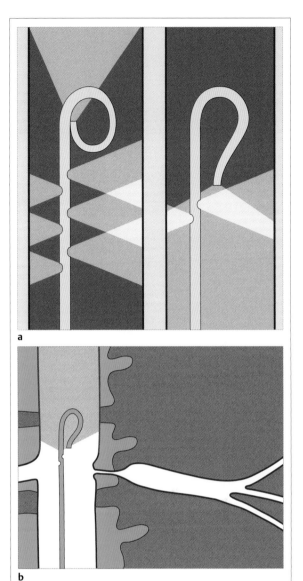

Fig. 4.13 How catheter shape influences quantity of contrast required.
a Contrast distribution patterns with pigtail and Omni-Flow catheter (Sos).
b Aortography with Omni-Flow catheter.

the renal artery origin is not known, then the side holes and end hole of the catheter should lie at the level of the T12–L1 vertebrae.

Sos and Trost (2008) recommend using contrast agent with 150 mg iodine/mL. The disadvantage of this is that blood invariably dilutes the contrast agent anyway. If half the volume of a contrast agent with 300 mg of iodine per mL is used, no greater contrast burden is placed on the kidneys but better contrast will briefly be achieved in the vicinity of the catheter tip.

The important thing is that at small contrast volumes (5 to 8 mL) one needs a high image frequency (4/s) and a summation image generated from a series of individual images.

The patient's position and the projection must remain unchanged during the intervention. Then an overlay image from the angiography performed beforehand is the most reliable guide for catheterizing the renal artery. Alternatively, an unsubtracted or partially subtracted image that clearly visualizes the skeleton can be displayed the whole time on a reference monitor for orientation purposes.

The aortography provides the basis for the final decision as to whether intervention is indicated. PTA or stent placement is generally regarded as indicated where a stenosis of over 70% (some authors say 80%) is

demonstrated (i.e., measured) on the image. Estimations according to the visual impression are unreliable and therefore inadmissible; in one experiment (Subramanian et al 2005) stenoses of 56.6 + 10.8% were estimated as 74.9 + 11.5%. The reference value for determining the severity of the stenosis is not the diameter in the region of the poststenotic dilation (**Fig. 4.14**)!

Measuring Pressure
If the indication cannot be determined unequivocally on the basis of morphological criteria, measurement of the pressure gradient can be the deciding factor. The measurement

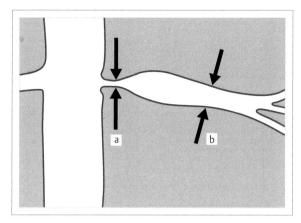

Fig. 4.14 Measurements to determine the severity of stenosis. a, diameter of the stenosis; b, reference diameter distal to the poststenotic dilation.

is performed simultaneously distal to the stenosis (preferably with a 0.014 in. pressure wire) and in the aorta (via the sheath). A gradient of > 10% at peak systolic pressure is regarded as conclusive; experiments have demonstrated increased renin production in the kidney above this gradient (Sos and Trost 2008).

Because the wire for the pressure measurement is expensive, operators usually use a 4 French catheter instead. Yet this leads to overestimation of the severity of the stenosis because the catheter itself occludes part of the cross section within the stenosis. The 4 French catheter will turn a 60% stenosis in an artery 5 mm in diameter into a stenosis of 70%. However, this will keep one on the safe side at least for excluding an indication for intervention.

The hemodynamic effectiveness of a stenosis depends on the flow rate and therefore on the peripheral resistance in the kidney. In advanced nephrosclerosis, it is possible that even a high-grade stenosis will not create a significant pressure gradient because of the low flow. Then intervention would be pointless (Sos and Trost 2008).

After Determining the Indication
- Select and introduce the appropriate sheath.
- Administer heparin (usually 5,000 IU).

To avoid spasms, 0.1 mg of nitroglycerin (short acting) is usually injected into the renal artery, or 2.5 mg of verapamil (longer acting). It is recommended to flush the sheath continuously during the intervention and to combine this with continuous blood pressure measurement. Otherwise the sheath must be flushed at least every 2 minutes.

Sos Flick Technique
The technique described by Thomas Sos employs a modified Sidewinder catheter (AngioDynamics, Latham, NY, USA) in combination with a 0.035 in. Bentson wire. The distal segment of the Sos Omni catheter (AngioDynamics)

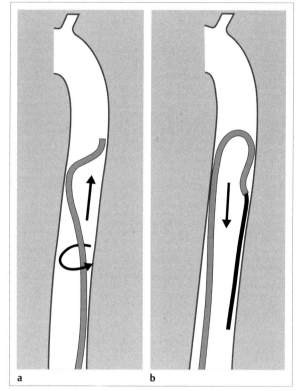

Fig. 4.15 Changing the direction of the Sos Omni catheter by advancing the catheter and simultaneously rotating it.
a Catheter is advanced and simultaneously rotated.
b Redirected catheter.

is shorter than that of the Sidewinder I. This makes it easier and less traumatic to pull it into the renal artery. It is also possible to turn the catheter by simultaneously advancing and rotating it within the aorta beneath the aortic arch (**Fig. 4.15**). This does not require catheterizing the subclavian artery.

The Bentson wire has a soft tip 16 cm long that does not reextend the catheter. When it projects several centimeters beyond the catheter tip, it makes it possible to pull the curved tip of the catheter tip smoothly downward. Below the ostium one withdraws the wire until just less than 1 cm projects out of the catheter (**Fig. 4.16b**). When the catheter is then slowly advanced past the ostium, the end of the wire snaps into the renal artery

Fig. 4.16 Sos flick technique. ▶
a Beneath the ostium withdraw the wire to < 1 cm.
b Slowly advance the catheter to the ostium.
c "Flick": The tip of the Bentson wire snaps into the renal artery.
d The wire is advanced further to secure its position.
e Carefully advance the catheter into the renal artery.
f The sheath is "parked" in the iliac artery.
g Once the wire and catheter lie securely within the renal artery, the sheath is advanced to the ostium under fluoroscopy (keep a grip on the wire and catheter!).

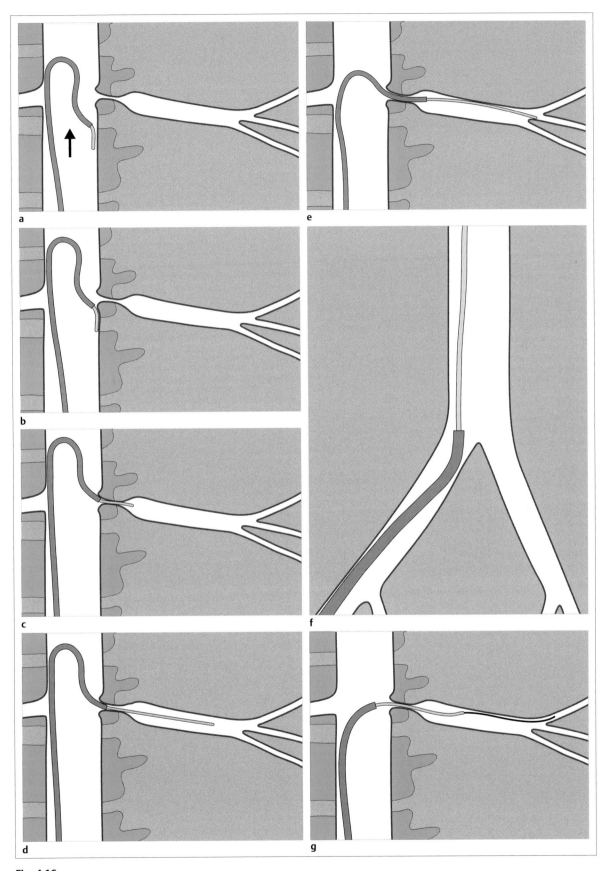

a

b

c

d

e

f

g

Fig. 4.16

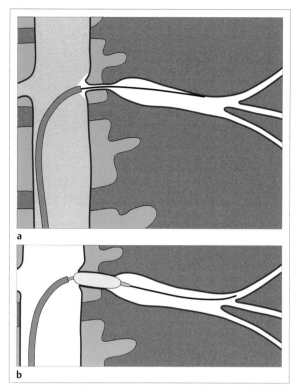

Fig. 4.17 Angiography, measurement, preliminary dilation.
a A suitable guidewire is inserted before the Sos catheter is removed. Angiography is performed and the vessel diameter measured.
b Perform preliminary dilation where indicated.

("flick"). Once the tip of the wire lies within the ostium, it is advanced further to secure its position (**Fig. 4.16d**). Then the catheter is carefully pulled into the renal artery (**Fig. 4.16e**).

Because the level of the ostium is apparent from the aortography (and visible on the overlay in applicable cases), one only needs to probe a very short segment of the aortic wall with the catheter and wire. After an unsuccessful passage, the procedure is repeated with a slight anterior or posterior change in direction. The curvature of the sheath can itself interfere with advancing the wire. For this reason the sheath is best left in the iliac artery during this phase (**Fig. 4.16f**). Once the wire lies securely within the renal artery, the sheath is carefully advanced over the immobilized catheter and wire to the ostium (**Fig. 4.16g**).

Before the Sos catheter is withdrawn, a guidewire suitable for PTA and stent placement must be inserted (**Fig. 4.17a**). For an over the wire system this will be a moderately stiff 0.035 in. wire (Sos recommends the Mallinckrodt TAD II [Abbott Vascular, Temecula, CA, USA]), for a monorail system the appropriate 0.014 in. wire.

Then angiography is performed via the sheath with precise measurement of the vessel diameter. Preliminary

dilation may be performed with a 4 mm balloon where indicated (**Fig. 4.17b**). Whether this is a good idea must be considered on a case by case basis. It makes it easier to introduce the stent, particularly in a very narrow stenosis. On the other hand, it also increases the risk of dissection and embolization compared with primary placement of a stent.

> **Rule:** Preliminary dilation is required for 90% stenosis and invariably for a narrow calcified ostium. If the patient feels pain during dilation, deflate the balloon and perform angiography!

Next, the balloon catheter (usually a monorail design) with the stent is introduced. Its position is verified by angiography and corrected as necessary. Then the stent is slowly deployed. This is done with the patient holding his or her breath after expiration (**Fig. 4.18**). Once the balloon has been deflated again, carefully advance the sheath into the end of the deployed stent and withdraw the balloon into the sheath. This safeguards the position of the stent as one withdraws the balloon. The sheath also has the optimal position for the contrast injection that follows.

The final step is to verify results by angiography. The entire kidney is visualized to exclude embolic vascular

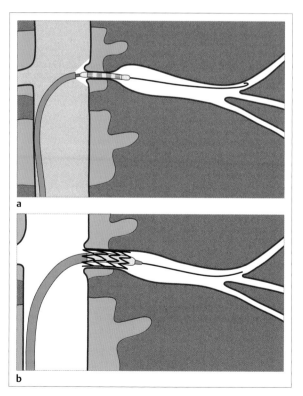

Fig. 4.18 Stent placement.
a Angiographic monitoring.
b The stent is deployed with the patient holding his or her breath after expiration.

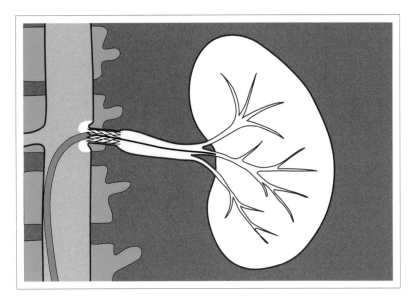

Fig. 4.19 A final angiographic examination is performed to exclude embolus or spasm.

occlusion and spasm (**Fig. 4.19**). The wire remains in the renal artery during this examination. It ensures that the sheath remains centered proximal to or within the ostium. It also provides an approach for performing any additional procedures that may become necessary, such as redilation with a larger balloon, thrombus aspiration, lysis, or embolization of a bleeding vessel.

Feldmann No-Touch Technique, <u>the Most Elegant and Least Invasive Method</u>

Here the sheath is introduced with a glide wire to just cranial to the renal artery (**Fig. 4.20a**). Then the dilator is removed and the glide wire withdrawn until only its soft tip projects from the sheath. This allows the sheath to regain its original bend and brings its tip close to the aortic wall. However, the wire keeps the tip from touching the wall.

A 0.014 in. wire is inserted into the sheath next to the glide wire (**Fig. 4.20b**). The glide wire prevents the sheath from rubbing against the aortic wall while the 0.014 in. wire is used to locate the ostium. This is done with the aid of an overlay wherever possible. Once the 0.014 in. wire lies within the renal artery, the glide wire is removed. Then angiography is performed to measure the renal artery (**Fig. 4.20c**).

The rest of the procedure is identical to the Sos technique: Where indicated, preliminary dilation is performed with a balloon appropriate for the 0.014 in. wire (4 mm). Next, a balloon catheter (usually a monorail design) with a stent is introduced. The correct position is verified, the stent is deployed, and the results are evaluated (**Fig. 4.21**).

Advancing a Sheath into the Renal Artery <u>(More Invasive, Not Recommended)</u>

This is a widely used technique in which the sheath itself is advanced past the ostial stenosis into the renal artery.

The stent is advanced into the stenosis within the sheath, and the sheath is then withdrawn. This technique is especially suitable for treatment with the stiffer 5 French systems. However, it is not the least invasive method. Considering that Schillinger and Zeller (2007) report that the 10 to 14% complication rate associated with the use of smaller systems (0.014 in. wire, monorail) can be reduced to less than 3%, one can hardly justify the use of 5 French systems.

To avoid shear effects on the arterial wall, the sheath should not be advanced into the stenosis without the dilator fully inserted. However, certain authors recommend simply advancing the sheath into the renal artery over the deflated balloon (Criado 1999, Henry et al 2008, Sos and Trost 2008). This is quick and convenient but increases the risk of cholesterol embolization.

Here, too, the first step is to obtain an aortogram. Then the appropriate sheath is selected according to the course and width of the aorta and the angle of the renal artery origins. The sheath initially remains within the iliac arteries (**Fig. 4.22**).

Various catheters are available for the initial catheterization of the renal artery. The choice again depends on the angle of the renal artery origin. The Levin catheter (like the Cobra catheter but without the reverse curve in the shaft) is suitable for many cases (**Fig. 4.22c**), or the Sos Omni (AngioDynamics) described above may be used. It is particularly suitable for acute-angle renal artery origins. (The distal segment of the similarly shaped Simmons I is too long.) Now angiography is performed to measure the renal artery.

The best choice of guidewire is a Teflon-coated wire with a soft tip ~ 5 cm long and a gradual transition to a shaft of medium stiffness. A relatively stiff straight wire (0.035 or 0.018 in.) will put the renal artery at a steep angle (**Fig. 4.23a**). This can make it very difficult to

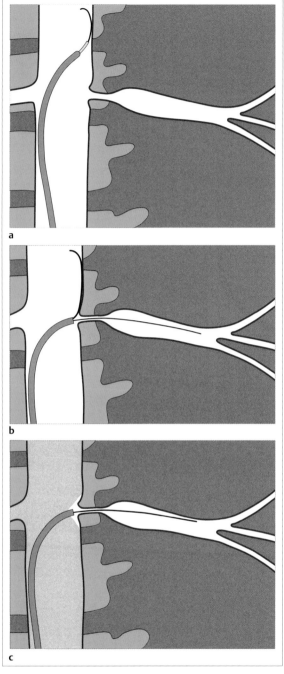

Fig. 4.20 Feldmann no-touch technique.
a Sheath with glide wire cranial to the renal artery.
b Dilator removed; glide wire protects the aortic wall; 0.014 in. wire probes the ostium.
c Remove glide wire, perform angiography.

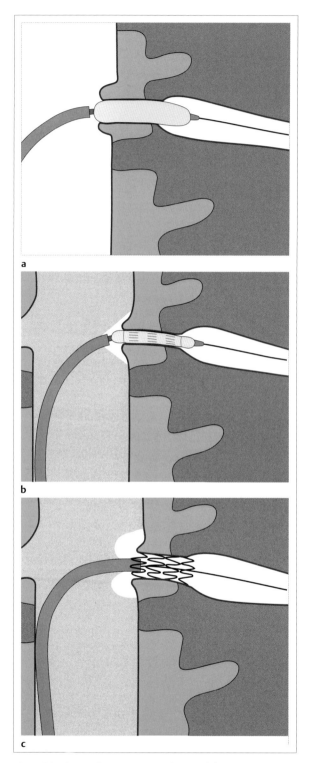

Fig. 4.21 Stent placement; completion of the intervention.
a Preliminary dilation (where indicated).
b Correct position is verified and stent placed.
c Result is evaluated.

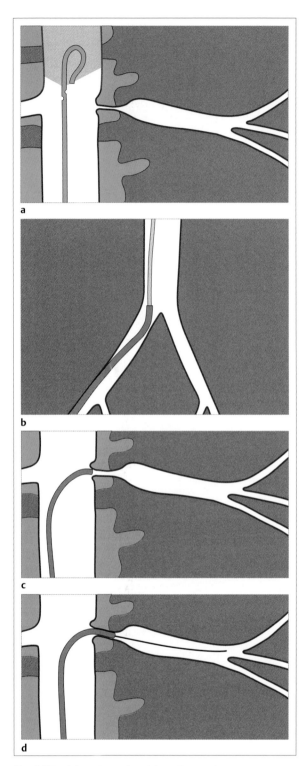

Fig. 4.22 Advancing a sheath into the renal artery.
a Aortography.
b Sheath still lies in the iliac artery.
c Advancing a Levin catheter into the renal artery; angiographic measurement of vessel diameter.
d Advancing a guidewire into the renal artery.

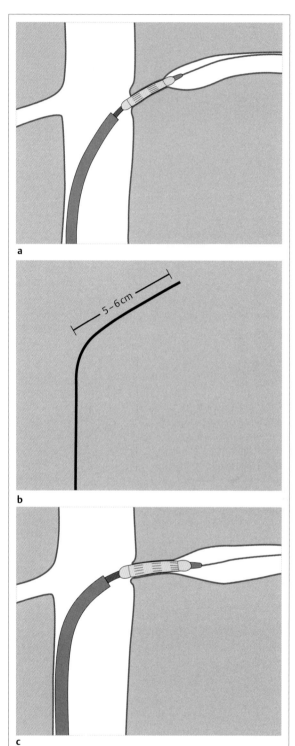

Fig. 4.23 A relatively stiff straight wire can put the renal artery at a steep angle, making it difficult to evaluate the position of the stent relative to the ostium.
a A relatively stiff straight wire puts the renal artery at a steep angle.
b A bend in the wire helps to alleviate this problem.
c More stable wire position and more precise placement of the stent.

reliably evaluate the stent's position relative to the ostium and aortic wall. Therefore it helps to give the wire a slight bend at the point that will lie in the junction between the aorta and the renal artery (**Fig. 4.23b**). This gives the wire a more stable position and facilitates precise placement of the stent (**Fig. 4.23c**).

> **Caution:** A j-shaped bend in the tip of the wire is problematic. Like a Rosen wire, a bend with a radius of only 1.5 to 2 mm can itself cause spasm or dissection, especially if it enters a segmental artery. It is best not to use glide wires because they can enter the peripheral branches more readily than Teflon-coated wires and can perforate the parenchyma.

Once the catheter and wire lie securely within the renal artery, advance the sheath to within a short distance of the ostium (**Fig. 4.24a**). Then, without changing the position of the wire, replace the catheter with a 4 mm balloon catheter to perform preliminary dilation (**Fig. 4.24b**). Before the sheath is advanced into the renal artery, one must insert the dilator into the sheath in place of the balloon catheter (**Fig. 4.24c**). The dilator allows one to guide the sheath through the stenosis without a significant step-off. Once the sheath lies within the renal artery, the balloon catheter can be reliably advanced into the correct position (**Fig. 4.24d**). Next withdraw the sheath and aspirate blood through the sheath to remove possible plaque material. Then inject a small volume of contrast to verify the correct stent position (**Fig. 4.24e**). Correct the position of the stent if necessary. The stent should project 1 to 2 mm into the aortic lumen.

Then the stent is slowly deployed with the patient holding his or her breath after expiration. It is all right for the patient to feel slight pressure, but stop inflating the balloon immediately if the patient reports any pain.

After removing the balloon catheter, perform angiography via the sheath. Visualize the entire kidney to exclude embolic vascular occlusion and spasm (**Fig. 4.25**). The wire remains in the renal artery during this examination. It ensures the sheath remains centered proximal to the ostium. It also provides an approach for performing any additional procedures that may become necessary, such as redilation with a larger balloon, thrombus aspiration, lysis, or embolization of a bleeding vessel.

Stenosis at a Proximal Bifurcation of the Renal Artery

Occasionally stenosis will occur in a proximal bifurcation of the renal artery at the point where a large branch arises from the artery. Such stenoses can affect both arterial branches. Dilating first one branch then the other risks pushing occluding material from one branch

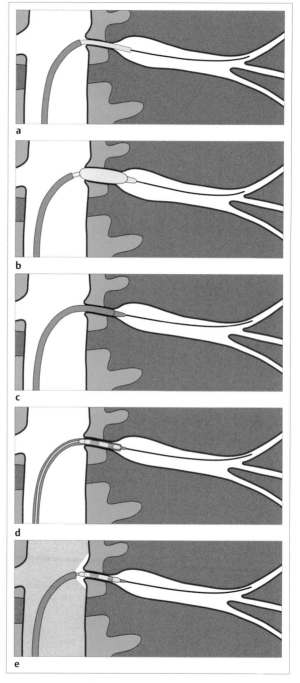

Fig. 4.24 Stent placement.
a Advance sheath up to ostium.
b Introduce balloon catheter; perform preliminary dilation.
c Introduce dilator; advance sheath through stenosis.
d Introduce stent-bearing balloon.
e Withdraw sheath and check position of stent (should project 1 to 2 mm into aortic lumen), correct if necessary.

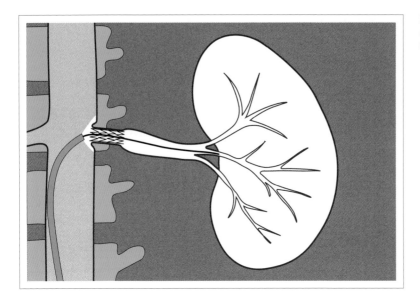

Fig. 4.25 Result is evaluated on angiogram of entire kidney; emboli and spasms are excluded.

into the other. This may make it difficult to pass a wire or catheter through the second branch.

In many cases it may be possible to insert two slender monorail systems side by side. Each catheter can then be advanced into a branch and both can then be simultaneously dilated (**Fig. 4.26**).

Bilateral Stenosis

Often both renal arteries will exhibit stenoses requiring treatment. In the past, operators were advised to refrain from treating both renal arteries in a single session. In light of today's high rates of technical success such misgivings are hardly justified. On the contrary, simultaneous treatment of both sides reduces the risk of injury to the access vessel (the common femoral artery) in which

there continues to be the highest share of complications. However, where kidney function is severely impaired it is probably better to distribute the required volume of contrast agent over two sessions. The general rule is therefore to treat both kidneys in one session in the absence of a higher-grade impairment of kidney function (Henry et al 2008).

Results of Stent Placement

Statistical compilation from studies published since 1995 (Henry et al 2008) reports the following:
- Technical success with 2,803 lesions: 98.5%
- Rate of restenosis: 14.7%; risk of recurrent stenosis is higher in smaller vessels than in large ones
- Effect on blood pressure in 1,245 patients: normalized in 15.5%, improved in 56% (together 71.5%)
- Effect on kidney function in 1,890 patients: improved in 25.3%, stabilized in 53.3%, worsened in 21.4% (the improvement from intervention increases with the severity of renal insufficiency, Sos and Trost 2008).

The complication rate in large series was once ~ 10 to 14%; since the introduction of guiding sheaths and smaller systems (0.014 or 0.018 in. wires, monorail) it is less than 3% (Schillinger and Zeller 2007).

Other Indications

Fibromuscular Dysplasia

FMD is usually observed in younger patients (median age: 33 years). Women account for over 75% of those affected by the disease. In about two thirds of all cases

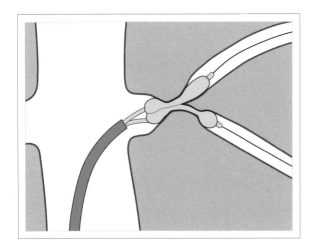

Fig. 4.26 Stenosis at a proximal bifurcation treated with two monorail systems as "kissing balloons."

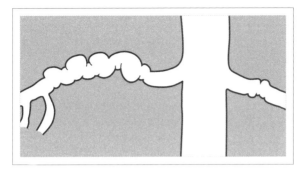

Fig. 4.27 Fibromuscular dysplasia.

FMD occurs bilaterally (also in other vessels such as the carotid, iliac, or leg arteries). The typical angiographic picture of fibromuscular dysplasia is present in ~ 80% of all cases: a sequence of short segments of ectasia alternating with narrow constrictions and resembling a string of pearls (**Fig. 4.27**). Medial hypoplasia and intimal fibroplasia are relatively rare (< 5% of all cases): Findings include long symmetrical stenoses in the middle segment of the renal artery, usually in very young patients.

The small aneurysms in medial fibroplasia are often projected over the stenoses, making it difficult to evaluate the degree of stenosis. For this reason measurement of blood pressure can help to confirm the indication. Often only minor changes are visible after PTA. This means that pressure measurement is the most reliable means of evaluating the success of treatment. On subsequent angiograms one will occasionally see smoothing of the contours with an expanded lumen.

Stents should be used in FMD only in emergencies and never in children. When the vessel grows, the stent can dislodge and migrate into the renal hilum, where it could later prevent a bypass operation.

Transplanted Kidney

Stenosis develops relatively often at the arterial anastomosis in transplanted kidneys. This too is amenable to interventional management. An end-to-side anastomosis of the iliac artery to the transplanted artery is best catheterized via an ipsilateral approach. A contralateral approach is better for an end-to-end anastomosis.

Aneurysms of the Renal Arteries

Aneurysms of the renal arteries are only amenable to interventional management if they are in a readily accessible location. Then they can be eliminated by a covered stent or treated by coil embolization. The risk of rupture is great; therefore, surgical treatment is preferable in many cases.

Visceral Arteries

The three major visceral arteries, the celiac trunk and the superior and inferior mesenteric arteries, are so closely connected that a proximal occlusion of one of the three arteries is invariably compensated for by the other two. It can even occur that occlusions of the two larger arteries are discovered as an incidental finding. The characteristic collaterals are usually visualized on posteroanterior (PA) aortography. They appear as prominent vessels along the head of the pancreas in occlusion of the celiac trunk (common), or as the long arterial arc of Riolan coursing along the transverse and descending colon where one of the mesenteric arteries is occluded (**Fig. 4.28**). The long course of the arterial arc of Riolan always indicates the direction of flow reliably during the course of the angiography series. This provides definitive evidence of where the causative occlusion lies.

The origins of the celiac trunk and the superior mesenteric artery can only be visualized in the normally supine patient using a horizontal-beam, cross-table lateral projection. The great depth of the object being imaged leads to relatively high amounts of scattered radiation. This means that a high degree of collimation is required to achieve acceptable image quality: The anterior margin of the spinal column is the posterior edge of the image. The patient's arms may remain on the table; they are outside the field of view.

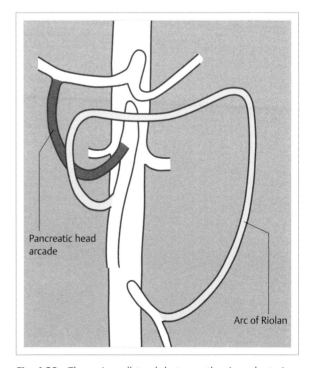

Fig. 4.28 The major collaterals between the visceral arteries (schematic diagram).

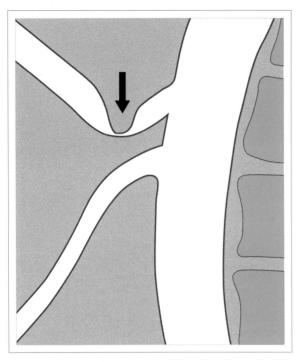

Fig. 4.29 Typical constriction of the celiac trunk by the crura of the diaphragm.

About 40% of all patients exhibit a cranial constriction of the celiac trunk (Glück et al 1983) that can be so pronounced as to produce occlusion (**Fig. 4.29**). This is caused by cranial compression of the arteries by the crura of the diaphragm. When in doubt, this can be confirmed by obtaining a series of images during deep inspiration. This typically alleviates the compression because the viscera are drawn away from the crus of the diaphragm. This finding is usually harmless and of course cannot be influenced by PTA or stent placement.

The condition known as **abdominal angina** (paroxysmal abdominal pain regularly occurring after meals) is in most cases the only indication for an interventional procedure. It is usually due to stenosis or occlusion of the superior mesenteric artery. There has been little experience with PTA and stent placement to date. Recurrences appear to be common. The treatment technique is similar to the one used for renal artery stenosis. The superior mesenteric artery normally arises from the aorta at an acute caudal angle. As a result, vascular access via the left brachial artery is indicated more often than it is for the renal arteries.

Abdominal Aorta and Bifurcation

About one in three cases of **peripheral arterial occlusive disease** occurs in the abdominal aorta and iliac arteries; in patients under 40 years old it is the most common location. The common iliac artery and aortic bifurcation are affected particularly often (typical smoker's disorder!). **Aneurysm** is by far the most common disorder in the abdominal aorta. In a significant number of cases, this disorder too is managed by endovascular intervention with placement of a prosthesis introduced via the inguinal arteries (see Chapter 7, Abdominal Aorta, p. 204).

Stenosis of the Infrarenal Abdominal Aorta

High-grade stenoses affecting only the aorta itself can occur within the abdominal aorta. Interventional management (usually with stent placement) has become the treatment of first choice within the last few years. Technical success rates of 95%, 3% complication rates, and a 5-year secondary patency rate of over 85% have been reported (Gross-Fengels et al 2010). Women between the ages of 30 and 50 years (smokers with hypercholesterolemia) are affected relatively often. Most times the aorta is narrow to begin with, measuring no more than 10 or

12 mm in diameter. Similar changes in a wide aorta do not easily lead to a hemodynamically significant stenosis.

The stenosis in a narrow aorta can be relatively easily dilated with a single balloon or treated with a stent of the appropriate size. Balloon-expandable stents (these are preferable because of their greater radial strength) are supplied ready to use, mounted on balloons in diameters up to 10 mm. Where indicated these stents can be expanded after deployment to 11 or 12 mm with a second balloon. In many cases this achieves sufficient width (**Fig. 4.30**).

For an aorta 13 mm or more in diameter, one can use a Wallstent (Boston Scientific [Natick, MA, USA]; see **Fig. 2.56**). These are available in diameters up 24 mm. However, the shortening that occurs when this stent is deployed can pose a problem if the stent has to be placed close to the bifurcation or immediately distal to the renal arteries. OptiMed (Ettlingen, Germany) supplies nitinol stents for the same purpose. These have a closed cell design that gives them sufficient stability (**Fig. 4.31**). They are less flexible, but this is not a disadvantage in a nearly straight aorta. These stents are available in various diameters between 16 and 34 mm and between 4 and 10 cm long (insertion system is 10 French).

The most important risk in an aortic dilation is the possibility of a **rupture**. This is most likely to occur in

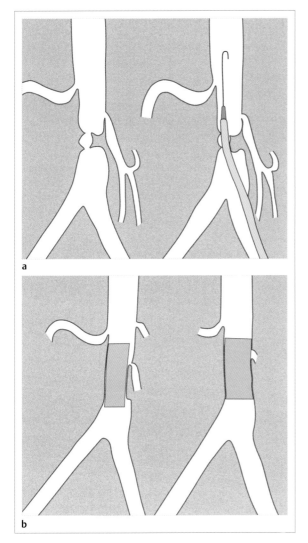

Fig. 4.30 Thirty-eight-year-old woman with bilateral stage IIb claudication and aortic stenosis.
a Sheath in the aortic stenosis.
b After therapy: left, with 10 mm stent in place; right, after dilation with 12 mm.

the presence of circular aortic wall calcifications. Therefore such calcifications must be excluded by CT prior to the intervention. In any case it is important to obtain a reliable measurement of the width of the aorta (with a sizing catheter where possible). The aorta should be dilated very slowly using a manometer (pressure values no higher than 3 to 4 bar), and the patient should be observed closely. Pressure must be reduced immediately if the patient reports any pain. If the pain persists, contact the surgeon and anesthesiologist and schedule a CT examination.

Where a rupture is suspected, it is advisable to keep the catheter in place within the stenosis to be able to tampon the bleeding aorta in an emergency. If this tamponade does not succeed, a latex occlusion balloon of the proper size will have to be placed at the level of the lesion until surgery. Anyone with sufficient experience can treat the leak directly by placing a covered stent (Klonaris and Katsargyris 2008).

Stenosis and Occlusion at the Aortic Bifurcation

In aortic stenosis close to the bifurcation, there is a risk that the balloon will injure the common iliac artery through which it is introduced into the aorta. This risk increases the closer the lesion lies to the bifurcation. Where such injury cannot be reliably excluded, one must treat even an isolated aortic stenosis like the far more common lesions that involve both the aorta and the iliac arteries. In this case a suitable balloon is introduced through each inguinal region and advanced into the bifurcation region. Then the two balloons are inflated simultaneously ("kissing balloons," **Fig. 4.32b**). Where percutaneous transluminal angioplasty has produced unsatisfactory results, this method is used to place two self-expanding stents in the distal abdominal aorta and in the iliac arteries and simultaneously redilate them (**Figs. 4.33** and **4.34**).

Stenoses at the bifurcation invariably involve the risk of the balloon simply pushing occluding material from one side into the other if only one side is dilated (**Fig. 4.35**). Therefore it is generally recommended to introduce a balloon on each side and inflate them simultaneously. The balloons lie within the aorta next to each other or crisscrossed (kissing balloons, **Figs. 4.35** and **4.36**).

Stenoses or occlusions of both common iliac arteries that require treatment are treated simultaneously (i.e., by simultaneous catheterization via the left and right inguinal regions). Where dilation only is planned, a balloon catheter is introduced into each side and advanced into the aorta

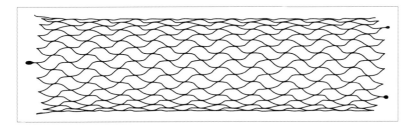

Fig. 4.31 Large-diameter nitinol stent with closed cell design (Sinus stent from OptiMed).

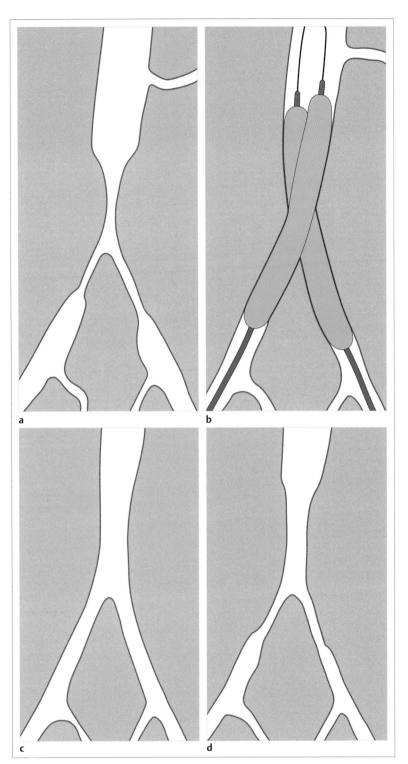

Fig. 4.32 Stenosis of the lower abdominal aorta and both common iliac arteries.
a Initial situation.
b Percutaneous transluminal angioplasty (PTA) with kissing balloons.
c Good result of PTA.
d Unsatisfactory result requiring treatment with stents (**Fig. 4.33**).

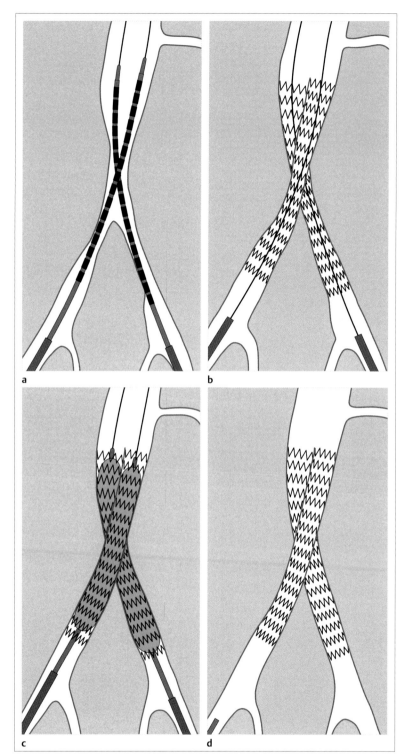

a

b

c

d

Fig. 4.33 Where results of percutaneous transluminal angioplasty are unsatisfactory, stents are placed.
a Placing the stents.
b Stents deployed and expanded; residual stenoses are present.
c Redilation.
d Good result.

Fig. 4.34 Sixty-one-year-old male smoker with stenosis of the aortic bifurcation. ▶
a Initial situation.
b Placement of two nitinol stents.
c Good result.

Fig. 4.35 Unilateral stenosis of the common iliac artery, plaque at the carina. ▶
a Initial situation.
b At the aortic bifurcation, the percutaneous transluminal angioplasty balloon can push plaque material to the contralateral side.
c Therefore simultaneous dilation with two catheters (kissing balloons) is indicated.

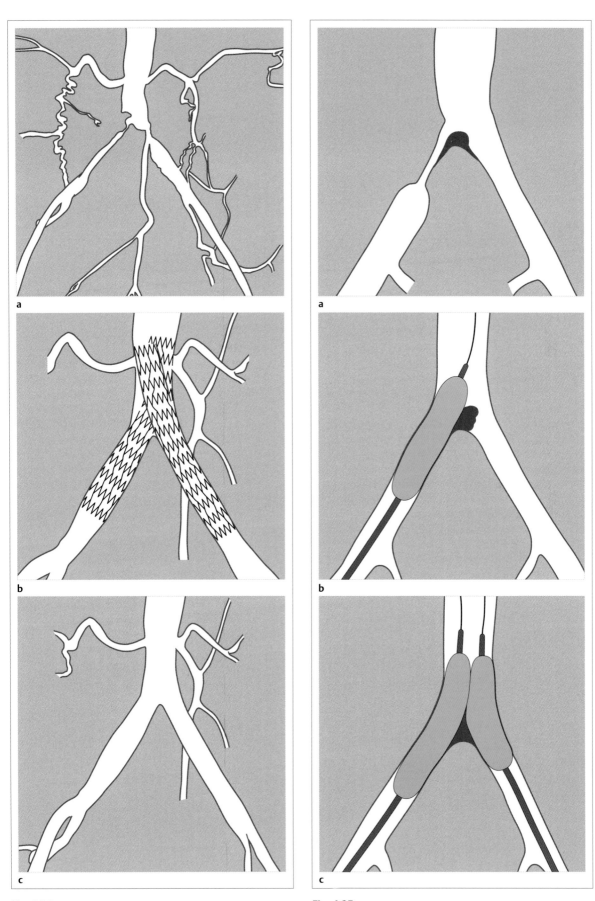

Fig. 4.34

Fig. 4.35

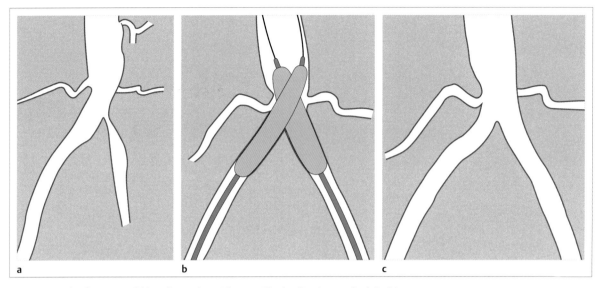

Fig. 4.36 Fifty-four-year-old female smoker with stage IIb claudication on the left side.
a Initial situation.　　　　　　　　**b** Kissing balloons, each 6 mm in diameter.　**c** Good result.

(**Fig. 4.36**). The dilation is then performed by inflating both balloons simultaneously with manometer syringes.

One will opt for **primary stent placement** where one or both common iliac arteries are occluded or the stenoses are severely calcified. For this purpose it is best to advance a sheath (25 or 30 cm long) from each side into the aorta. A balloon-expandable stent of the appropriate length and width is then advanced through each sheath to just above the bifurcation. Then each sheath is backed off the respective stent-bearing balloon (not too little or the balloon and stent will not expand sufficiently; not too much or it will compromise the quality of contrast injection via the sheath).

Next comes the most important phase of treatment: precise **placement of the stent**. The position of the distal ends is best evaluated by injecting contrast via the sheaths. However, the correct position of the proximal ends of the stents is more important. Where stenoses do not dictate treatment of the distal aorta as well, both stents should just touch each other at the bifurcation or project into the aorta at most 2 to 5 mm. This can be estimated sufficiently accurately by observing the visible ends of the stents before they are fully deployed. Mural calcifications in the iliac arteries are often helpful as well. When in doubt, visualize the distal abdominal aorta by injecting contrast through the lumen of one or both balloon catheters (after first withdrawing the wires).

> ⚐ **Important:** Stents that project too far into the aorta will hinder any subsequent crossover catheterization (Roffi and Biamino 2005)!

The position of the two stents relative to each other can be better evaluated when the balloons are inflated at

their proximal and distal ends. However, by this time it is usually no longer possible to correct their position. The balloons should be slowly inflated with two manometer syringes. In the absence of an assistant, one can inflate them a little at a time, alternating between left and right. Tell the patient to immediately report any sensation of pressure or pain (usually in the back).

When selecting the stents, always choose the narrower one when in doubt. If after placing the stent one has the impression that it should be 1 to 2 mm wider, remember that it is possible to redilate a balloon-expandable stent with a larger balloon. Steel stents can be placed with great precision. This is an important advantage at the bifurcation where both iliac arteries are to be stented right up to the bifurcation but any overlapping of the stents has to be avoided (**Figs. 4.37** and **4.38**).

Two stents that lie next to each other in the bifurcation should project far enough into the aorta that they lie against the aortic wall (**Fig. 4.39**).

Fig. 4.37　Placement of two stents at the bifurcation.　▶
a Precise placement of the stent-bearing balloons at the bifurcation.
b Balloons begin to inflate.
c Expanded stent in optimal position.

Fig. 4.38　Sixty-six-year-old male smoker with severely　▶
calcified stenoses of both common iliac arteries.
a Initial situation.
b Placement of two balloon-expandable stents.
c Good result.

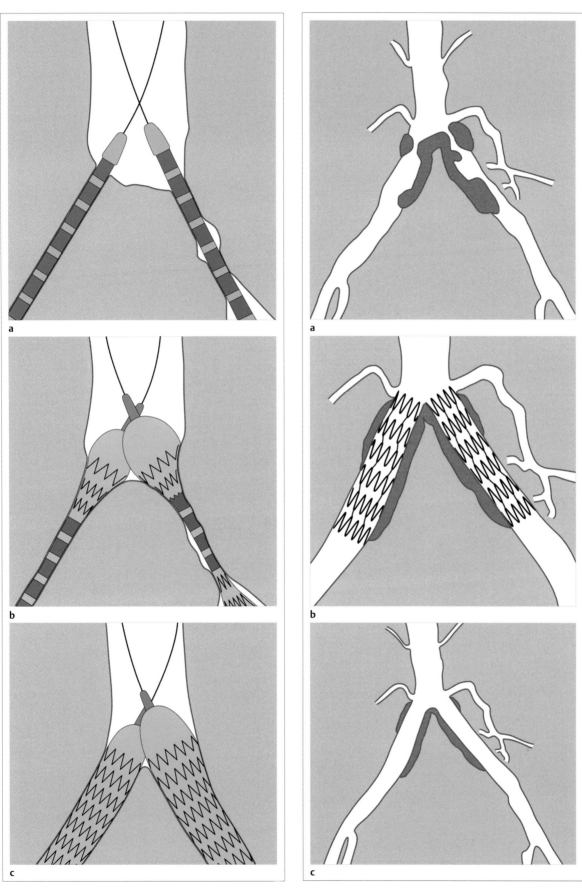

Fig. 4.37

Fig. 4.38

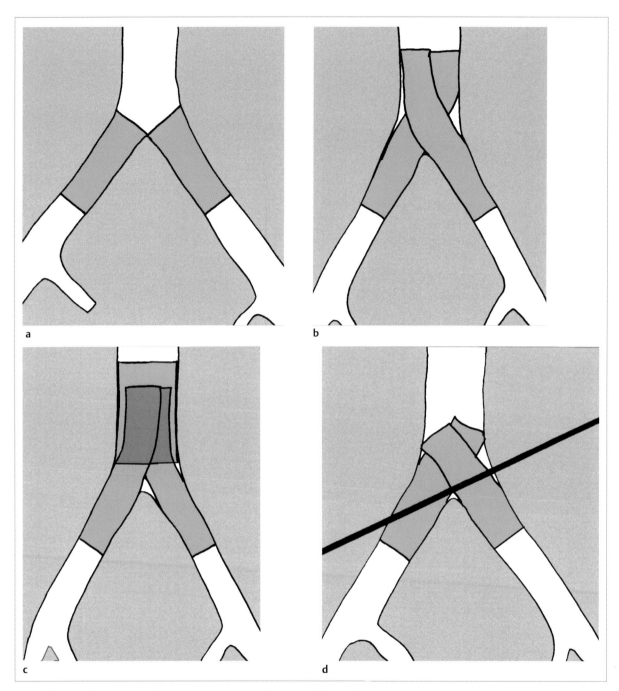

Fig. 4.39 Possible positions of the stents in stenoses of the aortic bifurcation.
a Stents extend precisely to the bifurcation.
b Proximal ends of the stents lie next to each other in the aorta.
c Stents in the aorta and both common iliac arteries.
d Ends of the stents impinge against the aortic wall—not recommended!

Iliac Arteries

The iliac arteries are probably the most intervention-friendly arteries the radiologist will encounter. They are readily accessible and usually wide enough that even stents are well tolerated. Because they are elastic vessels they are less likely to react to intervention with intimal hyperplasia than the arteries of the legs.

Results of interventional therapy. An extensive statistical compilation from 1989, before the advent of stents, showed a technical success rate of 92% and patency rates of 81% after 2 years and 75% after 5 years (Collins and McMullan 2008). However, the long-term results differ starkly (Roffi and Biamino 2005). In another statistical compilation (Bosch and Hunink 1997), the primary patency rate for stenoses after 4 years was ~ 65% (PTA) and 77% (stent). For occlusions it was 54% (PTA) and 61% (stent). In a recent series (Murphy et al 2004), a technical success rate of 98% was achieved; after 8 years the primary patency rate was 74%, the secondary patency rate 84%.

Catheterization

Advancing a wire or catheter into a stenosis or occlusion in the iliac arteries can be more difficult than in the superficial femoral artery because the iliac arteries often course in an arc. The attempt to steer the wire or catheter according to the fluoroscopic image often fails because the image lacks the third dimension; the operator cannot tell whether the vessel deviates anteriorly or posteriorly.

However, the relatively wide vessel is helpful because it often allows the operator to advance a curved glide wire through an unseen curve simply with a few random twists. Even in the case of an occlusion, the residual lumen that thrombosed last is often filled with relatively light thrombi as opposed to the harder plaque along the walls. As a result, it is often enough to "blindly" advance a curved glide wire. With any luck it will glide upward in this soft material without becoming stuck in the plaque, moving either straight ahead or with its tip bent back. Therefore one should always first try a curved glide wire. If this does not succeed, one can occasionally steer a catheter with a bend close to its tip in the direction that road mapping or mural calcification seems to indicate is correct. And in a really tight spot a straight wire can be better than a curved one.

Once the wire courses cranially within the aorta without any resistance, one has reliably passed the occlusion. However, in retrograde catheterization such attempts often steer the wire and catheter into the wall of the iliac artery and then into the aortic wall. When the wire courses in a spiral around the aortic lumen and cannot be advanced without resistance, then it most certainly lies outside the lumen. Then one can attempt to find a way within the lumen using another wire or with the aid of a slightly curved catheter. If this does not succeed, one still has the option of subintimal recanalization. Reentering the aortic lumen may require the use of an Outback catheter (Cordis, Miami, FL, USA) or a similar device (see p. 110, **Fig. 3.107**) because the changes to the intima of the aorta are so great that a wire alone cannot be passed through it (Bolia 2011).

In difficult cases (especially in the presence of a known long occlusion) it can be simpler to introduce a catheter into the lower abdominal aorta from the contralateral side and advance a glide wire (straight or curved) into the occlusion (**Fig. 4.40b**). A catheter of 5 French diameter will suffice (even without a sheath, curvature as in **Fig. 3.36**). Try to center the tip of the catheter at the beginning of the occlusion and attempt to push a straight guidewire into and through it. This will occasionally succeed. One can capture the wire with a snare distal to the occlusion or stenosis, pull it out through the sheath, and use it as a track for advancing a balloon catheter or stent applicator (**Fig. 4.40c**). Should one fail to capture the wire with the snare, then one should try to guide a slender balloon catheter into the occlusion over the wire already in place or over a 0.018 in. wire one has replaced it with. This catheter can be used to try to create a lumen that will be accessible from a distal approach.

In certain exceptional cases, the iliac arteries can also be treated via a **transbrachial** approach (**Fig. 4.40d**, see Chapter 3, Access via the Brachial Artery, p. 65). If only a wire is passed through the occlusion via this approach and the actual intervention is to be performed via the inguinal region, then a 4 or 5 French catheter with a slight bend near its tip will usually suffice. Yet if the entire intervention is to be performed via the brachial artery, then it is recommended to use a long sheath that can be advanced to just short of the bifurcation or even into an iliac artery.

Important: Thrombus deposition can occur on the long sheath. Withdrawing the sheath can then strip it off, allowing it to migrate into the left vertebral artery or the arteries of the arm. Immediate administration of heparin is indicated to address this risk. If the long sheath is not immediately withdrawn after the intervention has been completed, then it should be replaced with a shorter one.

What is most likely to fail is the attempt to pass a guidewire through a stenosis or occlusion of an iliac artery. Once the wire has safely passed the lesion, PTA or stent placement is rarely a problem.

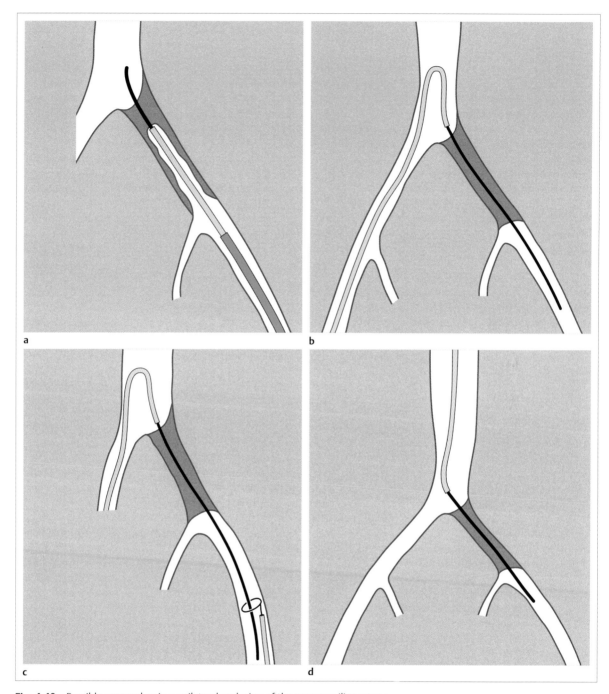

Fig. 4.40 Possible approaches in a unilateral occlusion of the common iliac artery.
a Retrograde catheterization.
b Antegrade catheterization from the contralateral side, preferable in an occlusion extending over a long distance.
c Capturing the wire with a snare distal to the occlusion.
d Transbrachial catheterization.

Contralateral Approach

Stenoses or occlusions of the common iliac artery can be dilated via a contralateral approach, whereas precise placement of a stent is practically impossible. If it is possible to advance a sufficiently stiff wire through the stenosis and far into the arteries of the pelvis or leg (see Chapter 3, Crossover Catheterization, p. 60), then it will usually be possible to advance a balloon catheter into the stenosis as well and then dilate the stenosis.

It is easier to achieve a symmetrical dilation of the ostium if one first creates a loop above the balloon as

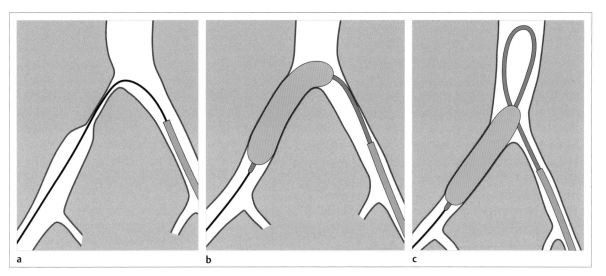

Fig. 4.41 Crossover percutaneous transluminal angioplasty of a stenosis of the common iliac artery: Creating a loop above the balloon allows more precise placement within the stenosis.
a Wire in the stenosis.
b Asymmetrical dilation at the bifurcation.
c Symmetrical dilation with catheter loop in the aorta.

shown in **Fig. 4.41**. Inflate the balloon far enough that it lodges in the stenosis and then advance the catheter into the aorta. It is not recommended to place a stent in a stenosis near the ostium of the common iliac artery from the contralateral side. This is because it is difficult to place the stent perfectly flush with the ostium via this approach (**Fig. 4.42**).

Lesions that are at least 2 to 3 cm distal to the aortic bifurcation can be treated using a crossover sheath advanced across the bifurcation into the affected side. The procedure is discussed in section Crossover Catheterization (p. 60). The self-expanding stents that are usually used in this situation lie protected within the applicator. This eliminates the need to advance the sheath into the stenosis or occlusion.

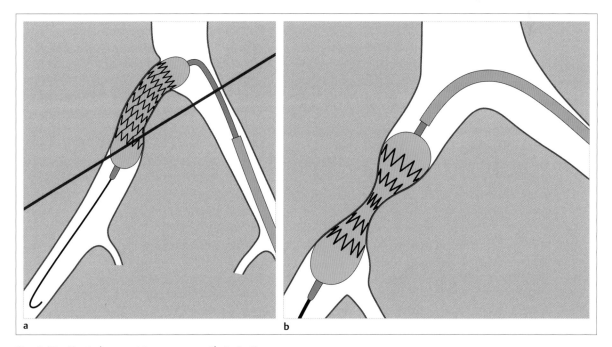

Fig. 4.42 Stent placement in crossover catheterization.
a Precise placement at the ostium of the common iliac artery is practically impossible.
b Further distal placement does not pose a problem.

Percutaneous Transluminal Angioplasty or Stent

The following principles have gained widespread acceptance:

- Where satisfactory results have been achieved with PTA alone (residual stenosis < 20 or 30%), then additional placement of a stent may be dispensed with.
- Significantly better results of recanalization of occlusions are achieved where stents are placed.
- Balloon-expandable stents are used in the treatment of lesions extending to the aortic bifurcation because only

these allow sufficiently reliable placement. They should be introduced via an ipsilateral approach because placement via a contralateral approach is rarely successful.

- Self-expanding stents are more suitable for all other locations because they can better adapt to the course and, in applicable cases, variable caliber of the iliac arteries.
- Lesions in the distal external iliac artery should be treated via a contralateral approach due to their proximity to the common femoral artery.
- When treating an occlusion, many authors feel that prior percutaneous transluminal angioplasty is not necessary if placement of a stent is planned.

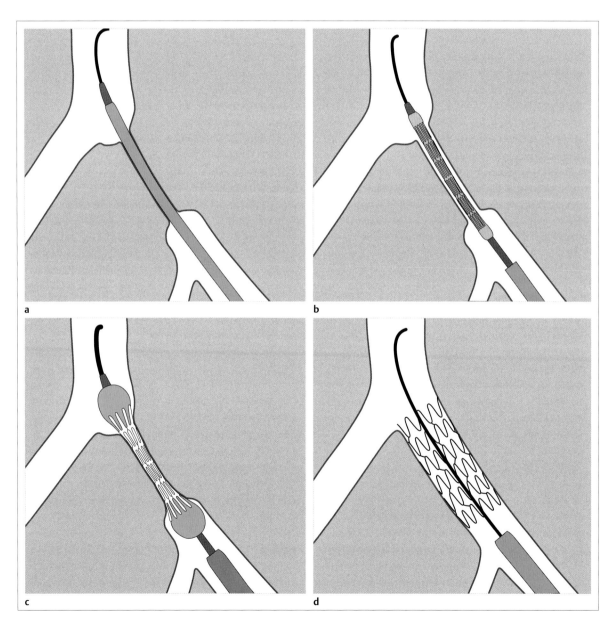

Fig. 4.43 Treatment of an occlusion of the common iliac artery with a balloon-expandable stent.
a Advancing a wire and sheath through the occlusion.
b Advance balloon catheter into correct position with sheath, then withdraw sheath.
c Inflate balloon.
d Remove balloon and evaluate result by angiography.

A possible rupture in an iliac artery is significantly more dangerous than in an artery of the leg. It is best avoided by precisely matching the balloon catheter to the **measured width of the vessel**. Additionally, the patient must understand that pain can occur and that this should be reported to the physician immediately. The patient should be observed closely as the pressure in the balloon is slowly increased. If the patient reports any sensation of pressure or pain one should immediately reduce the pressure and wait to see if the pain subsides. Persistent pain contraindicates further dilation: Keep the balloon in place and observe the patient!

Balloon-Expandable Stents

Primary stent placement is recommended for recanalizing occlusions of the iliac arteries. One reason for this is that potentially mobile thrombi may lie within the occluded segment; placement of a stent largely prevents them from entering the bloodstream. To facilitate placement of a balloon-expandable stent, a sheath at least 25 cm long is advanced into the aorta. The diameter of the sheath is one size larger than that required for the stent. This makes it significantly easier to inject the contrast agent needed to verify the position of the stent. The instruments and equipment are described in detail in Chapter 3, Stent Placement (p. 93).

Advance the stent within the sheath to the desired position or a bit further. Later it will be easier to withdraw it than advance it. Bone contours, road mapping, or an overlay may be used for orientation. Once the stent has reached the proper position (**Fig. 4.43**), the sheath is withdrawn far enough to expose the stent and balloon within the occluded lumen. The sheath must no longer cover the rear (proximal) end of the balloon either. Otherwise only the distal end of the balloon will expand when inflated, which could push the stent off the balloon. One can now verify the position of the stent again if necessary by injecting contrast through the sheath. Any necessary corrections to the position can be made as long as the balloon and stent have not been deployed.

Now slowly inflate the balloon with the aid of a manometer syringe to deploy the stent. Observe the procedure on fluoroscopy so that any errors can be immediately corrected. Once the balloon is fully inflated, the stent will disconnect from it. The balloon can then be deflated and withdrawn through the sheath (**Fig. 4.43d**). The wire remains in the stent for now. This will make it easier for one to introduce a larger balloon for redilation should this become necessary. Despite this precaution, a second balloon advanced to the site can still become caught on the stent. Usually it will be possible to separate the balloon from the stent by withdrawing the balloon while carefully rotating it.

Now one performs angiography via the sheath to evaluate results (inject the contrast close to the stent). Where residual stenosis is present or the stent is not fully in contact with the vessel wall one can introduce a suitable balloon catheter over the wire and redilate (see Chapter 3, **Fig. 3.87**, p. 96).

Self-Expanding Stents

Balloon-expandable stents should be used in the immediate vicinity of the bifurcation. Self-expanding stents are more suitable for all other locations because they can better adapt to the course and, in applicable cases, variable caliber of the iliac arteries. They are supplied on application systems in which they lie on an inner catheter covered by a thin-walled outer catheter. Once they have been introduced through a sheath and brought into the correct position, the outer catheter is withdrawn to deploy the stent (**Fig. 4.44**).

> **Important:** In this maneuver the inner catheter must not be moved and the outer catheter must not be immobilized (see also Chapter 3, Self-Expanding Stents, p. 93)!

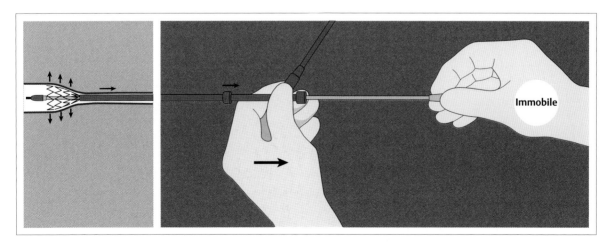

Immobile

Fig. 4.44 Deploying a self-expanding stent.

Most self-expanding stents can adapt very well to the curvature and variable caliber of the iliac arteries. This especially applies to stents with open cells and a modular design. Although such a stent does not shorten significantly when deployed, the vessel's curvature and the fact that its course is oblique to the imaging plane can make precise measurement of the required length difficult. In difficult cases it can be helpful to use a sizing catheter or a wire with markings.

The diameter of the fully deployed stent should always be 1 to 2 mm larger than the vessel in which it is placed. Otherwise it would not be in complete contact with the vessel wall and could be dislodged from its position. Subsequently inflating a balloon cannot expand a nitinol stent any further. For this reason it is not possible to use balloon dilation to fix in place a stent that has insufficient contact with the wall. On the other hand, the stent itself does not usually have the strength required to expand

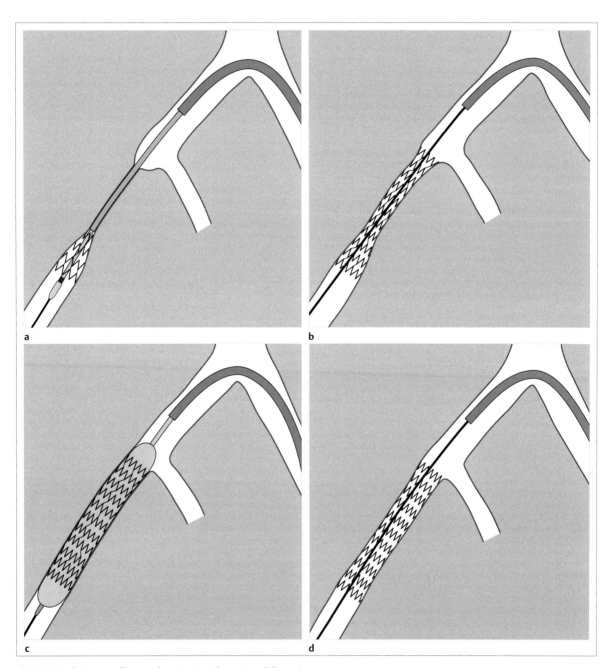

Fig. 4.45 Placing a self-expanding stent in the external iliac artery.
a Introducing and deploying the stent via a sheath.
b Deploying the stent.
c Redilate where indicated.
d Final result.

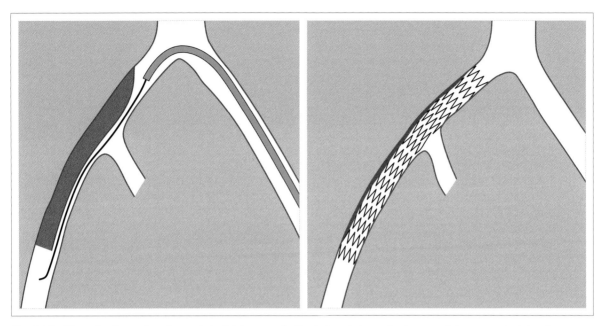

Fig. 4.46 Dissection from wire advanced via distal approach. Stent placed via proximal approach (crossover technique).

a stenosed segment of a vessel to the desired diameter. Therefore the stenoses must normally be redilated with a balloon catheter after a stent has been placed (**Fig. 4.45c**).

Nitinol stents do not show up very well on radiographs. Therefore it is recommended, especially in the iliac arteries, to use only stents with markings of gold, platinum, or tantalum on both ends. Where the length of the lesion or the varying caliber of the artery necessitates placing several stents in succession, they should overlap by at least 5 mm.

Wallstents (Boston Scientific) can be an interesting alternative to the nitinol stents used in most cases. Wallstents have greater radial strength, and their fine mesh structure covers the vessel wall particularly well. However, they have the disadvantage of shortening significantly when they are deployed. They also adapt less readily to variations in vessel caliber. This is because the elastic steel wires that make up the stent are continuous from one end to the other and are fixed to each other at any crossing.

Iatrogenic Dissection

A dissection of the iliac arteries requiring treatment is in many cases iatrogenic. In the attempt to advance a guidewire in retrograde fashion the wire becomes stuck on a piece of plaque and is diverted beneath the intima. If this is not noticed immediately, a catheter may be subsequently advanced through the dissection. In most cases such a dissection closes spontaneously. However, where bleeding occurs into the injury and thrombus develops within it, the result can be a stenosis extending over a considerable distance.

In this case, the true lumen is more easily catheterized from a proximal approach (**Fig. 4.46**). Once the guidewire lies safely within the true lumen next to the dissection, the true lumen can be recanalized with a self-expanding stent. The stent expands from distal to proximal, initially sealing the end of the dissection and preventing the thrombus material from being pressed into the lumen.

Peculiarities of the External Iliac Artery

The ipsilateral approach to the external iliac artery is simplest, provided the injury is far enough away from the common femoral artery. In far distal injuries, contralateral access (crossover catheterization, see Chapter 3, Crossover Catheterization, p. 60) is preferable and in some cases indicated.

The most important differences between the external iliac and common iliac arteries for the intervention are as follows:
- The external iliac artery is more mobile.
- Its course is often tortuous.
- Dilation of the artery can very easily lead to dissection.

Simple stenoses are treated by PTA (**Fig. 4.47**). Very careful measurement of the vessel diameter (rarely > 6 mm) is advisable due to the danger of dissection. If dissection occurs, repeat the PTA with low pressure (2 bar, intermittently) for 10 to 15 minutes with the intent of tacking down the intimal flap. If this does not succeed and a dissection that impedes blood flow remains, place a stent (a self-expanding stent due to the vessel's mobility and curvature).

Yet, where the stenosis will not have any significant hemodynamic effect, it is best to accept an initially suboptimal result without a stent: The intimal flap will often be completely absorbed over time and within a few months one will have a perfect result without a stent.

A stent in the external iliac artery should never extend past the junction with the common femoral artery for the following reasons (**Fig. 4.48**):
- The common femoral artery is mobile.
- Lesions of the common femoral artery are easily accessible by surgery.
- A stent will interfere with both subsequent surgery and subsequent interventional access.

Where the external iliac artery is severely elongated, stent placement must be adapted to the curves in the vessel. This is important because a stent (even a "flexible" one) severely alters the elasticity of the vessel wall. A stent that ends at the crest of a curve can cause kinking with a resulting high-grade stenosis that can only be eliminated by placing a second overlapping stent (**Fig. 4.49**). For this reason the stent should be short and should be placed only in a relatively straight segment wherever possible, or it should bridge the entire curve.

Occasionally a severely elongated external iliac artery will kink, producing a stenosis with a significant hemodynamic effect (**Fig. 4.50**). Naturally, such a situation cannot be influenced by PTA. All that will help here is a very flexible stent that symmetrically bridges the curve or surgery.

A membrane stenosis is another rare finding in the external iliac artery (**Fig. 4.51**). These lesions are usually very elastic and can be treated only with a stent.

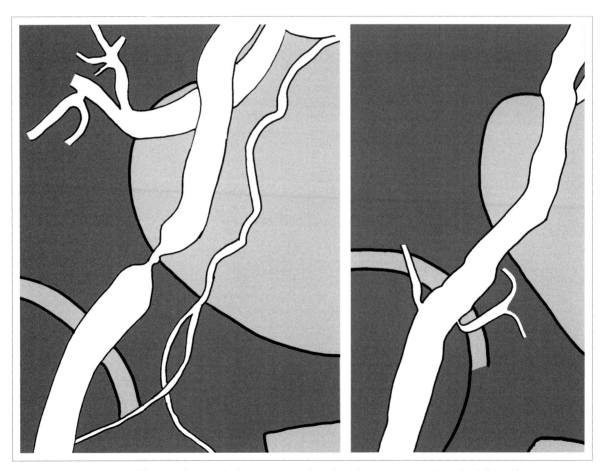

Fig. 4.47 Sixty-one-year-old man with stage IIb claudication on the right side: Crossover angiography followed by percutaneous transluminal angioplasty with dilation to 6 mm in same session eliminated symptoms.

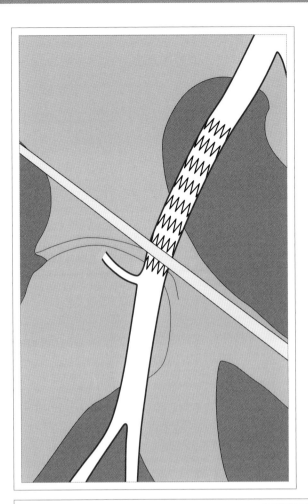

Fig. 4.48 A stent in the external iliac artery should stop short of the common femoral artery.

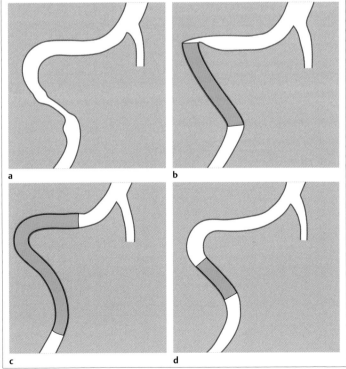

Fig. 4.49 Stenosis in the elongated external iliac artery.
a Stenosis in a severely elongated external iliac artery.
b An improperly placed stent can induce kinking and stenosis.
c The kink can be eliminated by placing a second, longer stent that splints the entire curve.
d A better alternative is to initially place a short stent.

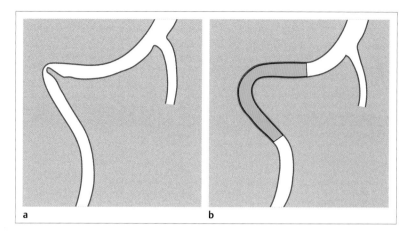

Fig. 4.50 Kinking and stenosis of the external iliac artery treated with a flexible stent.

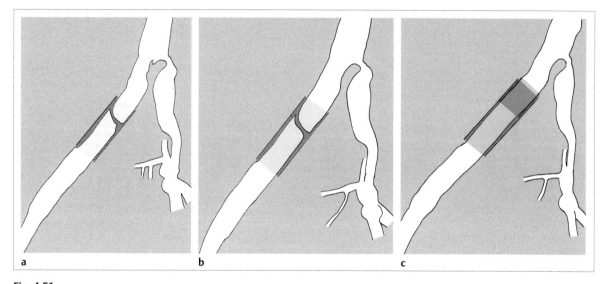

Fig. 4.51
a Membranous stenosis within a stent severely impairs the flow of blood into a newly created femoropopliteal bypass.

b Findings remain unchanged after percutaneous transluminal angioplasty.
c Short stent eliminates the stenosis.

Aneurysms of the Iliac Arteries

Some aneurysms in the iliac arteries represent an immediate extension of an aneurysm of the abdominal aorta. In such cases, the iliac artery aneurysm is treated in conjunction with the abdominal aortic aneurysm. In the case of endovascular management this involves extending the limb of the prosthesis.

The same type of aneurysm also occurs where the aorta is of normal width. The feasibility and type of endoprosthetic treatment are then determined by whether there is a neck proximal to the aneurysm where an endoprosthesis limited to the iliac artery can be connected. Treatment of

a **pseudoaneurysm** with a covered stent that seals the entrance to the aneurysm can be relatively simple (**Fig. 4.52**).

Eliminating an **aneurysm of the internal iliac artery** is much more challenging on the other hand, because here all arterial feeders must be embolized to preclude the risk of rupture (**Fig. 4.53**). The challenging part is to locate the feeders with the catheter where they drain into the aneurysmal sac. These arterial feeders are usually embolized with coils.

If it is long enough, the trunk of the internal iliac artery can also be embolized with coils or, a more elegant

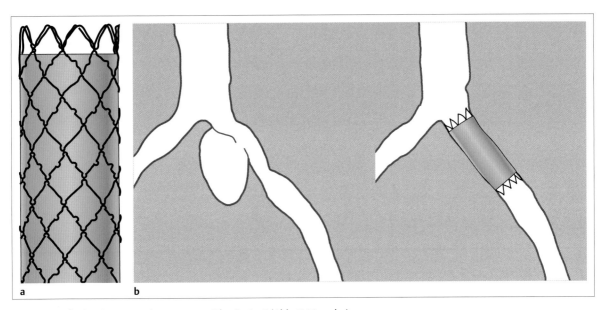

Fig. 4.52 Eliminating a pseudoaneurysm with a Jostent (Abbott Vascular).
a Dacron membrane between two balloon-expandable stents.   **b** Stent covers the mouth of the aneurysm.

solution, sealed with an occluder like the Amplatzer (St. Jude Medical, St. Paul, MN, USA). Where the trunk is very short, a covered stent is placed proximal to its ostium. The actual extent of these aneurysms cannot be evaluated by angiography alone if they are partially thrombosed. The preparation for the intervention must include computed tomography. Probably the most common lesions are anastomosis aneurysms after placement of an aortoiliac prosthesis. (For a detailed discussion of iliac artery aneurysms, see Uflacker [2008].)

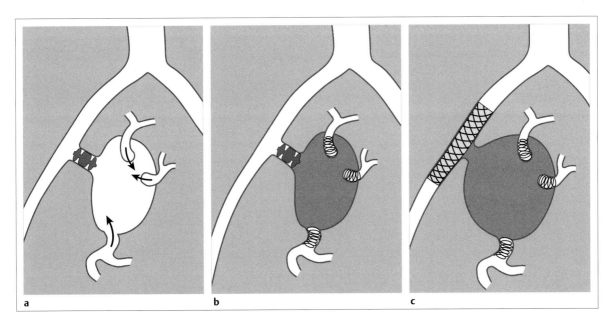

Fig. 4.53 Treatment of an aneurysm of the internal iliac artery depends on the length of the aneurysm neck. Occlusion of the branches arising from the aneurysm is crucial!
a Occluding the vascular trunk alone is not sufficient. Coil embolization of all branches of the internal iliac artery is necessary.
b Long neck: occlusion of the trunk with an Amplatzer occluder.
c Short neck: covered stent placed over ostium of the internal iliac artery

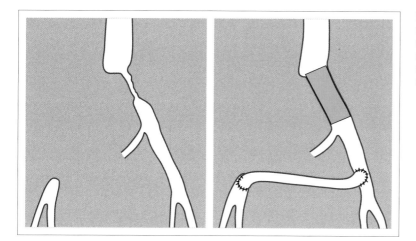

Fig. 4.54 Chronic occlusion of the right iliac arteries and stenosis of the left common iliac artery. The stenosis of the common iliac artery is managed with a stent; a transverse bypass is created to ensure arterial supply to the right leg.

Combination with a Surgical Intervention

Iliac artery occlusions that cannot be reliably recanalized by interventional means naturally represent an indication for surgery. This generally involves placement of an aortoiliac or an aortobifemoral prosthesis. In a unilateral occlusion there is also the option of a unilateral aortofemoral bypass. This can follow an extraperitoneal course, causing the patient fewer problems than an aortobifemoral prosthesis.

However, one will often encounter the situation where, in a patient who is a poor candidate for surgery, interventional recanalization of the iliac artery is successful on one side but fails on the other. Then it is important to restore the one side as well as possible so that from there the other side can also be supplied via a **transverse bypass**, a well tolerated procedure (**Fig. 4.54**).

References

Bolia A. The Bolia Technique. Munich: CIRSE; 2011

Bosch JL, Hunink MG. Meta-analysis of the results of percutaneous transluminal angioplasty and stent placement for aortoiliac occlusive disease. Radiology 1997;204(1):87–96

Collins T, McMullan PW Jr. Percutaneous transluminal angioplasty. In: Heuser R, Henry M, eds. Textbook of Peripheral Vascular Interventions. 2nd ed. London: Informa UK; 2008:39–44

Criado FJ. Techniques of renal artery intervention. In: Criado FJ, ed. Endovascular Intervention: Basic Concepts and Techniques. Armonk, NY: Futura; 1999:93–104

Glück E, Gerhardt P, Schröder J. Value of vascular morphology for the selection of catheters in selective celiacography and mesentericography [in German]. Rofo 1983;138(6):664–669

Gross-Fengels W, Wagenhofer K, Siemens P, Daum H. PTA und Stentversorgung von isolierten atherosklerotischen Stenosen der infrarenalen Aorta abdominalis. Berlin: Deutscher Röntgenkongress; 2010

Henry M, Henry I, Polydorou A, Polydorou A, Hugel H. Endovascular treatment of a renal artery stenosis: techniques, indications, and results. In: Heuser R, Henry M, eds. Textbook of Peripheral Vascular Interventions. 2nd ed. London: Informa UK; 2008:502–524

Klonaris C, Katsargyris A. Endovascular treatment of abdominal aortic occlusive disease. In: Heuser R, Henry M. Textbook of Peripheral Vascular Interventions. 2nd ed. London: Informa UK; 2008:467–472

Lenz T. Diagnostik renovaskulärer Veränderungen—Indikationen für revaskularisierende Verfahren. Berlin: Deutscher Röntgenkongress; 2010

Murphy TP, Ariaratnam NS, Carney WI Jr, et al. Aortoiliac insufficiency: long-term experience with stent placement for treatment. Radiology 2004;231(1):243–249

Patel VI, Conrad MF, Kwolek CJ, LaMuraglia GM, Chung TK, Cambria RP. Renal artery revascularization: outcomes stratified by indication for intervention. J Vasc Surg 2009;49(6): 1480–1489

Roffi M, Biamino G. Aortic, iliac and common femoral interventions. In: Casserly IP, Sachar R, Yadav JS, eds. Manual of Peripheral Vascular Intervention. Philadelphia, PA: Lippincott Williams & Wilkins; 2005:214–228

Sapoval M, Zähringer M, Pattynama P, et al. Low-profile stent system for treatment of atherosclerotic renal artery stenosis: the GREAT trial. J Vasc Interv Radiol 2005;16(9):1195–1202

Schillinger M, Zeller TH. Complications in renal and mesenteric vascular interventions. In: Schillinger M, Milnar E, eds. Complications in Peripheral Vascular Interventions. London: Informa UK; 2007:159–176

Sos TA, Trost DW. Renal angioplasty and stenting. In: Kandarpa K, ed. Peripheral Vascular Interventions. Philadelphia, PA: Lippincott Williams & Wilkins; 2008:287–314

Subramanian R, White CJ, Rosenfield K, et al. Renal fractional flow reserve: a hemodynamic evaluation of moderate renal artery stenoses. Catheter Cardiovasc Interv 2005;64(4): 480–486

Uflacker R. Interventions in iliac artery aneurysms. In: Kandarpa K, ed. Peripheral Vascular Interventions. Philadelphia: Lippincott Williams & Wilkins; 2008:341–364

5 Lower Extremities

Common Femoral Artery

Problems in the common femoral artery are treated primarily by surgery. The vessel courses superficially and is readily accessible. Surgery may be performed under local anesthesia if necessary. The often large eccentric plaques in the common femoral artery are poorly manageable by percutaneous transluminal angioplasty (PTA). Placement of a stent is contraindicated due to the motion in the groin and because a stent would prevent the use of the vessel for arterial access in any future endovascular procedures.

Superficial Femoral Artery

Anatomy and Indication for Treatment

The superficial femoral artery is an unusual vessel in many respects.

- It usually has only a few insignificant branches or none at all over a long distance. This means that a short stenosis can lead to thrombotic occlusion of the entire vessel (**Fig. 5.1**).
- Its distal segment is subject to mechanical stresses in the adductor canal. This may be why it is the peripheral artery most often affected by stenosis or occlusion (**Fig. 5.2**).
- Parallel to the superficial femoral artery there is the large deep femoral artery. In many cases this artery has such strong connections to the superficial femoral and popliteal arteries that it can fully assume the function of an occluded superficial femoral artery. If this succeeds it is the most reliable long-term resolution of claudication. One of the most important diagnostic tasks is to avoid missing a correctable stenosis at the origin of the deep femoral artery (**Fig. 5.3**).
- On the other hand in every intervention one must take care not to compromise the junction of the deep femoral artery collaterals with the superficial femoral artery. Correct evaluation of these collaterals can determine whether intervention in the superficial femoral artery is indicated. Yet there are certainly cases in which PTA in the superficial femoral artery helps to buy time until the deep femoral artery collaterals are fully developed (**Fig. 5.4a, b**).
- Stenoses distal to the junction of the deep femoral artery collaterals are of special importance. In contrast to stenoses located farther proximally, they cannot be compensated by the collaterals (**Fig. 5.4c**).

Long-Term Results

More than half of all cases of peripheral arterial occlusive disease involve the superficial femoral or popliteal artery.

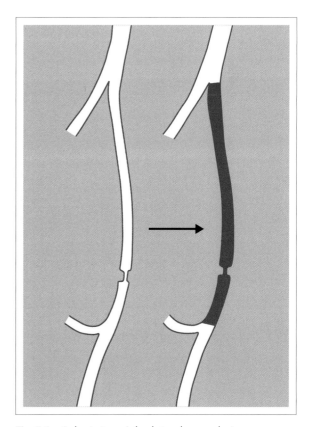

Fig. 5.1 A short stenosis leads to a long occlusion.

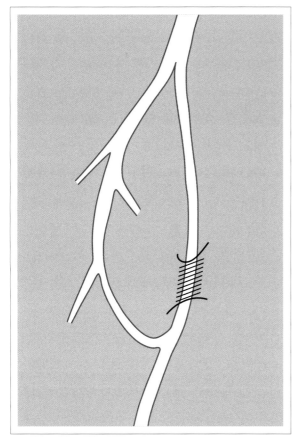

Fig. 5.2 Critical region of the adductor canal.

In spite of all the advances in interventional technique, the long-term results achieved with the venous bypass have been better than those of endovascular treatment. The results reported in the literature vary greatly. For example, a prospective study published in 2001 reported primary patency rates post-PTA of 87% after 1 year, 80% after 2 years, and 55% after 4 to 5 years (Clark et al 2001), whereas some authors observed primary patency rates of only 33 to 45% after 12 months (Dake 2011). Nevertheless, endovascular therapy remains the therapy of first choice for most cases. There are several reasons for this:

- The bypass operation represents a significantly more invasive procedure with higher mortality and associated risks, for example, those associated with harvesting the venous graft.
- Suitable veins are not always available and may also be required for coronary bypasses.
- Endovascular treatments can be repeated and do not exclude a subsequent bypass.

Approach

The most direct, quickest, and simplest approach to the leg arteries is the antegrade approach via the common femoral artery (see also Chapter 3, Antegrade Puncture of the Common Femoral Artery, p. 52). This applies to 80 to 90% of all cases. Even direct antegrade catheterization of the superficial femoral artery distal to the femoral bifurcation is an option in rare cases where the superficial femoral artery is wide enough. This may be the case in the presence of a high bifurcation of the common femoral artery or an abdomen that extends far caudally if crossover catheterization appears difficult or is unsuccessful. Obesity, a high bifurcation of the common femoral artery, or iliac arteries that also require treatment will necessitate crossover catheterization in 10 to 20% of cases (see Chapter 3, Crossover Catheterization, p. 60). The approach via the brachial artery (see Chapter 3, Access via the Brachial Artery, p. 65) or, very rarely, the popliteal artery is only occasionally required.

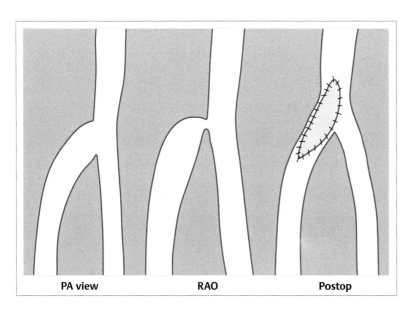

| PA view | RAO | Postop |

Fig. 5.3 Stenosis at the origin of the deep femoral artery, visualized only on an ipsilateral oblique projection (center). Posteroanterior view (left). Treatment by patch reconstruction (right).

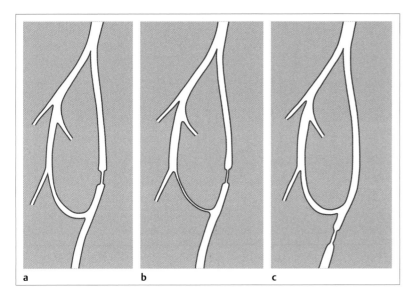

Fig. 5.4 Significance of deep femoral artery collaterals in stenosis of the superficial femoral artery.
a Superficial femoral artery stenosis compensated.
b Not compensated.
c Cannot be compensated.

Interventional radiologists will hardly question the use of an ipsilateral antegrade approach to the arteries of the leg as standard practice. However, some cardiologists who also perform peripheral interventions declare crossover catheterization to be the normal approach. They also find reasons to make this sound plausible:

1. The compression of the groin can lead to reduced flow and when applied on the treated side could increase the risk of an acute thrombotic recurrence of the occlusion. This objection is not consistent with everyday experience, and it does not apply when the access site is treated with a vascular closure system.
2. Stenoses of the superficial femoral artery close to its origin are easier to treat via a crossover approach. That is correct. However, these usually do not pose any real problem even with an antegrade approach (see later discussion).

Cardiologists' preference for crossover catheterization is understandable when one considers that cardiological interventions use only retrograde catheterization. In this setting the crossover approach naturally provides an opportunity to address stenosis in a leg artery as well.

There are several reasons why crossover catheterization should not be the technique normally used:

- It takes longer and requires significantly more material.
- The length of the approach through the iliac arteries renders manipulation difficult and limits one's options (e.g., thrombus aspiration, see Chapter 3, Aspiration of Thrombus, p. 105).
- A catheter bent at the bifurcation cannot be rotated around its longitudinal axis without resistance like an extended catheter can. In the bent segment of the catheter, the rotation causes internal deformation of the material. This consumes energy and is associated with resistance against the rotation (Schröder 1992).

- Unjustified irritation of the iliac arteries is associated with the risk of cholesterol embolization. This risk may be slight, but in most cases it is avoidable.

Performing the Procedure (Stenosis)

First select an appropriate sheath according to the following criteria:

1. Which instruments will be needed (guidewire, balloon catheter, stent)? When in doubt, check what is in stock.
2. Will it be possible to inject contrast through the sheath next to the balloon catheter?
3. How does one want to close the access site at the end of the intervention?

The decision is easy when you have already opted for a vascular closure system. Then select the sheath that fits the vascular closure system, for example, 6 French for Angio-Seal (St. Jude Medical, St. Paul, MN, USA). In this case one can use a 5 French PTA catheter and still inject contrast through the sheath for road mapping and angiographic monitoring. If it becomes necessary to introduce a stent one will not have to replace the sheath to do so.

Slender systems should be preferred where the access site is to be closed by external compression. Over the wire or monorail catheters that can be introduced over an 0.018 in. wire through a 4 French sheath are now available in all sizes commonly used in the superficial femoral artery. They are a good solution for all cases in which no difficulty in passing the wire or catheter is anticipated. In most catheters the shaft is so slender that it is also possible to inject contrast next to it.

Where one has the choice of 9, 10, or 11 cm lengths, one should always choose 11 cm for an antegrade procedure.

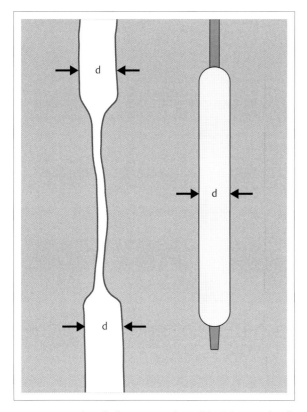

Fig. 5.5 Matching balloon size to the width of the vessel and length of the stenosis.

Then there will be less of a chance of the sheath slipping into the deep femoral artery from the superficial femoral artery when one changes the wire or catheter.

- Perform angiography down to and including the arteries of the lower leg.
- Administer a bolus of 5,000 IU of unfractionated heparin intra-arterially or intravenously. In small and very slender patients it may be advisable to reduce the dose to 3,500 or 4,000 IU. Do not administer heparin to patients with heparin-induced thrombocytopenia (HIT)!
- Measure the vessel diameter and the length of the stenosis.
- Select the appropriate balloon catheter: The diameter of the balloon should match the diameter of the vessel; the balloon should be 1 to 2 cm longer than the stenosis (**Fig. 5.5**).
- Place a wire in the flushed catheter and lock it within the catheter with the stopcock (**Fig. 5.6**): The wire should project out of the tip of the catheter ~2 mm to facilitate introducing it into the sheath.
- After introducing it into the sheath, advance the wire 1 to 2 cm further and again lock it (**Fig. 5.7**); advance the wire and catheter to within a short distance of the stenosis.
- Perform road mapping via the sheath.
- Introduce the wire and catheter into the stenosis under fluoroscopy (**Fig. 5.8**); remove the wire and flush the catheter and sheath with heparinized saline solution (flush intermittently during the entire treatment!).

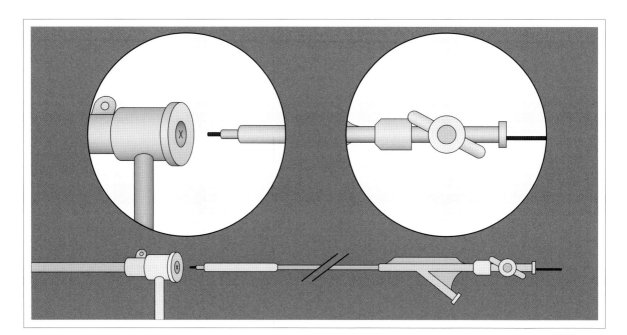

Fig. 5.6 Wire locked in place by stopcock.

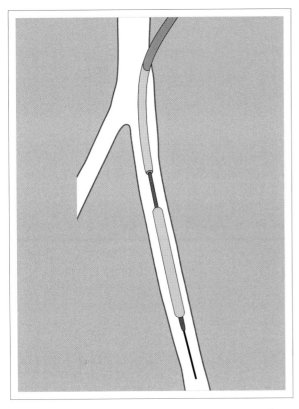

Fig. 5.7 Once the balloon catheter has passed through the sheath, the wire is advanced ~2 cm.

- Connect a manometer syringe (with contrast agent with 300 mg of iodine per mL, diluted 1:1) to the lumen of the balloon; slowly inflate the balloon under repeated fluoroscopic control (**Fig. 5.9**); slowly expanding the vessel reduces the risk of gross dissection.
- Increase pressure to 6 to 8 bar over a period of 30 to 60 seconds.

Why increase the pressure slowly?

If one wants to tear tissue, it is best done with a sharp tug. But if one wants to expand it, one must increase the tension slowly and steadily. This gives the fibers in the tissue time to rearrange themselves in response to the tension.

Dilating twice for 1.5 minutes is better than once for 3 minutes. This is because dilation creates a dead space proximal and distal to the balloon where the blood stagnates and can coagulate (**Fig. 5.10**).

If the balloon tends to slip out of the stenosis, advance it far enough in that it tends to slip out distally. Then keep tension on the catheter.

Some observations suggest that deformation and compression of the plaque material also contribute to the effect of PTA (Losordo et al 1992). For one thing, this would mean that moisture is being expressed. That is a process that takes time.

Anyone with the patience to try to improve the results of PTA with longer and repeated dilation using the same balloon and the same pressure can observe repeatedly

Fig. 5.8 Advancing a wire and balloon catheter through a stenosis.

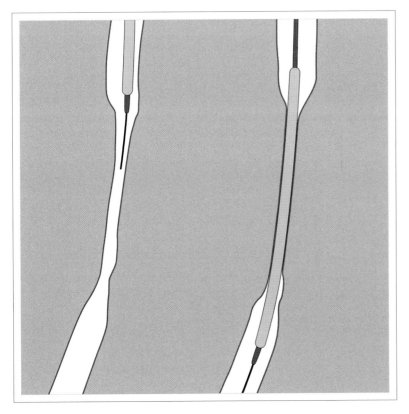

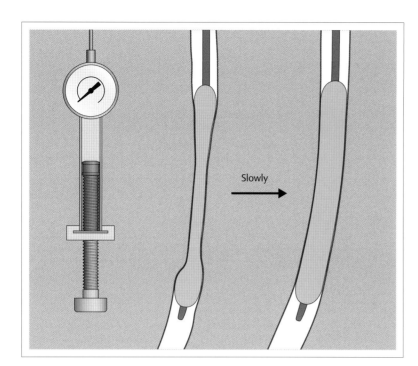

Fig. 5.9 Slow, controlled dilation.

Slowly

that this does indeed improve the results. Therefore, as a matter of course, it is best to dilate for longer than ~30 seconds. This spares all those patients requiring a second dilation unnecessary contrast administration. Moreover it spares them a second catheterization of the stenosis with the slight additional risk of dissection or thrombus mobilization (in the early days of PTA the watchword was "do not reenter!").

And cost-effectiveness is hardly the only reason why it is better to achieve a good result before having to switch to a larger balloon. Dilating for a little longer invests maybe an additional 3 minutes in the decisive phase of the treatment, which is hardly noticeable compared with the length of the procedure as a whole. Yet, to do so increases the probability of achieving good results and minimizes the risks.

- Maintain pressure for 1.5 minutes; flush the catheter. Compare the balloon diameter to the vessel diameter (road mapping), then deflate the balloon.
- When reinflating the balloon, observe whether it expands completely at low pressure (1 to 2 bar).
- Perform a second dilation at 6 to 8 bar over a period of 1.5 minutes.

Then the balloon catheter is withdrawn and results are evaluated by angiography performed via the catheter. Injecting contrast via the catheter will provide better image quality with the same amount of contrast agent.

Good results (residual stenosis <20%): Monitor lower leg arteries then finish intervention.

Residual stenosis >20%: Repeat PTA at a higher pressure (such as 14 bar) using a balloon with compliance, or repeat the dilation with a larger balloon (possibly a shorter balloon adapted to the length of the residual stenosis). Longer duration of PTA (5 to 15 minutes) will often help in the case of an irregular and calcified residual stenosis.

Another solution is to place a stent. Gross dissections that interfere with the flow of blood and residual stenoses >30% that do not respond to treatment justify placement of a self-expanding stent. Wherever possible the stent should be no longer than the lesion itself.

Caution: Only self-expanding stents should be used in the superficial femoral artery. Balloon-expandable stents can be permanently deformed by external pressure! Leg movement also causes changes in the length of the superficial femoral artery that only a self-expanding stent can adapt to.

Discussion of Catheterization Technique

The suggestion of introducing the balloon catheter with a straight wire in the very first step of the procedure deviates from the customary routine. Most authors recommend first advancing a straight or curved 0.035 in. glide wire or 0.018 in. guidewire with a hydrophilic tip (also straight or slightly curved). The wire should be fed through a diagnostic catheter (straight or slightly curved) with a Tuohy-Borst adapter at its proximal end (see **Fig. 2.45**). The adapter seals the catheter lumen against

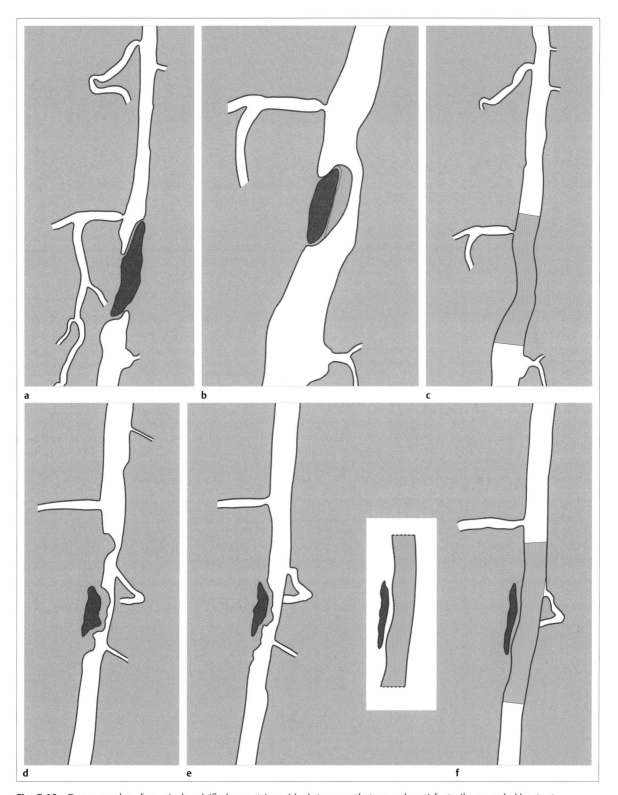

Fig. 5.10 Two examples of massively calcified eccentric residual stenoses that are only satisfactorily expanded by stent placement.
a Subtotal occlusion, massive calcification.
b Eccentric residual stenosis after percutaneous transluminal angioplasty (PTA).
c Good expansion with nitinol stent.
d Severely calcified eccentric stenosis.
e PTA fails to bring decisive improvement.
f Good result with nitinol stent.

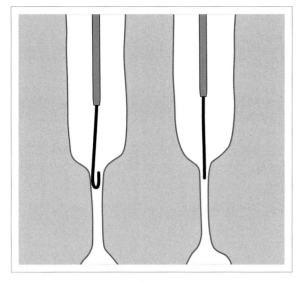

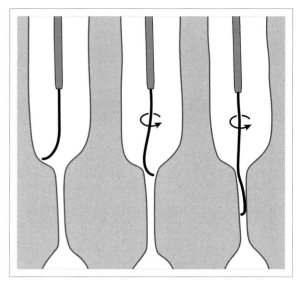

Fig. 5.11 Advancing through a concentric stenosis (left: curved wire; right: straight wire).

Fig. 5.12 Advancing a slightly curved wire.

the wire and at the same time allows contrast injections. These facilitate orientation by visualizing the current position of the wire and catheter. The balloon catheter is introduced only when the wire and diagnostic catheter have been successfully advanced through the stenosis.

My experience has shown that it is just as easy to advance a balloon catheter through the lesion as a straight or curved diagnostic catheter. The straight wire is in most cases clearly superior to the curved wire. It can better negotiate narrow stenoses than a curved wire, the tip of which usually becomes stuck at the beginning of the stenosis and then causes the wire to form a loop (**Figs. 5.11** and **Fig. 5.12**). For an eccentric stenosis one can give the wire a slight bend ~2 to 3 cm from its tip; this enables one to guide the otherwise straight tip of the

wire into the opening of the stenosis using road mapping (**Fig. 5.13**).

Occasionally one will encounter a very irregular stenosis through which the remaining lumen describes an irregular zigzag course. The lumen may contain dead ends that are only visualized on a different projection. It is practically impossible to formulate helpful general recommendations for catheterizing such stenoses. One can attempt to follow the lumen visualized by road mapping using a glide wire with a sharp bend immediately (2 mm) behind its tip (**Fig. 5.14**). If this is unsuccessful, you can best negotiate the stenosis by inflating the balloon to center the catheter within the lumen and then advancing the wire with the stiff end through the occlusion (**Fig. 5.14**).

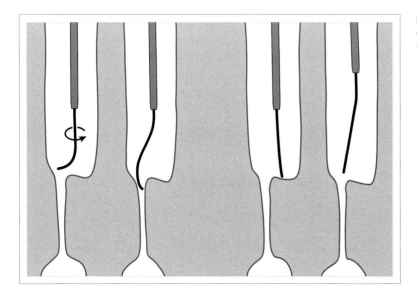

Fig. 5.13 Advancing through an eccentric stenosis (left: curved wire; right: straight wire).

Stenoses that are longer than the available balloon are dilated incrementally in overlapping segments from distal to proximal (**Fig. 5.15**). PTA with a balloon of sufficient length is quicker and better.

Very Narrow and Hard Stenosis

Occasionally a stenosis will be so narrow and rigid that a 5 French catheter cannot be advanced through it (**Fig. 5.16**). In this case leave the catheter in place and introduce an 0.018 in. wire. Over this wire advance a 3 or 3.5 French catheter into the stenosis.

This technique invariably works, and not only because of the smaller diameter of the balloon catheter. The 0.018 in. wire is also ~4 times as stiff as a normal 0.035 in. glide wire (see Chapter 2, Guidewires, p. 8).

Short Stenosis in a Superficial Femoral Artery with a Long, Narrow Segment

The risk of a superficial femoral artery measuring only **2 to 3 mm in diameter** becoming occluded over its entire length following PTA is relatively great (**Fig. 5.17**). This may change stage IIb disease to stage III, an indication for a femoropopliteal bypass. The excessively narrow recipient vessel could cause occlusion of the bypass, in turn causing the patient to lose the lower leg, unquestionably a very poor outcome.

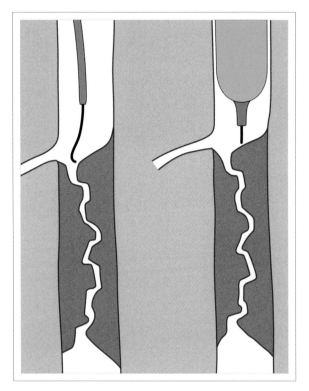

Fig. 5.14 Advancing a wire through a complicated stenosis is occasionally easier with the hard end of the wire centered in the lumen by the balloon catheter (right).

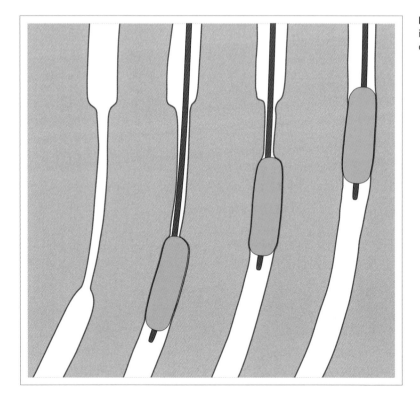

Fig. 5.15 Dilation with a short balloon in successive overlapping segments from distal to proximal.

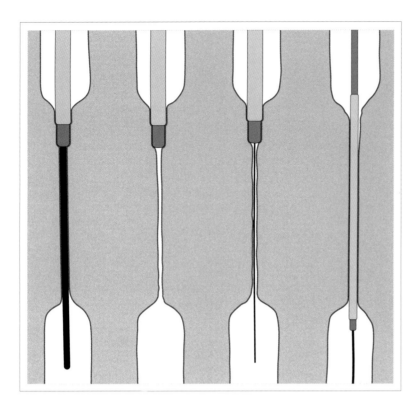

Fig. 5.16 Passing a wire through a very hard, narrow stenosis. From left to right: 0.035 in. wire and 5 French catheter, 0.018 in. wire, 3.5 French catheter.

Therefore, in the absence of pain at rest or peripheral emboli that would dictate active intervention, conservative management with gait training and supportive medical therapy is probably the better alternative. Convincing the patient of this will often require some effort. However, one will thus avoid a serious risk while giving collaterals from the deep femoral artery the chance to become strong enough that the symptoms finally disappear.

The indication is entirely different where a vessel with a **diameter of at least 4 mm** is present. Here the risk of an acute occlusion is significantly less and early elimination of the stenosis can prevent the imminent occlusion of a long segment of the superficial femoral artery (**Fig. 5.17**).

Blue Toe Syndrome

Thrombi can develop downstream of a stenosis or unstable plaque, become mobile, and occlude peripheral arteries as emboli. When this occurs, the patient presents with painful blue discoloration of sudden onset. This relatively rare clinical picture can be quickly eliminated by dilating the causative stenosis. In the case of an unstable plaque (note ultrasound findings), one may consider placing a covered stent. However, the search for the causative lesion can be difficult. When the toes of both feet are affected, one may expect to find the source of the embolism proximal to the aortic bifurcation.

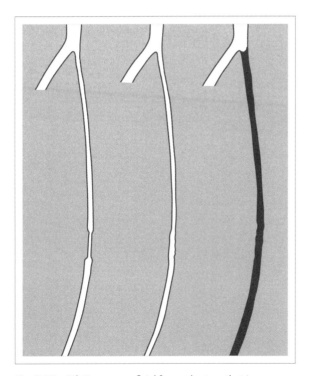

Fig. 5.17 Dilating a superficial femoral artery that is very narrow over a long distance can lead to occlusion.

Stenoses at the Origin of the Superficial Femoral Artery

PTA of a stenosis at the origin of the superficial femoral artery is difficult to perform via an antegrade approach due to the proximity of the access site in the common femoral artery. For this reason most authors use cross-over catheterization as a matter of course when treating the superficial femoral artery. The problem is that one must reliably avoid pulling the sheath out of the vessel and, more importantly, dilating the opening in the vessel wall as well. The solution is precision work guided by road mapping (**Figs. 5.18** and **5.19**).

Perform road mapping via the sheath using an ipsilateral oblique projection to visualize the femoral artery bifurcation.
- Inflate the balloon with low pressure and draw it up to the sheath.

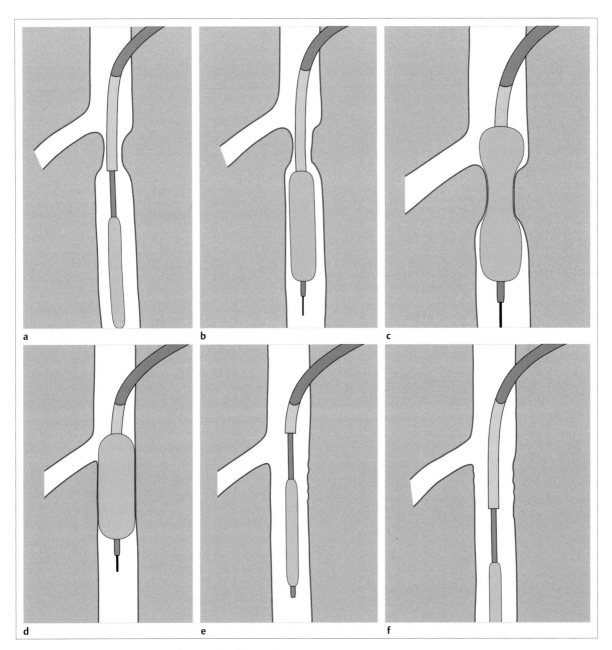

Fig. 5.18 Stenosis at the origin of the superficial femoral artery.
a Road mapping.
b Withdraw balloon back to sheath.
c Pull balloon into stenosis.
d Dilate.
e Angiography.
f Advance sheath.

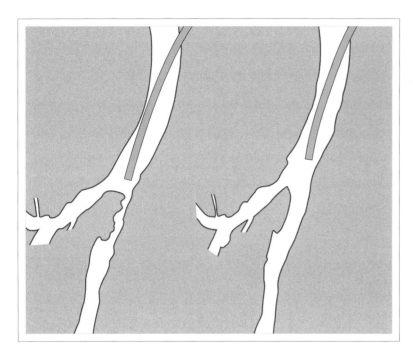

Fig. 5.19 Stenosis at the origin of the superficial femoral artery; 94-year-old woman with stage IV disease and erysipelas. Result of PTA (*left*).

- Withdraw the balloon and sheath under fluoroscopy (road mapping) until the balloon lies within the stenosis (yet with the sheath still in the vessel).
- Perform PTA (dilation).
- Deflate the balloon and push it away from the entrance to the sheath; perform angiography via the sheath to evaluate results.
- Advance sheath and catheter together until the sheath again lies securely within the superficial femoral artery.

Occlusions of the Superficial Femoral Artery

As to the question of how occluded segments of the superficial femoral artery should be catheterized, the literature provides a wide variety of opinions, some of them very imprecise. The most common recommendation is to use a wire with a hydrophilic coating, usually with a curved tip, guided by a straight or curved catheter.

It may be possible to maneuver a slightly curved wire tip first through the stenoses, now no longer visible, that have caused the occlusion. This requires the use of a torqueable wire like a 0.035 in. glide wire or an 0.018 in. steel wire with hydrophilic coating on its tip. More probably, the tip of the wire will usually become stuck proximal to the stenosis and a u-shaped bend must then be forced through the stenosis, or the wire will deviate from the lumen and enter the wall. A curved catheter makes it easier to correct the direction of the wire yet it also makes it difficult to advance the catheter in a straight line.

Catheterization Recommendations in the Literature

Most authors recommend initially advancing a **straight or curved glide wire** that is guided and steered by a catheter with a slight curve near its tip through an occluded segment (**Figs. 5.20** and **5.21**). Other authors reject the 0.035 in. glide wire in favor of an **0.018 in. wire with hydrophilic coating on its tip**, to which many of them give a slight bend.

The **"snowplow" technique**, advancing a van Andel catheter (Cook Medical, Bloomington, IN, USA) (straight, relatively stiff, tapered near the tip) from which projects the curvature of a Rosen wire (stiff steel wire, 1.5 mm radius of curvature), is somewhat similar to the technique the author suggests below. However, the disadvantage is that the curvature of a standard steel wire glides significantly less easily than the tip of a glide wire and certainly is more likely to deviate from the center of the vessel. These methods most often fail because the wire deviates into the vessel wall within the occluded segment. When advanced further, it usually spirals around the occluded lumen as the resistance increases (**Fig. 5.22**).

Correcting the direction of advance with the curved catheter can be difficult. This is because the occlusion obscures vision and because only right and left deviations are detectable, not anterior or posterior deviations.

Alternative Catheterization Technique

The superficial femoral artery courses for the most part in a straight line. If it is no longer possible to bypass impediments in an occluded segment, then it is safest

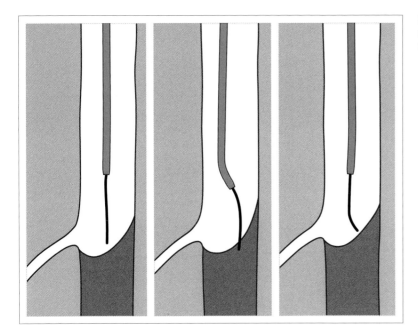

Fig. 5.20 Various combinations of wire and catheter for advancing through an occlusion.

to negotiate the occlusion by remaining in the center of the vascular lumen and advancing in a straight line. This means using a straight wire and straight catheter. It is best not to bypass local impediments. A relatively stiff catheter is preferable. The soft tip of the wire is kept in the center. It will be less likely to deviate into the wall if it projects only a few millimeters from the catheter. If one uses the balloon catheter for this initial step instead of the curved catheter, then one will already have a straight and relatively stiff system of catheter and wire that will tend to remain along the axis of the vessel (**Figs. 5.23** and **5.24**).

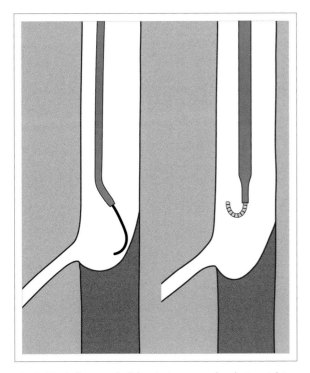

Fig. 5.21 Left: curved glide wire in a curved catheter; right: "snowplow" technique.

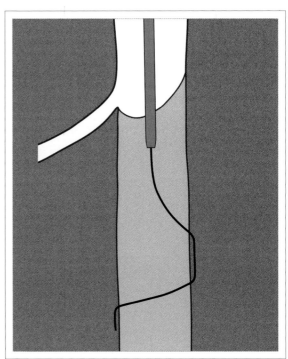

Fig. 5.22 Wire in subintimal space.

The author's experience has shown that the simplest and probably best instrument for catheterizing an occlusion of the superficial femoral artery is this system: an over the wire balloon catheter combined with a straight wire with hydrophilic coating. The two are securely connected together by a stopcock.

This simple stabilization of the system in the center of the vessel is at least a good compromise, and probably the optimal solution for routine clinical use:

- Very quick
- Involves minimal expense
- Yields good results

The balloon catheter also offers the option of recentering the system in the vascular lumen when it appears to be deviating from it. One should use the hard

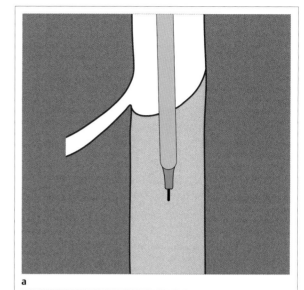

a

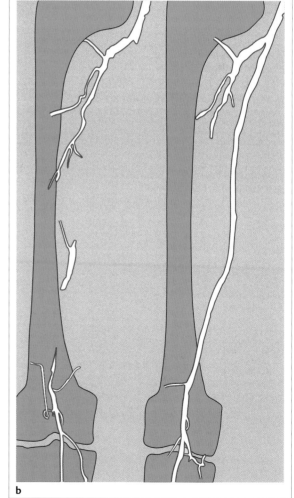

b

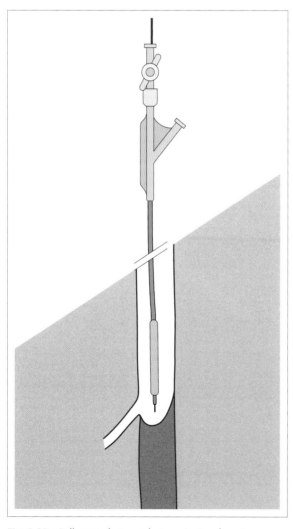

Fig. 5.23 Balloon catheter and wire prior to advancing through an occlusion. The wire is locked within the catheter with a half-closed stopcock.

Fig. 5.24 Advancing a straight wire and balloon catheter.
a Wire and balloon catheter are advanced into the occlusion together.
b Example of a long occlusion recanalized by percutaneous transluminal angioplasty (83-year-old woman with stage IV peripheral arterial occlusive disease).

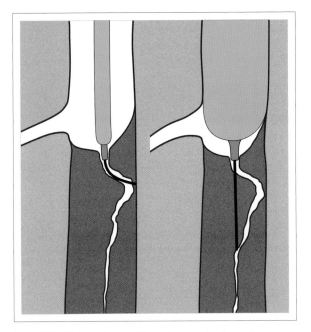

Fig. 5.25 If the soft end of the wire deviates from the center of the vessel (left), use the hard end and center the wire and catheter with the balloon.

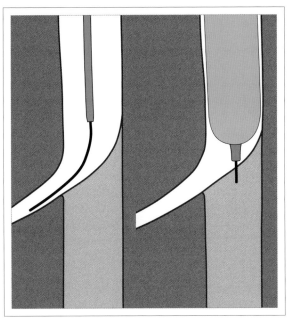

Fig. 5.26 Stiff end of wire centered by balloon prevents deviation into branch artery (or false lumen).

end of the wire if one encounters too much resistance and the tip of the wire deviates (Sharafuddin et al 2010). If necessary one can advance this hard end a short distance by itself after having inflated the balloon to optimally center and immobilize the system (**Fig. 5.25**).

One can proceed in the same manner where the wire deviates into a branch artery or into the wall at the very beginning of the occlusion. The same applies where one has already created a false lumen with the catheter into which the wire and catheter continually deviate (**Fig. 5.26**). In such cases, inflate the balloon, center the wire with it, and then force the stiff end of the wire through the impediment.

While advancing through an occlusion, the system deviates into the wall (Figs. 5.27 and 5.28):
- Withdraw wire and catheter until both are again straight and presumably lie in the center of the vessel.
- Carefully inflate the balloon to shift the catheter lumen into the center of the vessel.
- Advance the stiff end of the wire, deflate the balloon, and advance it after the wire.
- Reinflate the balloon, again advance the wire, and so on, and continue to move forward in small steps until the end of the occlusion is reached.

Successful catheterization. When the wire and catheter have passed through the occlusion, the wire will glide forward along the course of the vessel without resistance. When in doubt, remove the wire and inject contrast through the catheter: If the contrast agent flows away rapidly, the catheter lies within the lumen of the vessel.

Short Occlusion (~1 to 5 cm)
Short occlusions can usually be reliably catheterized. Where PTA has produced unsatisfactory results, a stent may be indicated: The often calcified wall is usually so hard that the stent cannot further impair its elasticity.

Long Occlusion (5 to 20 cm)
Passing a wire and catheter through a long occlusion is often difficult. Once this has been done successfully, satisfactory to good results can regularly be achieved with PTA alone or with PTA and stent placement.

We are now able to recanalize even long occlusions of the superficial femoral artery. Where patency cannot be restored within the physiologic lumen, there is always the option of subintimal recanalization. The prognosis is essentially determined by the quality of the peripheral drainage and the length of the recanalized segment. The better the outflow and the shorter the treated occlusion, the better the prognosis.

Recurrent stenosis due to intimal hyperplasia is a major problem after stent placement but also after simple PTA. Recent studies indicate that local application of a cytostatic agent (paclitaxel) will become an effective means of

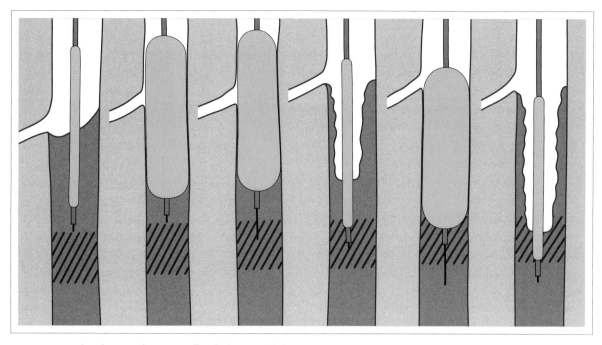

Fig. 5.27   Hard occlusion: advancing stiff end of wire and balloon catheter incrementally.

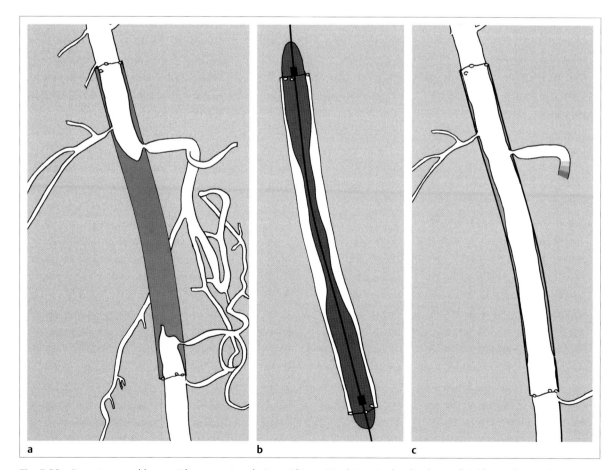

Fig. 5.28   Seventy-year-old man with recurrent occlusion within a nitinol stent in the distal superficial femoral artery 2 years postoperatively.

a Initial findings. Very hard occluding material. Instruments advanced as in **Fig. 5.27**

b Early phase of dilation. Fig. 5.28

c Result after four 2-minute dilations at 14 bar maximum.

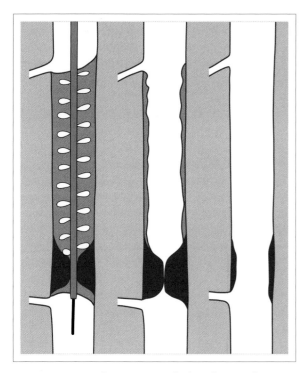

Fig. 5.29 Primary lysis in a primarily thrombotic occlusion (left: lysis; center: result of lysis; right: after percutaneous transluminal angioplasty).

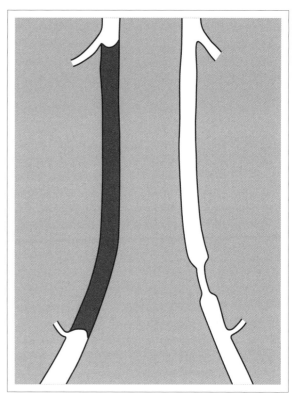

Fig. 5.30 This constellation of findings suggests that an isolated stenosis is the cause of the occlusion on the right side.

controlling intimal hyperplasia. The cytostatic agent can be applied to the surface of the PTA balloon or used as a coating on stents that are then pressed against the vessel wall. Close monitoring of the patient during aftercare is also of paramount importance so that recurrent stenoses can be detected and treated before they lead to occlusion of the vessel.

The superficial femoral artery gives off only a few minor branches in its long segment between the groin and the adductor canal. Therefore even a very short occlusion can lead to acute thrombosis along this entire segment. The appropriate therapy in such a case would be local lysis followed by PTA or stent placement (**Fig. 5.29**, see also Chapter 3, Local Thrombolysis, p. 97; Tran 1998). However, this is rarely done in practice for several reasons. This particular type of occlusion is often not recognized in time, and local lysis itself would require several hours to perform.

The following criteria suggest a primarily **thrombotic occlusion:**
- Wire and catheter pass through it easily.
- The vessel is wide.
- Collaterals are poorly developed.
- The lumen of the corresponding segment of the contralateral artery is largely patent (**Fig. 5.30**). (Arterio-

sclerotic changes are often distributed symmetrically in the peripheral arteries.)

When Is a Stent Indicated?

The prognosis for a residual stenosis of no more than 20 to 30% will usually be no worse if a stent is not placed. Intimal flaps that lie within the flow of blood but do not obstruct it often disappear spontaneously. The unfavorable experience with early model stents in the superficial femoral artery is no longer applicable to the newer, vastly improved designs in current use. Some trials (Schillinger et al 2007, Laird et al 2012) demonstrated better results of femoropopliteal lesions treated with primary nitinol stent implantation compared with balloon angioplasty alone at 2 and 3 years after treatment. Partly in contrast Nguyen et al (2011) found that stenting resulted in long-term outcomes equivalent to those with balloon angioplasty when stratified by indications. The overall 5-year primary patency was 41% for stenting and 36% for balloon angioplasty. However, primary patency was significantly higher at 5 years after stenting of TASC II C and D lesions (34% vs 12%).

Self-expanding stents should be used in the thigh as a matter of course. Wherever possible they should not be significantly longer than the residual stenosis. The longer the stent, the greater the risk of recurrent stenosis and occlusion.

Optimally matching the stent diameter to the diameter of the vessel (1 mm greater than the measured vessel diameter) is also thought to play an important role. A stent that is too wide will be subject to permanent compression within the artery. This can lead to material fatigue and stent fracture. Stretching the stent when it is deployed has an equally detrimental effect. A stent in the superficial femoral artery is stretched and compressed by the motion of the leg. If it was already stretched when deployed, these deformations will be more likely to exceed its load limit (Bosiers 2010).

Whenever possible stents should end before the first popliteal segment. This is the most important recipient segment for a femoropopliteal bypass. An anastomosis is no longer possible with a stent in place. Exception: a femoropopliteal bypass to the first popliteal segment can be safely ruled out. The use of covered stents or stent prostheses is very problematic in an area where important collaterals can join or arise from the artery.

Recent experience with stents coated with the cytostatic agent paclitaxel have led to a complete reevaluation of stent placement in the superficial femoral artery. The patency rates achieved with this treatment are clearly superior to those of bare stents and also to the results achieved with PTA alone. Another contributing factor is presumably the fact that the risk of stent fracture, a possible cause of recurrent occlusion, is significantly less with newer products.

Subintimal Recanalization, Excimer Laser, and Atherectomy

These three options are discussed as fully fledged methods of recanalization in Subintimal Recanalization, Atherectomy, and Excimer Laser (from p. 109 on). Subintimal recanalization is by far the most important of these three methods. This is due in part to the fact that it is largely free of complications and can be performed anywhere without any additional expense.

Simultaneous Treatment of Pathology in the Arteries of the Lower Leg

More than a few patients not only have stenoses or occlusions of the superficial femoral artery but also problems in the popliteal artery and arteries of the lower leg. Since the advent of reliable methods of treating the arteries of the lower leg as well, the prevailing view has been that hemodynamically significant lesions should be treated even if current symptoms appear to be adequately addressed by treatment limited to the superficial femoral artery. Improving peripheral drainage also improves the long-term results of treatment of the superficial femoral artery.

DeRubertis et al (2007) state in their survey of the treatment of the leg arteries that 46.2% of all interventions involved two levels and a further 14.9% three levels. Goodney et al and Egorova et al see the fact that endovascular procedures are used earlier and are often combined with interventions at other levels (pelvis and lower leg) as the main reason for a 25 to 38% reduction in amputation rates over a 10-year period (Egorova et al 2010, Goodney et al 2009).

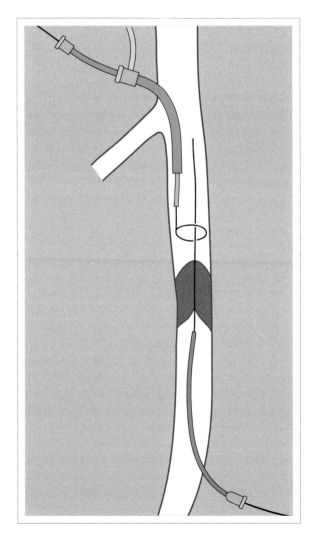

Fig. 5.31 Retrograde catheterization of the popliteal artery, pull-through technique.

Completing the Intervention

Unless renal insufficiency dictates the extremely sparing use of contrast, we finish up the intervention with **angiography**. This examination documents the results of treatment and always includes the arteries of the lower leg to exclude a peripheral embolus. In the presence of renal insufficiency, a duplex ultrasound scan is preferable to angiography.

If it has not already been done in an earlier phase of the procedure, the **position of the sheath** in the common femoral artery is visualized angiographically (lateral oblique projection, short forceful injection through the sheath, high image frequency because the contrast only flows back briefly to proximal of the access site). This angiogram is used to determine whether a vascular closure system can be used.

Most closure systems require a vascular lumen 4 or 5 mm in diameter. They should not be used in the presence of calcified plaques on the anterior wall of the common femoral artery. Angio-Seal (St. Jude Medical) or Perclose (Abbott Vascular, Temecula, CA, USA) may not be placed in the immediate vicinity of the origin of the deep femoral artery.

Access via the Popliteal Artery

Retrograde catheterization of the superficial femoral artery via the popliteal artery primarily comes into consideration where proximal catheterization of an occlusion of the superficial femoral artery is not feasible.

Usually this is preceded by antegrade catheterization via the common femoral artery. Cover the inguinal region with a sterile drape and position the patient prone. Prep and drape the popliteal fossa for the puncture.

Then the popliteal artery (collimated view) is visualized using road mapping by contrast injection through the sheath in the inguinal region. Administer local anesthesia! It is usually easy to perform the puncture with road mapping. To minimize the size of the access wound in the popliteal artery, introduce only a 4 French catheter without a sheath. Then attempt to advance a straight 0.035 in. glide wire into the occlusion. Once this wire has passed through the occlusion, together with the catheter if possible, cover the popliteal fossa with a sterile drape and carefully reposition the patient supine. Taking care to maintain sterility, ensure that the end of the catheter in the popliteal artery is placed on the sterile drapes covering the patient's anterior aspect.

Now one can capture the wire from the groin with a snare (see Chapter 3, Extracting Foreign Bodies and Pull-Through Technique, p. 118), pull it out through the sheath, and use it as a track for PTA (**Fig. 5.31**). Then you can advance the same catheter or a better fitting balloon catheter of a different size to the puncture site in the popliteal artery. Next, compress the puncture site with the balloon from within the artery for ~3 minutes (Huppert et al 2010, see Chapter 3, Treatment of the Access Site, p. 66).

The retrograde catheterization of the first popliteal segment (using road mapping) can also be performed anteriorly. This spares the patient the prone position and having to be repositioned a second time.

Deep Femoral Artery

A stenosis is often present at the origin of the deep femoral artery. This stenosis is important because it can interfere with or prevent the deep femoral artery functioning as a collateral of a stenosed or occluded superficial femoral artery (see **Figs. 5.3** and **5.4**). Here, the radiologist's most important task is to avoid neglecting to visualize the stenosis. This almost always requires a lateral oblique projection (30 to 40°).

Treating the stenosis is invariably the surgeon's job:
- The origin of the deep femoral artery, like the common femoral artery, is readily accessible for the surgeon.
- Surgical reconstruction with endarterectomy and patch angioplasty is more effective than PTA.
- The open procedure does not involve the risk of pushing plaque material out of the origin of the deep

femoral artery and into the origin of the superficial femoral artery.

Naturally placement of a stent is also contraindicated in the origin of the deep femoral artery.

For the radiologist, the deep femoral artery is first and foremost a diagnostic problem. However, situations can arise in which it seems advisable to dilate the origin of the deep femoral artery as well within the scope of an intervention in the arteries of the leg (Egorova et al 2010). Where the common femoral artery access site is at a sufficient distance to the origin of the deep femoral artery, this may also be done via an ipsilateral approach like the one described earlier for PTA of the origin of the superficial femoral artery (see **Figs. 5.18** and **5.19**).

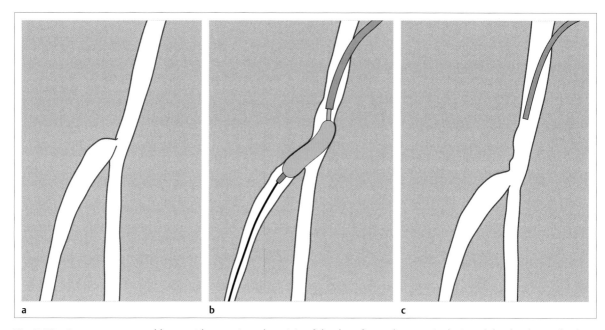

Fig. 5.32 Seventy-two-year-old man with stenosis at the origin of the deep femoral artery. Occlusion of the distal superficial femoral artery was recanalized in the same session.
a Typical stenosis at the origin of the deep femoral artery.
b Dilation.
c Sufficient expansion without impairment of the superficial femoral artery.

As **Figs. 5.32** and **5.33** show, the results are not always optimal.

Perhaps it is more important that there may be an indication for PTA in the trunk of the deep femoral artery distal to the origin. This is a region that is significantly less accessible to surgery than the inguinal region. Another possible indication in the setting of critical ischemia of the extremities is a situation in which findings include not only a chronic occlusion of the superficial femoral artery but also a high-grade stenosis of the trunk or a major branch of the deep femoral artery.

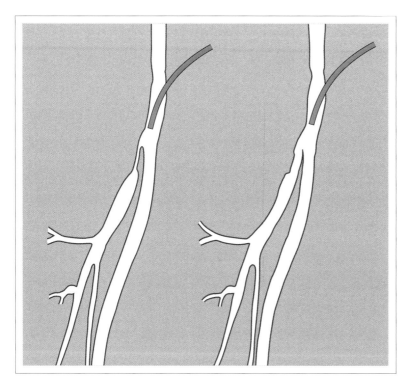

Fig. 5.33 Fifty-four-year-old man with filiform stenosis at the origin of the deep femoral artery.

Popliteal Artery

Differences to Intervention in the Femoral Arteries

The risks of intervention in the superficial femoral artery are limited. If angioplasty is unsuccessful, the situation can almost always be saved by placing a stent. Even an unsuccessful intervention does not decisively worsen the situation because definitive occlusion of the artery is the natural progression of the disorder anyway. Collaterals from the deep femoral artery normally ensure that the leg will be preserved, and the chances of improving the situation with a bypass are good in most cases.

The situation of the popliteal artery is entirely different (**Fig. 5.34**):
- Natural collaterals are largely absent.
- Even slight worsening (such as occlusion of a stenosis after PTA) can acutely endanger the lower leg.
- The bypass options are significantly more limited than in the thigh.

> Interventions in the popliteal artery have a greater risk than those in the superficial femoral artery. Yet at the same time the lack of collaterals increases the urgency of treating stenoses and occlusions (consult a vascular surgeon about alternatives).

All these arguments oblige one to proceed with the utmost caution and diligence in the popliteal artery. One must fully exploit the limited possibilities that are available here, especially the possibility of longer dilation (**Figs. 5.35** and **5.36**).

Therefore:
- To avoid dissections, carefully match the balloon diameter to the width of the vessel.
- Where the results of PTA are unsatisfactory, dilate longer (with the same balloon, **Figs. 5.35** and **5.36**).

- In the presence of eccentric plaques, atherectomy should be considered.

The earlier reservations against the use of stents in the popliteal artery have for the most part been addressed by new developments in stent design. The stents with a modular design are not as susceptible to kinking and fractures, which represent the greatest risks in the highly mobile popliteal artery.

A new stent design marketed under the name SUPERA (IDEV Technologies, Webster, TX, USA) is particularly well suited to the popliteal artery. This stent consists of 2×6 nitinol wires arranged in a spiral pattern resembling crisscrossed left-handed and right-handed threading (see **Fig. 2.59**). This structure gives the stent extraordinary flexibility and ~4 times the radial strength of standard nitinol stents. No fractures of this stent have yet been observed (**Fig. 5.37**).

The SUPERA stent is extended while in the applicator system; it reaches its definitive width only by shortening significantly. As it is deployed it is pressed together incrementally with the aid of the catheter containing it. The stent will expand to its full width only if the stenosis has been dilated beforehand.

Naturally we have the risk of **recurrent stenosis** in the popliteal artery as well. And because the popliteal artery is such a critical vessel, this would be the site where the prophylactic use of **drug-eluting balloons** would most likely be indicated.

Disorders Specific to the Popliteal Artery

Certain clinical pictures in the popliteal artery rarely or never occur elsewhere in the leg or even the entire vascular system.
- Aneurysm (often acutely thrombosed)
- Embolus, especially in the third segment
- Cystic degeneration of the adventitia
- Entrapment (popliteal artery compression syndrome)

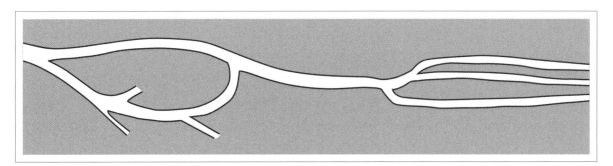

Fig. 5.34 In the thigh there are two parallel arterial systems that can mutually compensate for each other, whereas in the lower leg there are three. However, at the level of the knee there is only the popliteal artery.

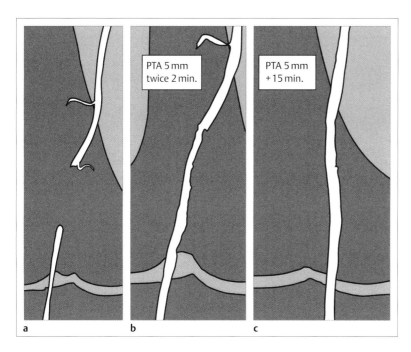

Fig. 5.35 Improvement in the result of percutaneous transluminal angioplasty (PTA) by longer dilation (over 15 minutes).
a Occlusion (initial finding).
b PTA 5 mm, twice for 2 minutes.
c PTA 5 mm, over 15 minutes.

Aneurysm

Aneurysm is the most common of these disorders (**Fig. 5.38**). In any occlusion of the popliteal artery, one must consider an aneurysm and confirm or exclude it with ultrasound.

The presence of an aneurysm normally contraindicates endovascular intervention. Yet the possibility of bridging the popliteal artery aneurysm with an endovascular prosthesis has repeatedly been mentioned in the literature. No long-term results are yet available. And in any case there is still the risk of embolic occlusion of the arteries of the lower leg.

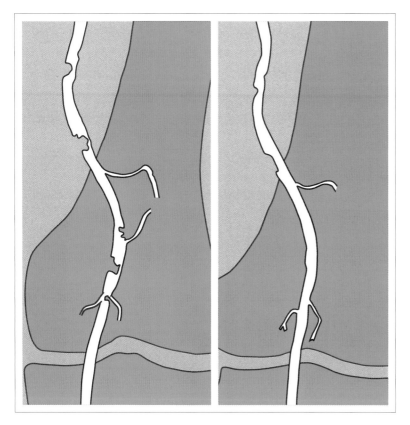

Fig. 5.36 Longer percutaneous transluminal angioplasty can produce satisfactory results even with eccentric plaques.

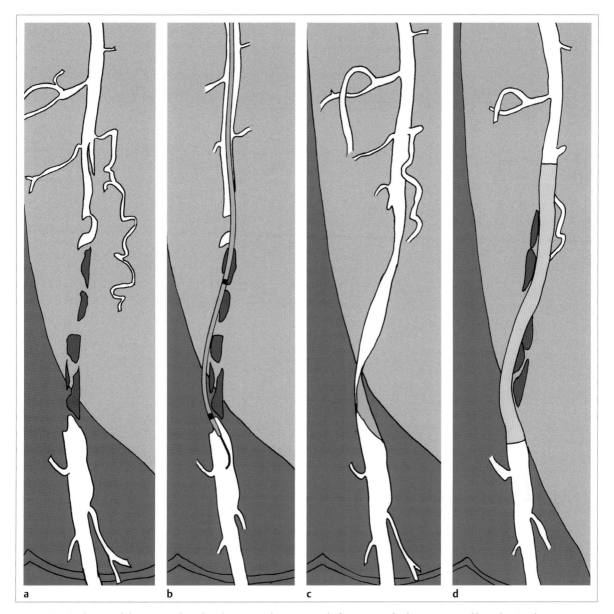

Fig. 5.37 Occlusion of the proximal popliteal artery with massive calcifications in the lumen. Treated by subintimal recanalization and SUPERA stent (IDEV Technologies).
a Initial findings.
b Subintimal catheterization.
c After dilation.
d With SUPERA stent.

Once one has demonstrated a popliteal artery aneurysm, one must search carefully for aneurysms on the contralateral side and in the abdominal aorta. These aneurysms often occur bilaterally and in association with aortic aneurysms.

Emboli

The distal popliteal artery is the site in the leg that is most frequently occluded by **emboli** (**Figs. 5.39** and **5.40**). The trifurcation of the distal popliteal artery into the three arteries of the lower leg is a narrow point at which emboli measuring 2 to 6 mm lodge. This often represents an indication for thrombus aspiration, and occasionally for thrombolysis. Alternatively, surgical embolectomy may be considered. Every attempt at PTA is hazardous because thrombus fragments can occlude the arteries of the lower leg.

Cystic Adventitial Disease

Cystic adventitial disease (**Fig. 5.41**) appears on the angiogram as an oval, smoothly demarcated filling defect

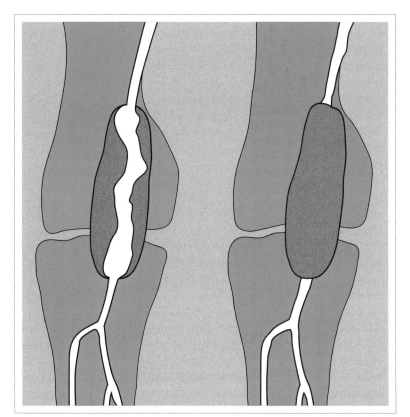

Fig. 5.38 Partially and fully thrombosed popliteal artery aneurysm.

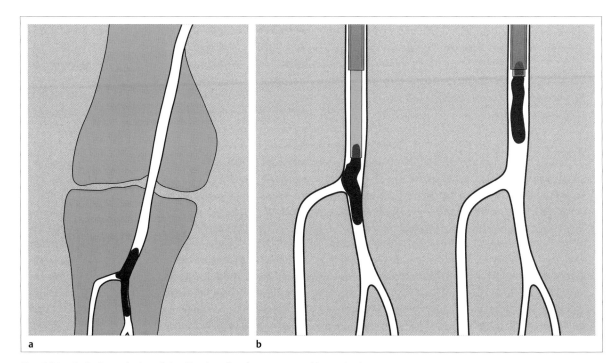

a

b

Fig. 5.39 Embolic occlusion of the distal popliteal artery treated by aspiration.
a Initial situation.
b Thrombus aspiration.

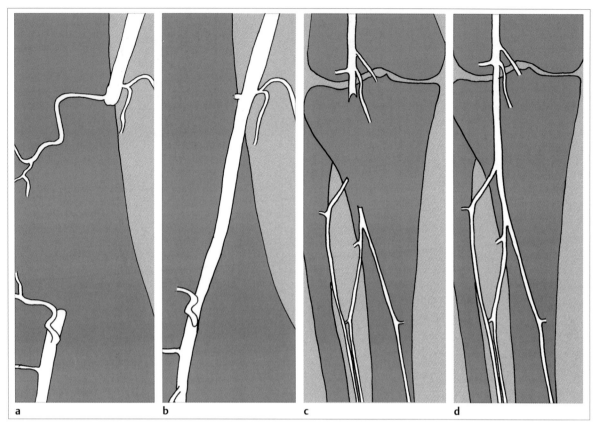

a   b   c   d

Fig. 5.40 Recanalization of a segmental occlusion of the distal superficial femoral artery by percutaneous transluminal angioplasty (PTA). This led to embolic occlusion of the distal popliteal artery. Successful aspiration thrombectomy.
a Segmental occlusion of the distal superficial femoral artery.   **c** Resulting embolic occlusion of the popliteal artery.
b Recanalization by PTA.   **d** Result after aspiration embolectomy.

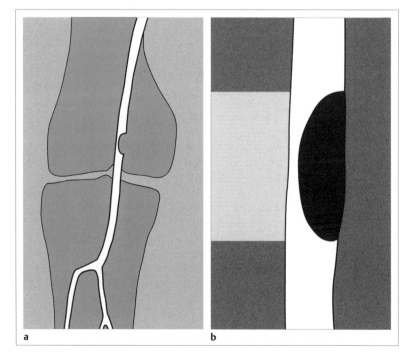

a   b

Fig. 5.41 Cystic adventitial disease.
a Angiography.
b Ultrasound.

along the wall, invariably near a joint. It is presumably caused by ectopic seeding of synovial tissue (in which case the name would be inaccurate). The disorder is diagnosed by color Doppler imaging: It shows a smoothly demarcated filling defect along the wall without a flow signal (Gardiner and Wagner 2006).

Treatment is surgical; the lesion cannot be managed by PTA. (The author once attempted PTA at the surgeon's request because a catheter had already been placed at the site. The patient was asymptomatic after treatment but the claudication reappeared the next morning.)

Entrapment

Entrapment (popliteal compression syndrome) appears on the angiogram as a medial shift of the popliteal artery and possibly the vein as well (**Fig. 5.42**). This is caused by an atypical insertion of the medial head of the gastrocnemius muscle. There are several variants. This is best evaluated with magnetic resonance imaging (MRI) with the foot in dorsiflexion and plantar flexion. Treatment is surgical (Rich 1998).

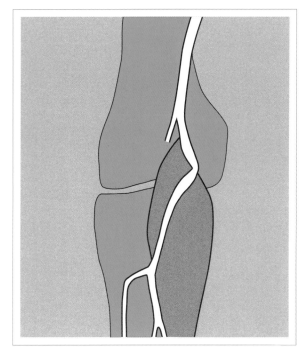

Fig. 5.42 Entrapment. Medial head of the gastrocnemius muscle is shown in blue.

Arteries of the Lower Leg

Clinical Presentation and Indication

Occlusions of the arteries of the lower leg with pain at rest or trophic disorders in the foot and lower leg with an ankle-brachial index (ABI) <0.5 require surgical or interventional treatment. The alternative would be amputation. Any treatment that helps to avoid major amputations is also a reasonable treatment in economic terms.

If, as in most cases, surgical intervention is not an option, then attempting interventional treatment is justified even if the chances of success may not be good. Because better results can be achieved by surgery under certain circumstances, this alternative must first be given consideration. This decision will usually have to be based on precise angiographic images.

The prospects for a favorable clinical outcome are good where uninterrupted blood flow to the foot can be restored. The best long-term results are achieved with **venous bypasses** to the peripheral posterior tibial or dorsalis pedis arteries, or even the plantar artery under the following conditions:

- The patient's general health permits a long operation.
- A long vein is available for the bypass.
- The recipient region is at a sufficient distance from any gangrenous or infected areas.

- The surgeons are sufficiently experienced in this challenging technique (Friedman and Safa 2002).

These conditions are rarely fulfilled. Two thirds of all patients seeking treatment of occluded arteries of the lower leg are diabetics. The problem here is rarely claudication. On the contrary, these patients suffer from trophic disorders such as gangrene and infected ulcers, often in the setting of critical ischemia of the extremity. Additionally, they are often in poor general health. This means that many of these patients will tolerate only a minor intervention. One will have to settle for defining success as restoring patency to an artery of the lower leg long enough for an ulcer to heal. Especially in older patients the improvement in the symptoms seems to persist even when the treated vessels have again become occluded (Atar et al 2005).

Healing trophic disorders requires large quantities of oxygen and nutrients, which normally can be delivered only where at least one vessel is permanently open. Once the wound has healed, the need for oxygen decreases. Under favorable circumstances this need can even be covered when the main vessel has again become occluded.

PTA can be repeatedly performed in the arteries of the lower leg. Even in patients in poorer health, it is quick and reliable.

PTA to treat hemodynamically significant stenoses in the arteries of the lower leg is often performed as a supplementary procedure following PTA in the thigh: Improving peripheral drainage also improves the prognosis for patency of the femoral artery (Egorova et al 2010, Goodney et al 2009, Varty et al 1995).

General Conditions

Goal of Treatment
The objective is to restore patency to at least one of the major arteries of the lower leg as far as the foot, wherever possible even two or three. Only precise analysis of the angiographic findings can determine in which of the vessels there is a chance of restoring patency. Therefore the first step must be **exact angiography** of the arteries of the lower leg, where possible as far as the plantar arch.

Preparation
- Clopidogrel at least 6 hours before the procedure, an initial dose of 600 mg, thereafter 75 mg daily
- Aspirin >2 hours before the procedure, 100 mg orally or 500 mg IV
- Nifedipine 10 mg orally
- Possibly 100 to 200 mg of nitroglycerin intra-arterially before and after PTA
- Heparin, 5,000 IU

Approach
Wherever possible an ipsilateral antegrade approach is used with a long sheath extending to the popliteal artery. This ensures good quality angiography with minimal use of contrast. Many of these patients are diabetics with impaired kidney function. If the indication is not yet clear, angiography is initially performed via a long 18 gauge plastic cannula or a 4 French dilator.

In the rare case of chronic occlusion of the superficial femoral artery over a long segment, one may consider antegrade catheterization of the popliteal artery with the patient prone to treat the arteries of the lower leg (Schroeder 1989). Catheterization via the distal anterior tibial, posterior tibial, or dorsalis pedis artery has also been described several times within the last few years (Huppert et al 2010). This is best done with slender "low profile" systems: a 3 or 4 French catheter with a 0.014 or 0.018 in. wire.

Results
Over the last few years results have been published of larger groups of patients receiving endovascular treatment of the arteries of the lower leg. Bosiers et al (2006) reported on 443 patients (primarily with type 4 disease according to the Rutherford classification). A primary patency rate after 1 year of 68.6% was achieved for PTA alone, 75.5% for PTA and stent placement, and 75.4% for excimer laser treatment. Conrad et al (2009) reported on 144 very high risk patients (74% were in categories C and D according to TASC II; see Chapter 1, TASC II, p. 3). They registered a primary patency rate of 62% after 40 months, whereby only five patients received a stent.

Complications
- Thrombosis (acute occurrence therapy): lysis (see Chapter 3, Local Thrombolysis, p. 97).
- Embolization of plaque or organized thrombus: aspiration with a 5 or 6 French catheter (see Chapter 3, Aspiration of Thrombus, p. 105).

Catheterization

It is not generally recommended to steer the guidewire into one of the arteries of the lower leg with the aid of a catheter and then introduce a balloon catheter over the same wire. It is a lot quicker and easier to choose among the three arteries with the aid of a curved wire. The wire over which the balloon catheter will later be introduced is first given an appropriate bend.

The fibular artery is most easily reached with a straight wire via the tibiofibular trunk. To enter the posterior tibial artery, the wire needs only a slight bend ($\sim$20°). The angle of the anterior tibial artery origin can be as large as 90° (**Fig. 5.43**). This origin is often the site of a stenosis that is clearly visualized only on a medial oblique (30°) projection. The vessel arises from the popliteal artery in an anteromedial direction (**Fig. 5.44**).

A wire with the proper curvature for entering the origin of the anterior tibial artery will tend to continue on into the anterior tibial recurrent artery. That artery arises proximally at the level of the next bend.

If the wire cannot be advanced past this artery, advance the catheter to just short of this bend (**Fig. 5.45**). This effectively shortens the curved part of the wire, and the remaining end is easier to steer within the narrow vessel.

Percutaneous Transluminal Angioplasty
The literature does not provide any consistent recommendations for catheterizing the arteries of the lower leg. Yet everyone agrees that recanalization should be performed with very slender systems: 3 to 4 French catheters and 0.014 or 0.018 in. wires.

Over the wire catheters have significant advantages over monorail catheters in the lower leg. One can better exert axial pressure to push the catheter through a

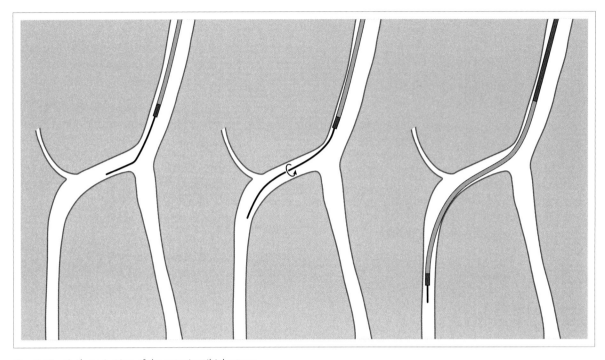

Fig. 5.43   Catheterization of the anterior tibial artery.

stenosis or occlusion because the entire length of the catheter is splinted by the wire. And with minimal injections of contrast through the catheter, it is always possible to determine the exact location of the tip of the catheter and to visualize the further course of the vessel.

Calabrese (2008) advances the 0.014 in. wire only a few millimeters out of the tip of the catheter and then immediately advances the catheter after it. Other authors (Jagust and Sos 2006) recommend initially advancing a 0.035 in. Bentson or 0.035 in. glide wire (Silver and Ansel

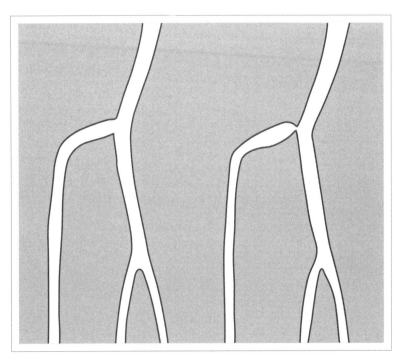

Fig. 5.44   Stenosis at the origin of the anterior tibial artery, visualized only on a contralateral oblique projection.

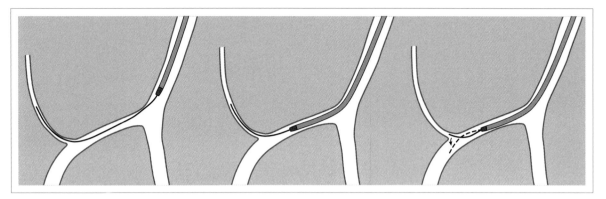

Fig. 5.45 The wire tends to deviate into the anterior tibial recurrent artery.

2005; within a 4 French catheter) and then switching to a 0.014 or 0.018 in. wire with a 4 French PTA catheter.

Usually it is possible to treat **focal stenoses** or **occlusions of the proximal arteries of the lower leg** without great difficulty. Carefully advancing a guidewire with the proper bend and then performing PTA produces satisfactory to good dilation results in the majority of cases (**Figs. 5.46** and **5.47**).

In contrast the recanalization of **arteries occluded over a long distance** can be a very challenging task. This again requires precise angiographic visualization. Based on these images a decision must be made as to where there is the best chance of restoring the continuity of arterial supply to the plantar arch or to the dorsalis pedis artery. First, the appropriate catheter must be steered around any curves in the vicinity of the trifurcation. After that, one advances more or less in a straight line (**Fig. 5.48**). My experience has shown a slender balloon catheter (3 to 4 French in diameter) in conjunction with the appropriate guidewire (preferably a wire with a nitinol core, e.g., the

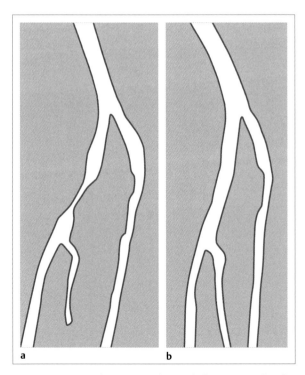

Fig. 5.46 Proximal stenosis without calcification. Results of dilation are usually good.
a Initial situation.
b Findings after dilation.

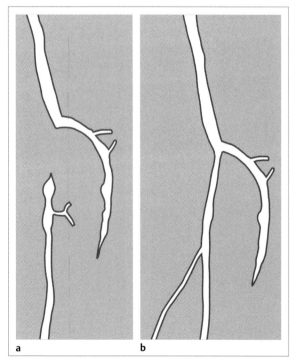

Fig. 5.47 Eighty-two-year-old man with stage IV disease. Recanalization of the tibiofibular trunk by percutaneous transluminal angioplasty (3 mm).
a Occlusion of the tibiofibular trunk in stage IV disease.
b After recanalization, antegrade filling of the posterior tibial artery is again observed.

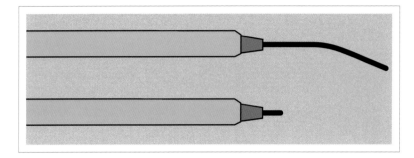

Fig. 5.48 A bent wire has a straight tip again once it has been withdrawn into the catheter.

Terumo Glide Wire Advantage [Terumo Interventional Systems, Somerset, NJ, USA]) to be a suitable instrument combination. Where resistance is slight, one may advance the wire alone as long as it does not deviate from the axis of the vessel. When in doubt, inject a small amount of contrast through the catheter, either via a Tuohy-Borst adapter with the wire in place or through the open catheter after removing the wire.

Then the direction is marked as far as possible using **road mapping**. Often visible mural calcifications will aid in orientation. As long as the catheter and guidewire remain along the axis of the vessel, one may continue to advance them carefully under fluoroscopic control. Where great resistance is encountered, either a hard plaque lies within the vascular lumen or the tip of the guidewire has entered the wall or a branch artery (**Fig. 5.49**). Usually the guidewire must be withdrawn slightly before the next attempt. If one is certain one has not deviated from the lumen (verified by fluoroscopy, possibly in a second plane, with contrast injected through the catheter), one may have hit an intraluminal obstruction.

In such cases one may succeed with the aid of a so-called support catheter that has increased pushability and a tapered low profile tip for ease of lesion entry. It is best used with 0.014 or 0.018 in. wires with varying tip thicknesses (such as the CMW–14 series, 6–25 G, Cook Medical). They are each designed for a different "tip load," meaning the maximum resistance (gram) the straight wire can encounter without bending. One uses the low tip load for soft occlusions and the high tip load for hard resistance.

The extremely long balloons (up to 28 cm) that are now supplied for the arteries of the lower leg have the advantage of shortening the treatment time for an artery with lesions extending over a long segment. They also eliminate the need for double dilation at overlapping sites as is necessary when working with a shorter balloon.

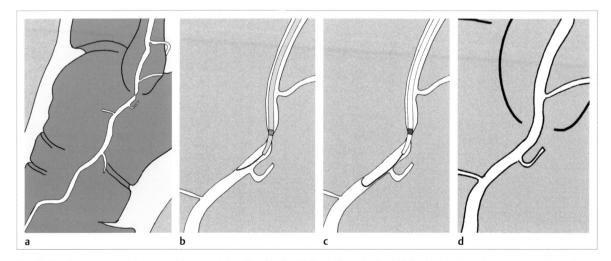

Fig. 5.49 Seventy-year-old man with a poorly healing forefoot injury. The anterior tibial artery is the only artery supplying the forefoot. This vessel exhibits a high-grade stenosis at the level of the ankle.
a Initial findings.
b Catheter cannot be advanced into the stenosis because the guidewire becomes caught on the wall distal to the stenosis.
c A 0.014 in. wire with a tight ⌡-shaped bend allows passage of a balloon catheter through the stenosis.
d After percutaneous transluminal angioplasty with 2 mm.

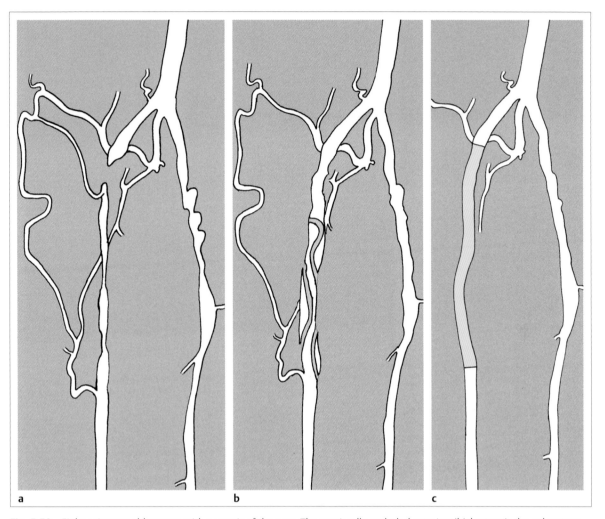

a   b   c

Fig. 5.50 Eighty-six-year-old woman with necrosis of the toes. The proximally occluded anterior tibial artery is the only artery supplying the forefoot.
a Initial findings. Subintimal passage through the occlusion with spontaneous reentry into the true lumen.
b Findings after dilation with a 2 mm balloon.
c After placement of a 2.5 × 57 mm balloon-expandable stent (cobalt-chrome).

After the dilation, the balloon catheter is withdrawn back into the popliteal artery but the wire is left in place within the treated segment until one has performed **angiography** via the sheath and has documented satisfactory to good results. If necessary one can then easily advance the catheter back into position and repeat PTA or introduce a different catheter.

An experienced operator can achieve good results with subintimal recanalization (**Fig. 5.50**) even in the arteries of the lower leg (Bolia et al 1994).

Stents

Stents in the arteries of the lower leg are handled in a variety of ways. However, the consensus now is that better patency rates in short stenoses and occlusions can be achieved with balloon-expandable stents than with PTA alone (**Fig. 5.50**; Calabrese 2008, Zeller 2010). In longer lesions, special nitinol stents have made it possible to achieve results similar to those in the femoral arteries (Zeller 2010). Smaller studies have also demonstrated that drug-eluting stents are superior to standard stents (Zeller 2010). In any case, only stents specially designed for use in small-caliber vessels should be used in the arteries of the lower leg. Otherwise too much metal would further narrow the small vascular diameter. Recurrent in-stent stenoses may be treated by balloon angioplasty with good results (**Fig. 5.51**).

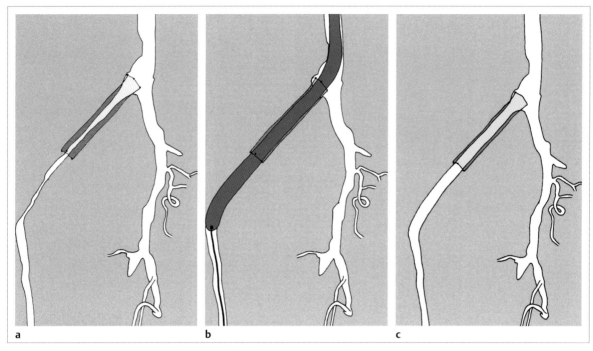

a   b   c

Fig. 5.51 Seventy-seven-year-old man with a stent in the proximal anterior tibial artery.
a Recurrent stenosis.
b Dilation with a 3.5 mm balloon.
c Result after percutaneous transluminal angioplasty.

References

Atar E, Siegel Y, Avrahami R, Bartal G, Bachar GN, Belenky A. Balloon angioplasty of popliteal and crural arteries in elderly with critical chronic limb ischemia. Eur J Radiol 2005;53(2):287–292

Bolia A, Sayers RD, Thompson MM, Bell PR. Subintimal and intraluminal recanalisation of occluded crural arteries by percutaneous balloon angioplasty. Eur J Vasc Surg 1994;8(2):214–219

Bosiers M. The use of dedicated self-expanding stents and potential effects of deployment on clinical outcome. Interventional Course; Leipzig, Germany; 2010

Bosiers M, Hart JP, Deloose K, Verbist J, Peeters P. Endovascular therapy as the primary approach for limb salvage in patients with critical limb ischemia: experience with 443 infrapopliteal procedures. Vascular 2006;14(2):63–69

Calabrese E. Infrapopliteal arterial diseases: angioplasty and stenting. In: Heuser RR, Henry M, eds. Textbook of Peripheral Vascular Interventions. 2nd ed. London: Informa UK; 2008:633–638

Clark TW, Groffsky JL, Soulen MC. Predictors of long-term patency after femoropopliteal angioplasty: results from the STAR registry. J Vasc Interv Radiol 2001;12(8):923–933

Conrad MF, Kang J, Cambria RP, et al. Infrapopliteal balloon angioplasty for the treatment of chronic occlusive disease. J Vasc Surg 2009;50(4):799–805

Dake MD. How Good Are Drug Eluting Stents? Munich, Germany: CIRSE; 2011

DeRubertis BG, Pierce M, Chaer RA, et al. Lesion severity and treatment complexity are associated with outcome after percutaneous infra-inguinal intervention. J Vasc Surg 2007;46(4):709–716

Egorova NN, Guillerme S, Gelijns A, et al. An analysis of the outcomes of a decade of experience with lower extremity revascularization including limb salvage, lengths of stay, and safety. J Vasc Surg 2010;51(4):878–885, 885

Friedman SG, Safa TK. Pedal branch arterial bypass for limb salvage. Am Surg 2002;68(5):446–448

Gardiner GA, Wagner SC. Angiography of lower extremity peripheral vascular disease. In: Baum S, Pentecost MJ, eds. Abrams Angiography Interventional Radiology. 2nd ed. Philadelphia, PA: Lippincott Williams & Wilkins; 2006:312–327

Goodney PP, Beck AW, Nagle J, Welch HG, Zwolak RM. National trends in lower extremity bypass surgery, endovascular interventions, and major amputations. J Vasc Surg 2009;50(1): 54–60

Huppert P, Mueller W, Bauersachs R. Alternative Zugangswege bei der Rekanalisation von Extremitätenarterien. Berlin: Deutscher Röntgenkongress; 2010

Jagust MB, Sos TA. Infrapopliteal revascularization. In: Baum S, Pentecost MJ, eds. Abrams Angiography Interventional Radiology. 2nd ed. Philadelphia, PA: Lippincott Williams & Wilkins; 2006:348–361

Laird JR, Katzen BT, Scheinert D, et al. Nitinol sent implantation vs. balloon angioplasty for lesions in the superficial femoral and popliteal arteries for patients with claudication: three-year follow-up from the RESILIANT randomized trial. J Endorasc Ther 2012;19:1–9

Losordo DW, Rosenfield K, Pieczek A, Baker K, Harding M, Isner JM. How does angioplasty work? Serial analysis of human iliac arteries using intravascular ultrasound. Circulation 1992;86(6): 1845–1858

Nguyen BN, Conrad MF, Guest JM, et al. Late outcomes of balloon angioplasty and angioplasty with selective stenting for superficial femoropopliteal disease are equivalent. J Vasc Surg 2011;54(4):1051–1057

Rich MR. Popliteal entrapment an adventitial cystic disease. In: Perler BA, Becker GJ, eds. Vascular Intervention: A Clinical Approach. Stuttgart, New York: Thieme; 1998:231–237

Schillinger M, Sabeti S, Dick P, et al. Sustained benefit at 2 years of primary femoropopliteal stenting compared with balloon angioplasty with optional stenting. Circulation 2007;115(21): 2745–2749

Schroeder J. Catheter lysis and percutaneous transluminal angioplasty below the knee via the popliteal artery in a patient with femoral artery obstruction: technical note. Cardiovasc Intervent Radiol 1989;12(6):344–345

Schröder J. Control of catheters in coronary angiography—resistance to torsion in the aortic arch [in German]. Z Kardiol 1992;81(8):449–452

Sharafuddin MJ, Hoballah JJ, Kresowik TF, Nicholson RM, Sharp WJ. Impact of aggressive endovascular recanalization techniques on success rate in chronic total arterial occlusions (CTOs). Vasc Endovascular Surg 2010;44(6):460–467

Silver MJ, Ansel GM. Infrapopliteal intervention. In: Casserly IP, Sachar R, Yadav JS, eds. Manual of Peripheral Vascular Intervention. Philadelphia, PA: Lippincott Williams & Wilkins; 2005:252–264

Tran VK. Perkutane Rekanalisation bei Verschlüssen von Beinarterien. Inauguraldissertation Kiel, 1998

Varty K, Bolia A, Naylor AR, Bell PR, London NJ. Infrapopliteal percutaneous transluminal angioplasty: a safe and successful procedure. Eur J Vasc Endovasc Surg 1995;9(3):341–345

Zeller T. PTA und Stents im Bereich der Unterschenkelarterien. Berlin: Deutscher Röntgenkongress; 2010

6   Upper Extremities

Stenosis or Occlusion of the Left Subclavian Artery

There is only one intervention in the branches of the aortic arch (supra-aortic branches) that is largely free of the risk of a cerebral insult, that is not particularly demanding from a technical standpoint, and that has been performed since the beginning of interventional radiology: **percutaneous transluminal angioplasty (PTA) of the left subclavian artery**. A stenosis develops relatively often between the origin of the subclavian artery on the aortic arch and the origin of the left vertebral artery. This stenosis can progress to an occlusion in the further course of the disorder. This leads to reduced blood pressure and, in advanced cases, weakness in the left arm.

The only major collateral that can mitigate the problem for the left arm is the **left vertebral artery**. The posterior portion of the cerebral circulatory system is supplied by two arteries that join together to form the trunk of the basilar artery. Stenosis of the left subclavian causes blood pressure to decrease in the left vertebral and brachial arteries until blood flow in the left vertebral artery reverses. Where the condition has progressed to complete occlusion of the subclavian artery, the left arm is supplied nearly exclusively via the vertebral artery.

The simple **flow reversal**, which can be well visualized angiographically (see Chapter 3, Angiography of the Upper Extremities, p. 88) is referred to as subclavian steal or subclavian steal phenomenon (**Fig. 6.1**). One refers to a **subclavian steal syndrome** when this tapping of the vertebral artery by the left arm triggers symptoms of cerebral ischemia. The typical symptom of vertigo occurs when physical exertion increases the blood required by the left arm.

Intervention is regarded as indicated where the typical symptoms of the subclavian steal syndrome are present, or at least the weakness of the arm represents a significant impairment, and when a stenosis of at least 70 to 80% in the left subclavian artery suggests that the intervention will eliminate the symptoms.

The technical success rate for stenosis is close to 100%. In the presence of an occlusion, catheterization may fail. The flow reversal invariably present in the vertebral artery largely excludes any cerebral complications from the intervention. Because the subclavian artery is an elastic vessel, the rate of recurrence is relatively low at 5 to 7% (Kedhi et al 2008).

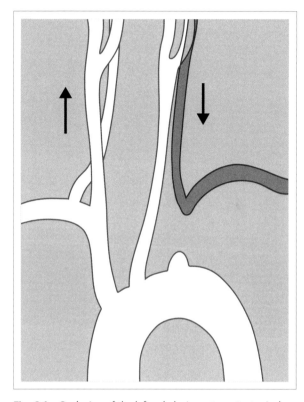

Fig. 6.1 Occlusion of the left subclavian artery at a typical location with flow reversal in the left vertebral artery. Early phase (*arrow up*); late phase (*arrow down*).

Performing the Procedure

A thoracic aortogram is obtained via a transfemoral approach to visualize findings. Then one usually advances an 80 to 90 cm sheath up to the origin of the left subclavian artery. In most cases a **vertebral artery catheter** (straight with a slight bend close to the tip) is suitable for catheterizing the subclavian artery. Place the tip of this catheter into the origin of the subclavian artery and then advance a straight glide wire through this catheter into the stenosis or occlusion (**Fig. 6.2**). If the wire is not able to pass through an occlusion, attempt to find a better approach by changing the position of the catheter tip. One can also try a slightly curved glide wire or an 0.018 in. guidewire with a short flexible tip (preferably one with

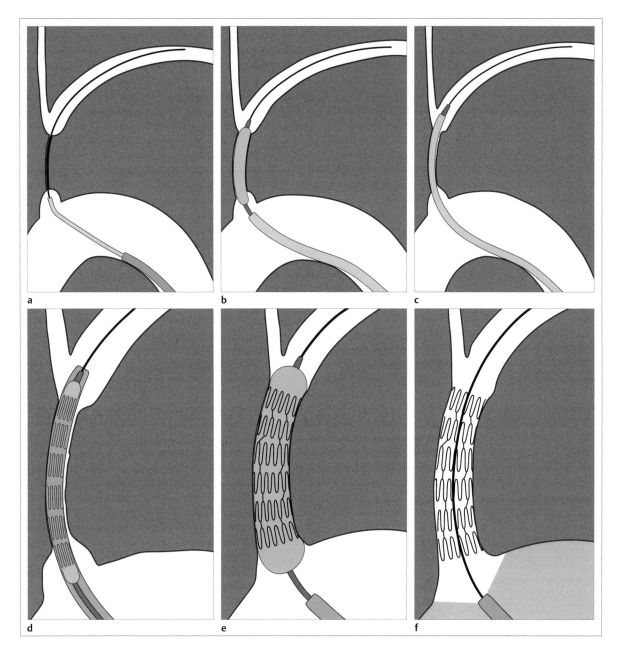

Fig. 6.2 Recanalization of an occlusion of the left subclavian artery.
a Advance wire.
b Preliminary dilation.
c Advance sheath into occlusion.
d Place balloon-expandable stent within sheath in the occlusion.
e Withdraw sheath, dilate.
f Evaluate results with angiography.

a core of nitinol, e.g., the Terumo Glide Wire Advantage, Terumo Interventional Systems, Somerset, NJ, USA).

Access via the Brachial Artery

Access via the left brachial artery is an alternative. (In the absence of a palpable arterial pulse, a Doppler probe should be used to locate the artery for the puncture.)

Many times it is possible to pass a wire from the arm through an occlusion that cannot be penetrated from the aortic arch. One can capture the long wire with a snare, pull it out through the sheath in the common femoral artery, and then use it as a track for advancing the balloon catheter (**Fig. 6.3**). Naturally, the entire intervention may be performed via the brachial artery. However, then it is not as easy to place a stent with great precision.

Because of the more favorable results, the method generally preferred today is to treat not only occlusion but also stenosis by placing a stent. Stenoses are more often encountered close to the origin of the vessel, where **precise placement** is crucial. For this reason balloon-expandable stents are preferable. To select the correct stent one must measure both the width of the vessel and the length of the lesion. The stent should not cover the origins of the vertebral and internal thoracic arteries. In an ostial stenosis the stent should project 1 to 2 mm into the aorta as in the renal arteries. In a stenosis distal to the origin of the vertebral artery (which does not lead to a subclavian steal syndrome), a self-expanding stent is of course preferable.

Stenoses and Occlusions in Other Branches of the Aortic Arch

Stenoses in the right subclavian artery are encountered much less frequently than in the left subclavian artery. Endovascular management of these lesions is riskier and far more challenging. The same applies to stenoses in the brachiocephalic trunk and left carotid artery.

Except in the hands, arteriosclerotic stenoses and occlusions occur relatively rarely in the arteries of the arm. Primarily in elderly women one will occasionally encounter chronic occlusions in the axillary artery and upper arm in the setting of giant cell arteritis. Thickening of the vascular wall is a typical ultrasound finding. These disorders are treated with immunosuppressants. Careful dilation can bring relief of symptoms in certain cases when the inflammation is well controlled.

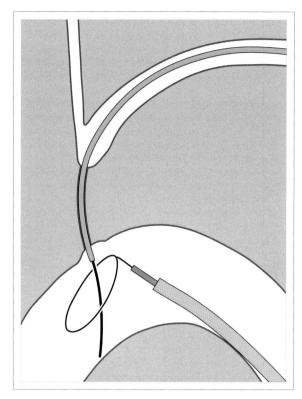

Fig. 6.3 Advance wire via brachial artery, capture wire with snare.

In the usual case of catheterization via the groin only, advance the wire into the brachial artery prior to PTA so that there is a sufficiently reliable track for overcoming resistance.

Dialysis Shunt

General

There are two common types of arteriovenous dialysis shunts: the Cimino-Brescia **arteriovenous fistula** and a polytetrafluoroethylene (PTFE) graft interposed between an artery and vein. The arteriovenous fistula is usually created between the radial artery and the cephalic vein at a distal location in the nondominant arm. It is usually created as a side-to-end anastomosis (**Fig. 6.4**). This shunt must "mature" over a period of 3 to 4 months (i.e., the vein must increase significantly in width due to the increased pressure and flow volume and its wall must

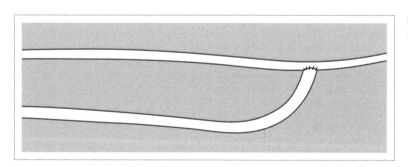

Fig. 6.4 Arteriovenous fistula between radial artery and cephalic vein.

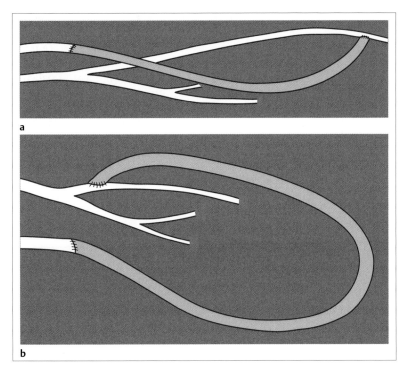

a

b

Fig. 6.5 Two options for placing polytetrafluoroethylene graft in the forearm.
a Interposed graft between distal radial artery and vein in the proximal forearm.
b Interposed graft between proximal radial artery and vein in the proximal forearm (loop).

become thicker before it can be used for dialysis). The interposed PTFE graft (**Fig. 6.5**) has the necessary width right from the start and can therefore be used within 2 weeks of implantation.

The average duration of initial patency for arteriovenous fistulas is 3 years, for PTFE grafts only about 1 year. Interventional measures or surgical corrections can extend these periods (secondary patency) to 7 and 2 years, respectively (Calabrese and Yasin 2008). This shows the importance of the task entrusted to the interventional radiologist along with the surgeon.

> Repeated interventions can double the useful life of a dialysis shunt!

Symptoms

A variety of symptoms can indicate the necessity of intervention. These are the most important ones:
- Decreased pulse or absence of flow sounds at the anastomosis.
- Insufficient pressure (vein collapses) and flow in the shunt (normal values: 500 mL/min in an arteriovenous fistula and 700 to 800 mL/min in a PTFE graft).

These are usually sequelae of stenoses or kinks in the arteriovenous anastomosis (**Fig. 6.6**). Abnormally **high venous pressure** and swelling in the forearm or hand are indicative of a problem in the venous tract. Where the entire arm is swollen one must expect to find stenoses in the central veins. Yet **isolated swelling** of the hand can also be attributable to abnormally high venous pressure as a result of an overly wide anastomosis.

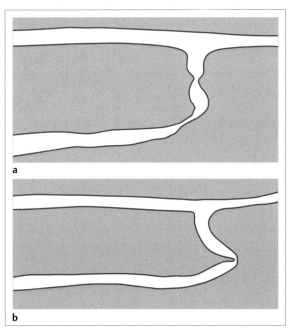

a

b

Fig. 6.6 Stenoses at the arteriovenous fistula.
a Scarred stenosis.
b Kink.

> **Important:** Known stenoses (stenosis grade > 40 to 50%) should be eliminated promptly so that they cannot lead to thrombosis in the shunt.

However, stenoses in the anastomosis can only be dilated 1 month postoperatively at the earliest. Otherwise the sutures could be torn out, causing major bleeding.

Diagnostic Workup

The clinical examination is extraordinarily helpful for planning intervention in a dialysis shunt. In many cases one will be able to see and feel the entire length of the shunt beneath the skin. One can palpate the flow of blood behind the arteriovenous fistula, feel the pressure in the vein, and see the aneurysms.

In an arm that has repeatedly undergone surgery, it is not often easy to determine the direction of blood flow through the shunt. Press one end of it shut. If the vein then empties, then one is on the arterial side. If it fills up, then one has compressed the venous end.

Ultrasound, preferably in the form of color Doppler imaging, permits very precise evaluation. In the case of a stenosis requiring treatment, the referring nephrologist can now often provide very detailed information based on ultrasound studies and pressure measurement. Where this is the case, one can occasionally puncture the shunt in the direction of the stenosis right away in an effort to minimize the extent of the intervention (**Fig. 6.7**).

Yet as a rule **angiographic visualization of the entire system** from the supplying artery to the superior vena cava should be the first step. To do this the cubital artery is typically catheterized in retrograde fashion with a 22 gauge plastic cannula (connected to a perfusor line) or a 3 French catheter. The patient is positioned to permit visualization of the entire arm and upper chest region. At the same time, care must be taken so that the shunt remains accessible proximally and distally for punctures. This is not always easy. The forearm and hand are initially imaged in supine position (palm facing up). The forearm must be rotated as required to visualize the anastomosis optimally. Here, palpation findings can be very helpful.

Thrombosis in a PTFE shunt is usually total. This can be reliably verified by ultrasound. Angiography prior to thrombolysis will not provide any additional information (Vorwerk 2007). The causative stenosis in a PTFE shunt is usually at the venous anastomosis.

Percutaneous Transluminal Angioplasty and Stent Placement

The vascular access for intervention is invariably established via the shunt vein. The sheath (usually 6 French) is introduced at a sufficient distance from the lesion. In the more common stenoses close to the arteriovenous fistula, the wire over which the balloon is guided into the stenosis should be advanced in retrograde fashion far enough into the radial artery so that its stiff section expands the curve at the anastomosis.

A poorly palpable vein can be filled with the aid of a tourniquet. A Doppler probe can also be helpful during the puncture. Occasionally it will not be possible to advance a wire from the shunt vein through a stenosis in the arteriovenous fistula. In this case, there is the option of catheterizing the brachial artery in antegrade fashion at the level of the elbow. From there a wire can be advanced through the stenosis. This wire can then be captured with a snare in the shunt vein and used as a track for dilating the shunt from the venous side (Vorwerk 2007).

Stenosis in a dialysis shunt is usually **stenosis from scarring**. Scar tissue is significantly harder, is less compressible, and has higher tensile strength than the plaque material one encounters in arteries. Therefore one needs balloons that are able to withstand **very high pressure** (up to 20 bar; **Fig. 6.8**). It will occasionally be possible to achieve better initial results with a **cutting balloon** (see p. 29). However, a study by Vesely and Siegel (2005) has shown that the long-term results achieved with cutting balloons are no better than those that can be achieved with high-pressure balloons.

Placement of a stent is recommended wherever a stenosis collapses after dilation. On the other hand, it

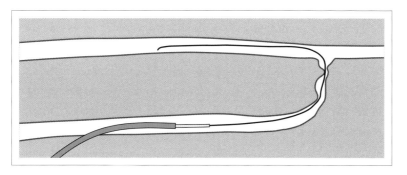

Fig. 6.7 Where the location of the stenosis is known, one may choose an approach leading directly to the stenosis.

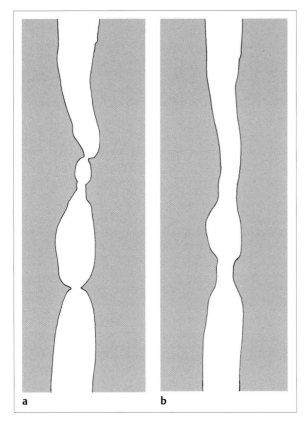

Fig. 6.8
a Sixty-nine-year-old man with shunt vein in upper arm and two stenoses.
b Findings after percutaneous transluminal angiography with 7 mm and 20 bar.

is not advisable to place a stent in a stenosis that cannot be dilated with high pressure. Balloon-expandable stents should not be used in the arm because they can be deformed by external pressure.

Kinking, as is likely to occur in the vicinity of the arteriovenous anastomosis (see **Fig. 6.6b**), cannot be corrected by dilation. Placement of a stent is not recommended either because it fails to address the cause, namely that the vessel is too long. Straightening the vein at one point along its course can produce a kink at another point nearby. Therefore kinks should always be corrected surgically.

Central Veins

Prior dialysis via a central venous catheter can lead to **stenosis or occlusion in the central veins**. Such findings require treatment (with PTA or even stent placement **Fig. 6.9**) where they cause increased venous pressure and possibly swelling of the entire arm. In a stenosis, the first step should always be dilation with high pressure and a balloon whose diameter precisely matches that of the vessel.

A stent is only indicated where an occlusion is recanalized or where a stenosis collapses after dilation.

When implanting a stent, take care to avoid placing it so that it crosses the junction of the internal jugular vein. Otherwise this could interfere with subsequent catheterization (**Fig. 6.10**). Whether in a central or peripheral vein, the size of the stent should always be selected so that it securely adheres to the vessel wall and cannot migrate toward the right heart and pulmonary artery. Remember that in the veins, unlike in the arteries, blood flows toward the larger vessels!

Where there is a known central venous stenosis at the time the AV fistula is created or the PTFE graft implanted, it may be advisable to eliminate this stenosis in the same session by PTA or stent placement. This reduces the risk of early thrombosis of the AV fistula (Shemesh et al 2004).

Thrombosis and Thrombolysis

Often the dialysis shunt will only be treated when the shunt vein or the graft is already occluded by thrombosis. Then the thrombi must be eliminated by thrombolysis or by a mechanical thrombectomy procedure before treatment of the causative stenoses is possible.

The thrombotic occlusion in arteriovenous fistulas can be very short. In this case it will usually be sufficient to carefully advance a catheter through the occlusion and dilate it with a balloon. This eliminates the stenosis, fragments the thrombus, and dissects it off the wall so that it can be transported by the bloodstream and lysed in the lung. If the lesion lies close to the arteriovenous fistula, one should make sure that the tip of the PTA balloon lies within the artery. This will prevent thrombus fragments from being pressed into the artery (Vorwerk 2007).

In many cases the entire segment through which the catheter is introduced is thrombosed. In this situation, unlike arterial thrombosis, one cannot reach the entire thrombus from one side. Here it is necessary to introduce two systems that then cross on the middle of the shunt vein or interposed graft (**Fig. 6.11**).

The most suitable method of thrombolysis is **pulse-spray lysis** (see Chapter 3, Pulse-Spray Lysis, p. 99). If one leaves a short plug of thrombus at the venous anastomosis, one will often find that within an hour sufficient thrombolysis will have been achieved. Residual thrombus fragments along the wall can be pulverized and mobilized with the PTA catheter without any significant risk. One will not occlude any peripheral arteries in this case. On the contrary, one may safely assume that such small thrombus fragments will not exceed the thrombolytic capacity of the lung.

Careful dilation of the causative stenosis or stenoses completes the treatment.

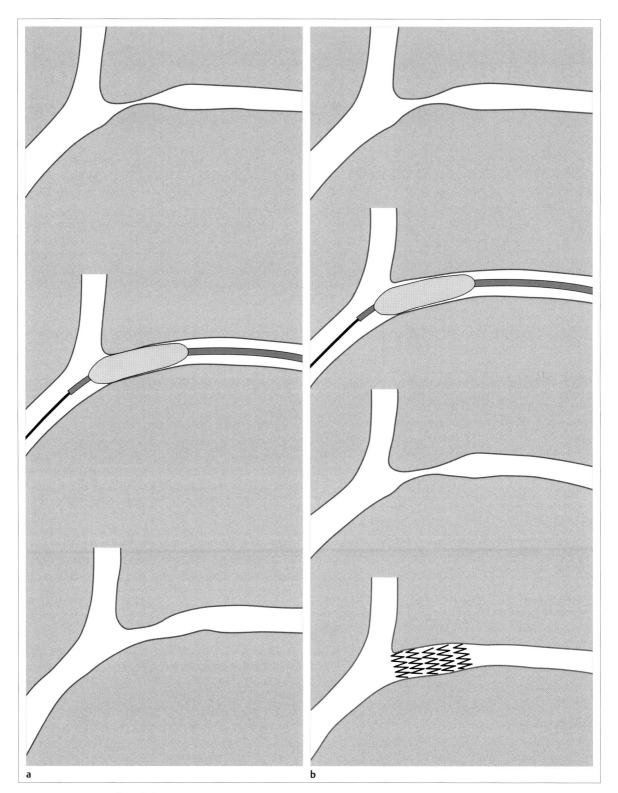

Fig. 6.9 Stenosis in the subclavian vein.
a Treatment with percutaneous transluminal angiography (PTA).   **b** Where PTA results are unsatisfactory, stent is placed.

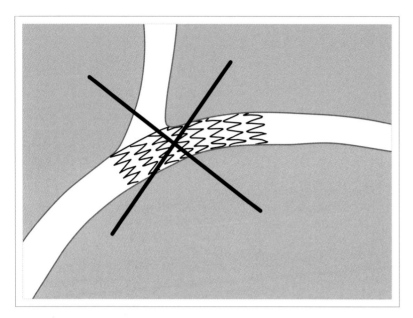

Fig. 6.10 A stent that covers the junction of the internal jugular vein could prevent subsequent placement of a central venous catheter, even for dialysis.

Contrast Agents

Where some residual kidney function is still present, one should use contrast very sparingly.

Dialysis patients are usually experienced in compressing the puncture site themselves. However, one can spare the patient another puncture if one makes arrangements with the dialysis department to replace the sheath with a dialysis catheter (Kessel and Robertson 2005).

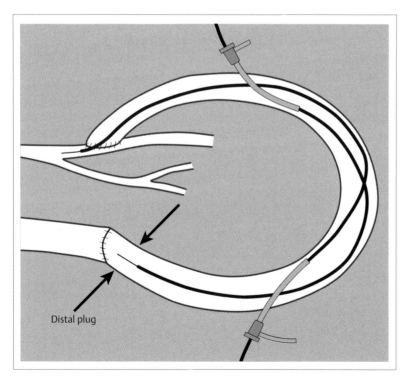

Distal plug

Fig. 6.11 Thrombolysis in a polytetrafluoroethylene loop with two crisscrossed catheters.

Superior Vena Cava Syndrome

Superior vena cava syndrome with swelling of the arms and face, shortness of breath, and pain in the head and chest is attributable to malignant tumors in ~90% of all cases. Bronchial carcinomas in turn account for ~90% of these tumors (Pisco and Duarte 2008). In most cases, interventional treatment can bring immediate relief of symptoms in cases where it is possible to advance a wire and catheter through the stenosis and place a stent. Symptoms can be expected to resolve completely within 3 to 4 days (Wagenhofer et al 2010). Because of their limited life expectancy patients usually do not experience any recurrence of symptoms.

Immediate treatment is desirable to preclude the development of thrombi, which could complicate the procedure significantly. Risks that warrant mention include pulmonary emboli, perforation of the vein, and, rarely, right heart decompensation.

There is a certain lack of consensus as to what sort of diagnostic preparations are required. Superior vena cavography via the veins of both arms can fail for several reasons. Venous puncture is difficult in swollen arms, the flow in the veins of the arms is extremely slow, and contrast agent can dissipate into collaterals in the upper mediastinum. The author has found that meticulous analysis of the contrast computed tomographic (CT) images was nearly always sufficient, and such images were always available. However, it may be that the CT images do not allow complete evaluation of the inflow tract. In that case, superior vena cavography is recommended with simultaneous contrast injection via both cubital veins (20 mL of contrast agent with 150 mg of iodine per mL in each) and with a blood pressure cuff on both upper arms.

Vascular access is normally established via the right femoral vein. However, Kessel and Robertson (2005) have good reasons for preferring the approach via the right internal jugular vein (see Chapter 3, Catheterization of the Internal Jugular Vein, p. 79). If this vein is patent, it provides the shortest route for diagnostic access and stent placement. A stent introduced via the jugular vein has another advantage. As it widens from caudal to cranial, the stent traps any thrombi that may be present before they can be mobilized and carried toward the right heart.

Normally the **residual lumen of the superior vena cava** can be accessed and visualized on angiography via a catheter introduced through the femoral vein. However, this may require a slightly curved catheter and various different guidewires. Even the passage through the right atrium can require a slightly curved catheter to steer the guidewire. Catheterization may be deemed successful once the lumen of the right internal jugular vein has been reached (**Fig. 6.12**).

Replacing the catheter with the stent application system requires a wire at least 180 cm long, or even 200 or 220 cm in the case of long application systems. Normally a 14 mm wide **self-expanding stent** is used (nitinol, with closed cells wherever possible due to the greater radial strength, or a Wallstent [Boston Scientific, Natick, MA, USA]). There are of course occasions when one would appreciate the greater radial strength of a balloon-expandable stent. Yet one must also allow for a possible decrease in the severity of the tumor-induced stenosis under chemotherapy or radiation therapy. In such a case the stent, to maintain its position, must be sufficiently elastic to adapt to the receding wall of the vein.

The stent must at least **cover the entire stenosis**; slightly greater length is desirable to adapt to possible tumor growth. The caudal end of the stenosis is not usually well visualized on angiography when contrast is injected cranial to the stenosis. Yet this is possible using a long sheath (45 cm). To do so the sheath must be advanced through the right atrium into the superior vena cava. The sheath should not be longer than 45 cm if a length of 80 cm is to be sufficient for the standard stent application system. It is very easy to inject contrast through the sheath when using a 7 French sheath and a 5 French catheter.

The stenosis must almost invariably be **redilated** after the stent has been placed. Even then it is practically impossible to expand the stenosis completely (**Fig. 6.13**).

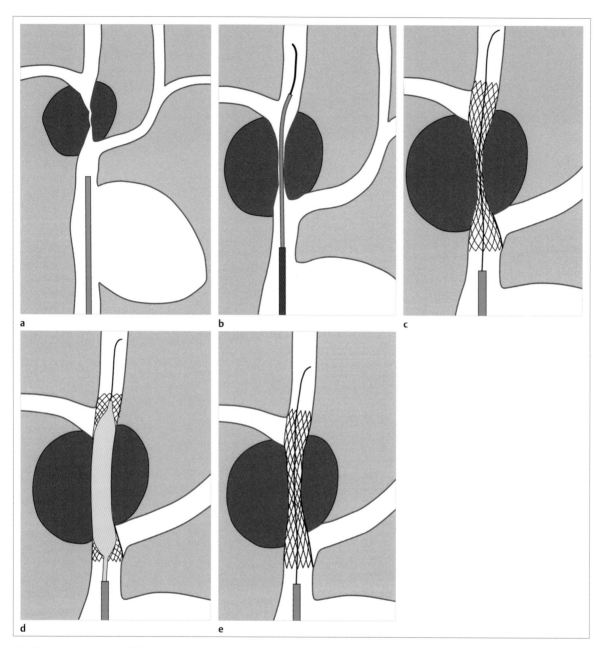

Fig. 6.12 Compression of the brachiocephalic vein by a tumor. Transfemoral catheterization.
a Sheath introduced via femoral approach distal to the tumor stenosis.
b Advancing glide wire and catheter through the stenosis.
c Unsatisfactory result with self-expanding stent.
d Redilation.
e Satisfactory expansion.

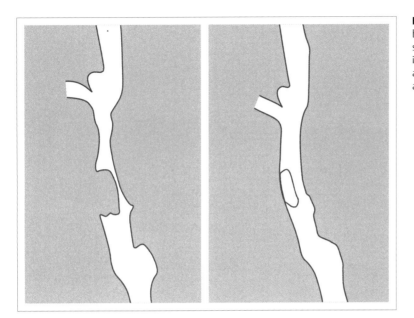

Fig. 6.13 Fifty-one-year-old man with bronchial carcinoma and high-grade stenosis of the superior vena cava. Tumor impression remains after stent placement and percutaneous transluminal angioplasty (PTA).

References

Calabrese E, Yasin B. Hemodialysis access intervention. In: Heuser RR, Henry M, eds. Textbook of Peripheral Vascular Interventions. 2nd ed. London: Informa UK; 2008:699–702

Kessel D, Robertson I. Interventional Radiology: A Survival Guide. London: Elsevier; 2005

Kedhi E, Tanguay JF, Bilodeau L. Pathophysiology of restenosis. In: Heuser RR, Henry M, eds. Textbook of Peripheral Vascular Interventions. 2nd ed. London: Informa UK; 2008:763–769

Pisco J, Duarte M. Superior and inferior vena cava thrombosis. In: Heuser RR, Henry M, eds. Textbook of Peripheral Vascular Interventions. 2nd ed. London: Informa UK; 2008: 858–863

Shemesh D, Olsha O, Berelowitz D, Zaghal I, Zigelman CZ, Abramowitz HB. Integrated approach to construction and maintenance of prosthetic arteriovenous access for hemodialysis. Vascular 2004;12(4):243–255

Vesely TM, Siegel JB. Use of the peripheral cutting balloon to treat hemodialysis-related stenoses. J Vasc Interv Radiol 2005;16(12):1593–1603

Vorwerk D. Haemodialysis shunts. In: Lanzer P, ed. Mastering Endovascular Techniques. Philadelphia, PA: Lippincott Williams & Wilkins; 2007:386–395

Wagenhofer K, Siemens P, Kugler C, et al. Interventionelle Therapie der (malignen) oberen Einflussstauung—Material und technische Durchführung. Berlin: Deutscher Röntgenkongress; 2010

7 Other Endovascular Interventions

The methods presented here are either performed only in special facilities or they require extensive experience or a specific clinical environment. They are described briefly to provide a comprehensive overview of the capabilities of endovascular interventions.

However, this discussion is neither intended nor sufficient to serve as a practical guide for performing these procedures.

Note: Neuroradiologic and cardiological interventions are not discussed here.

Carotid Stents

Stent placement in carotid artery stenoses has been the subject of more discussion in recent years than any other vascular intervention. This has not been because of technical difficulty but because of the specific risks and because its indication is defined in competition with established surgical therapy. As elastic arteries with a low rate of restenosis (5 to 8%), the carotid arteries provide a favorable setting for endovascular treatment. The crucial problem lies in the risk of acute complications from embolism or spasm.

Balloon dilation was initially the predominant procedure (Mathias 1981). Today self-expanding stents are normally used. In the majority of cases they are placed across the origin of the external carotid artery. Some are therefore supplied in a specially adapted design. Following angiography a sheath is introduced into the common carotid artery over a stiff glide wire (the end of the wire lies in the external carotid artery). Next the internal carotid artery is catheterized. Preliminary dilation is performed in applicable cases, and then the stent is placed (**Fig. 7.1**).

A **protection system** in place of the 0.014 in. guidewire can provide a track for introducing the balloon catheter and stent. This system consists of a wire with an umbrella-like or saclike filter that is expanded cranial to the region being treated. Its purpose is to capture any plaque or thrombus material from the stenotic region that may be mobilized during treatment.

The comparative studies available to date suggest that stent placement is not inferior to surgical treatment in terms of quality of results and complications. Particularly in this sensitive region, thorough and conscientious deliberation is crucial in determining the indication. Equally crucial is good cooperation with vascular surgeons and neurologists.

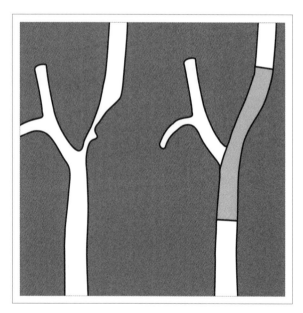

Fig. 7.1 Stenosis of the internal carotid artery. Treatment with a stent.

Endovascular Aortic Prostheses

Abdominal Aorta

The surgical treatment of aortic aneurysms essentially consists of placing a synthetic tube or a γ-shaped bifurcation prosthesis in the aneurysmal sac. The tube or prosthesis is then joined to the nondilated connecting vessels by proximal and distal sutures.

Similar synthetic prostheses can be advanced into the aneurysmal sac through sheaths of sufficient width and length via the femoral arteries, obviating the need to open the abdomen (**Fig. 7.2**). Elastic wire constructions incorporated into the prosthesis create a tight connection to the abdominal aorta proximal to the aneurysm and to the iliac arteries distal to it. Hooks attached to the outer circumference are pressed into the aortic wall with a large balloon.

The prosthesis with its two "legs" can only be introduced from one side. This means that the limb for the contralateral side must be pulled down from the contralateral side and usually lengthened. The width of the prosthesis body must be precisely measured and ordered beforehand. The length of each limb is often adapted to the individual anatomy only during the procedure itself. In some cases one must forgo this type of treatment because certain anatomical conditions are not met.

The important thing is that there are **no leaks** at the junctions between the prosthesis and the vessels and also at the joints between the sections of the prosthesis. Otherwise the blood pressure would continue to act against the wall of the aneurysm and the risk of a rupture would not be eliminated.

An equally dangerous risk is posed by vessels arising from the aneurysm that communicate with the arterial system outside the aneurysm via other vessels such as the inferior mesenteric or lumbar arteries. Such vessels can be occluded beforehand by embolization. Or one may attempt to occlude them later if the computed tomographic (CT) scan demonstrates inflow of contrast into the treated aneurysm.

The monoiliac prosthesis is an interesting option. Its simplicity makes it well suited for treating a ruptured aneurysm (**Fig. 7.3**). It can quickly bridge the aneurysm (eliminating the need to open the abdominal cavity). A suprapubic transverse bypass is then created to reestablish the connection to the contralateral side. The procedure also requires closing the contralateral common iliac artery with an occluder.

Thoracic Aorta

Aneurysms and dissections of the thoracic aorta are less common than in the abdominal aorta. However, they are more likely to rupture. Moreover, open surgical treatment has a high mortality rate (10 to 30%, Ohki and Malas 2005). Implantation of endovascular prostheses for aneurysms of the descending aorta (**Fig. 7.4**) and for Stanford type B dissections (DeBakey 3, **Figs. 7.5** and **7.6**) is a viable alternative. Patients tolerate the procedure far better, and it is associated with significantly lesser mortality.

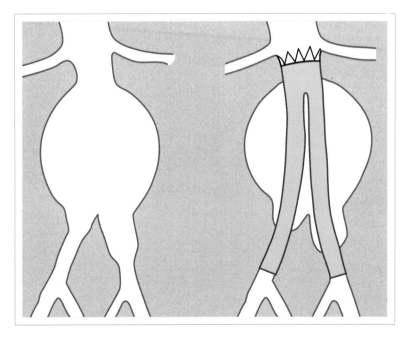

Fig. 7.2 Abdominal aortic aneurysm, endovascular prosthesis.

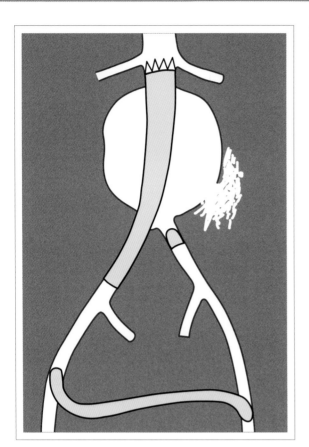

Fig. 7.3 Treatment of a ruptured aneurysm with a monoiliac prosthesis.

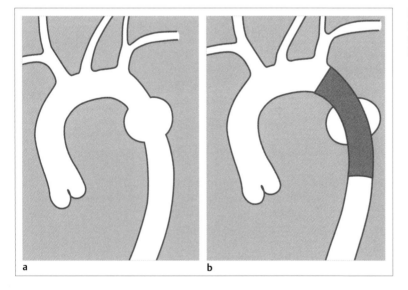

Fig. 7.4 Aneurysm of the descending thoracic aorta.
a Initial findings.
b Treatment with an endovascular prosthesis.

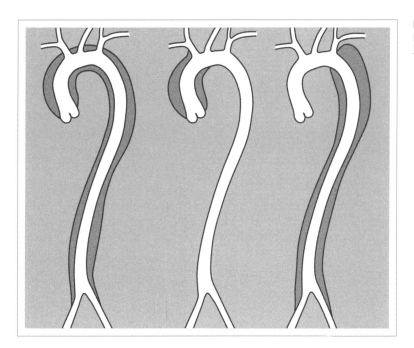

Fig. 7.5 Types of aortic dissection. Left: DeBakey 1, Stanford A; middle: DeBakey 2, Stanford A; right: DeBakey 3, Stanford B.

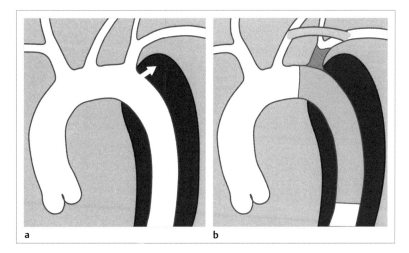

Fig. 7.6 Treatment of a type B (DeBakey 3) aortic dissection with an endovascular prosthesis.
a Initial findings: Dissection begins directly after the origin of the subclavian artery.
b The prosthesis covers the origin of the left subclavian artery, requiring a bypass from the left common carotid artery to the subclavian artery.

Arteriovenous Malformations

Pulmonary Arteriovenous Malformations

Pulmonary arteriovenous malformations appear on the chest radiograph as dense focal shadows with a characteristic pedicle in the direction of the pulmonary hilum. These malformations can become quite large and can occur singly or multiply. They can result in such a large shunt volume that they produce the clinical symptoms of a cyanotic heart defect.

Treatment consists of embolizing the feeder branches of the pulmonary artery with large Gianturco coils (Cook Medical, Bloomington, IN, USA) or more simply with an Amplatzer occluder (St. Jude Medical, St. Paul, MN, USA). Given the great width that these fistulas can attain, the major risk of treatment is that a coil could pass through the fistula into the left heart and from there enter the systemic circulation.

Renal Arteriovenous Malformations

Congenital arteriovenous fistulas occasionally occur in the kidney as well. Here too the shunt volume can become high enough to cause cardiac problems and create a steal phenomenon that impairs the blood supply to the renal

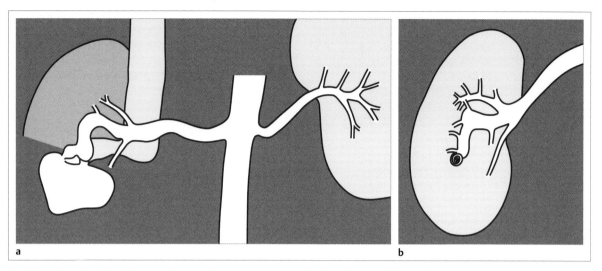

Fig. 7.7 The patient is a 34-year-old man with an arteriovenous fistula in the right kidney with a venous aneurysm, strong contrast enhancement of the vena cava, and a steal effect in the caudal portion of the kidney.
a Initial findings.
b Fistula is occluded with a coil.

parenchyma (**Fig. 7.7a**). The fistula can be occluded by one or more coils of the appropriate size.

The risk of losing a coil through the fistula is most effectively addressed by using coils (**Fig. 7.7b**) or an Amplatzer occluder that must be actively disconnected from the introducer system. The devices are only deployed when it is obvious that they will lodge proximal to the fistula.

Vascular Malformations in the Extremities

There is a broad spectrum of vascular malformations. Arteriovenous shunts can render surgical treatment difficult or even impossible. Where only varicose vessels are excised and the arteriovenous shunts are preserved, recurrence is inevitable.

This is the advantage of angiographically guided intervention. Where they are of the necessary size, shunts can be catheterized and occluded with cyanoacrylate. However, it is often only possible to catheterize the feeder vessel and not the arteriovenous fistula itself. This involves a risk of damage to adjacent normal tissue as well, such as skin. Therefore even interventional treatment should be used sparingly. On the other hand, targeted occlusion of specific arteriovenous shunts after precise angiographic analysis can be very helpful.

Intestinal Bleeding

Since the relationship between gastric ulcers and *Helicobacter pylori* has been known, the prevalence of **upper intestinal bleeding** has greatly decreased. Advances in endoscopy have also largely eliminated the indications for angiographic demonstration of bleeding and treatment by embolization or vasopressin infusion in the upper gastrointestinal tract.

Arterial bleeding in this region most often occurs in the area supplied by the left gastric artery. Such hemorrhages are often difficult to detect but can be treated relatively safely by embolization. This is because there is normally good collateral supply to the stomach. Where selective catheterization of the left gastric artery is not possible, vasopressin infusion via the celiac trunk will also produce the desired effect (Baum 2006).

Even in the **lower intestinal tract** most arterial bleeding can now be managed endoscopically. The main causes of massive hemorrhages are diverticula and vascular dysplasia in the ascending colon. Exact angiographic localization is only possible during the active bleeding phase. In applicable cases one will have to wait for this and closely observe circulation. Positive evidence of bleeding will depend both on its intensity and on the concentration of contrast agent achieved in angiography (superselective contrast injection is therefore indicated). Demonstration of a deposit of contrast agent that persists past the venous phase is diagnostic.

The most reliable treatment is embolization with minicoils. To minimize the risk of intestinal infarction, they should only be used far peripherally. Infusion of vasopressin (0.2 IU/min) may be considered as an alternative. Results are evaluated by angiography after 20 to 30 minutes. Where bleeding persists, the dose may be temporarily increased to 0.4 IU per minute. If this is unsuccessful, other methods of treatment will have to be explored. Once hemostasis has been obtained, treatment continues in the intensive care unit with 0.2 IU per minute for 12 to 24 hours, and then with 0.1 IU per minute for 24 hours (Baum 2006, Görich 2001).

There are also **other sources of bleeding** in the abdomen that can be treated by embolization. These include aneurysms or hemorrhages in pancreatic pseudocysts in the setting of arterial erosion.

Embolization of Solid Organs

Embolization of Hepatic Tumors

With its dual vascular supply (25% via the hepatic artery and 75% via the portal vein), the liver provides an interesting setting for embolization. Embolic occlusion of its feeder arteries can cause necrosis in a hypervascular tumor such as a hepatocellular carcinoma that is supplied only arterially. This treatment can be performed without causing any significant damage to the normal liver parenchyma.

Chemoembolization is often used in the liver. The treatment employs a mixture of oily contrast medium and cytostatic agents, which allows very high concentrations of active ingredient. Radioactive yttrium-90 seeds are also used for certain types of tumors.

Embolization of the Spleen

In the spleen, embolization can be used to treat traumatic bleeding and alleviate symptoms of hypersplenism from a variety of causes.

Embolization of Renal Tumors

Since the 1970s preoperative embolization of hypervascular renal tumors has been common practice. Today this is still done where a tumor has invaded the renal vein or the inferior vena cava. Embolization in the kidneys may also be used as a palliative measure for inoperable bleeding tumors. Benign angiomyolipomas can also be embolized if bleeding occurs.

Embolization of Uterine Myomas

Embolization of uterine myomas has become common in the last few years. Microspheres are used for this purpose, often introduced selectively into the uterine artery (usually bilaterally) via a microcatheter using a coaxial technique.

Other Embolizations

Traumatic bleeding in the region of the **internal iliac artery** is often life threatening but is difficult to reach by surgery. For radiologists experienced in interventional techniques, this is a relatively straightforward task. Embolic materials that permit subsequent recanalization (Gelfoam, Pfizer, New York, NY, USA) are preferable here.

Inoperable bleeding tumors often occur in the true pelvis (in the bladder, uterus, prostate, or rectum [see Fig. 2.44]). Here, embolization can usually achieve hemostasis as a palliative measure.

Varicocele

Like the greater or lesser saphenous vein, the spermatic and ovarian veins course vertically for a longer distance without surrounding muscles that pump the blood cranially from valve to valve and could prevent ectasia. As a result these veins are susceptible to varices. Varicosis of the spermatic vein develops in the scrotum (pampiniform plexus) and can be a possible cause of male infertility because it leads to elevated temperature in the testes.

The vein can be surgically exposed in the pelvic region and ligated. The interventional alternative involves catheterizing the vein from a femoral or the right jugular vein (on the left via the renal vein and on the right directly from the inferior vena cava). The vein is then occluded with coils at several levels according to the angiographic findings (**Fig. 7.8**). This is necessary to prevent recurrence via the collaterals that are usually present. Coil embolization can be combined with the use of a sclerosing agent (Reiner et al 2008).

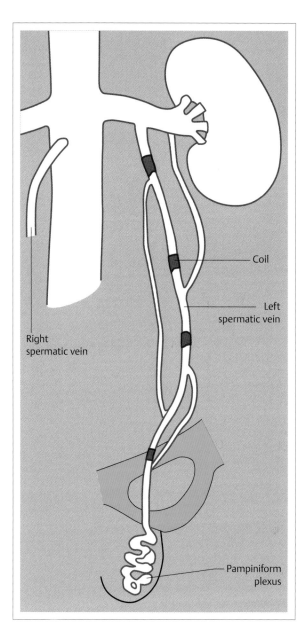

Fig. 7.8 Left varicocele treated by coil embolization.

Coil

Left
spermatic vein

Right
spermatic vein

Pampiniform
plexus

Transjugular Intrahepatic Portosystemic Shunt

Cirrhosis of the liver is the most important cause of portal hypertension. It leads to diffuse stenosis of the intrahepatic branches of the portal vein and thus increases the pressure throughout the portal venous system. Collaterals develop via the gastric and esophageal veins. The most well known sequela is massive variceal bleeding. It was once common to surgically create shunts between the portal vein and the inferior vena cava to decompress the portal venous system and relieve these collaterals. Such connections included portocaval or splenorenal anastomoses.

Transjugular intrahepatic portosystemic shunt (TIPS) is an elegant alternative that has largely made these operations obsolete. A shunt is created within the liver between a branch of the portal vein and a liver vein (**Fig. 7.9**). A catheter is introduced into a hepatic vein via the right jugular vein. A long, sharp cannula similar to those used in percutaneous transhepatic cholangiography (PTC) is advanced through this catheter. The hepatic parenchyma is punctured in several directions (done under ultrasound guidance) until a large branch of the portal vein is located. The path between the hepatic vein and the portal vein is secured by a wire, dilated with balloon catheters, and finally held open by a stent.

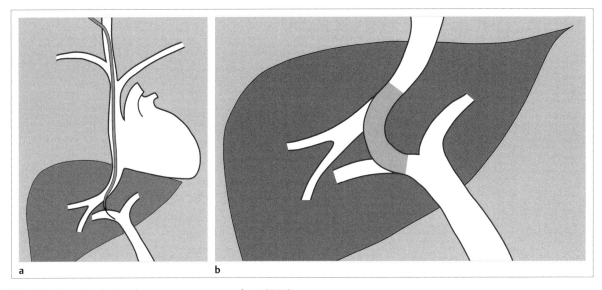

Fig. 7.9 Transjugular intrahepatic portosystemic shunt (TIPS).
a Catheterizing a branch of the portal vein via the right jugular vein, vena cava, and a hepatic vein.
b A stent keeps the intrahepatic shunt open.

Inferior Vena Cava Filter

Inferior vena cava filters are fine metal constructions that are inserted through a peripheral vein, folded tightly together. They are deployed and secured in the infrarenal inferior vena cava to trap emboli there (**Fig. 7.10**). In rare cases such as in thrombosis of the renal vein, they are deployed cranially to the renal veins, occasionally even in the superior vena cava.

Indications and Prognosis

Indications for an inferior vena cava filter include recurrent pulmonary emboli despite adequate anticoagulation and deep venous thrombosis contraindicating anticoagulation. There are also a few relative indications.

After a few years of frequent use, vena cava filters have fallen from favor in recent years. This reflects the lack of convincing evidence that they actually reduce the incidence of fatal pulmonary embolism. Even the alternative of a temporarily deployed filter that is later removed after the critical phase has failed to gain widespread acceptance. Long-term results are not available because patients receiving an inferior vena cava filter generally have a very short life expectancy (Hoppe and Kaufman 2008).

Performing the Intervention

Inferior vena cava filters are introduced via the femoral vein (on the normal side where possible) or, in the case of bilateral thrombosis or involvement of the inferior vena cava itself, via the right internal jugular artery. Correctly deploying the filter just caudal to the renal veins is the critical step. These must be located precisely before the filter is placed. This requires inferior vena cavography. Cavography is also used to measure the width of the vena cava to ensure a good fit.

The filter is deployed by withdrawing the sleeve within which it is introduced over a wire. The deployed filter is fixed in place by small hooks that press into the wall of the vein. When the filter is to be removed (some designs allow this), it is grasped with a hook and held in position while a sleeve is pushed over it. This pulls the hooks out of the wall, mobilizing the filter so it can be withdrawn from the vein in the sleeve.

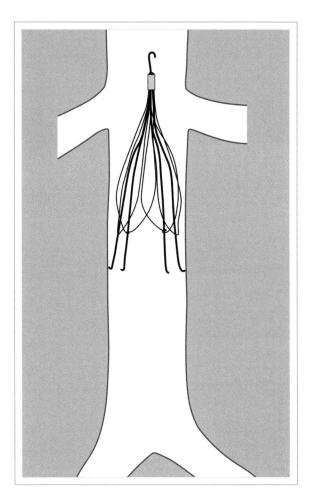

Fig. 7.10 Günther Tulip filter in the inferior vena cava (Cook Medical).

Port Implantation

Patients undergoing long-term therapy with cytostatic agents or pain medication or who are receiving parenteral nutrition require a central venous access site that is impervious to infection. These patients are treated with an implantable port device. This is a capsule with a thick silicone membrane that can be punctured through the skin with special cannulas (**Fig. 7.11**). Connected to the capsule is a catheter that conducts the injected medication into the superior vena cava via a vein such as the subclavian vein or the internal jugular vein.

Performing the procedure. The course and patency of the subclavian vein are evaluated by ultrasound. The vein is then punctured percutaneously with the aid of ultrasound or using road mapping (contrast is injected via the cubital vein). Next a guidewire is advanced into the superior vena cava. Then the port catheter is introduced over the wire and advanced up to the right atrium. Then the sheath is removed without withdrawing the catheter. A subcutaneous pocket is then created

by blunt dissection under local anesthesia, admittedly a rather unfamiliar technique for radiologists. The port, filled with heparinized saline solution, is then placed in this pocket and connected to the catheter. The catheter is shortened to the required length and fixed in place with a suture if required. The pocket is then closed.

Most port devices are implanted by surgeons. Originally they exposed the vein (usually the subclavian vein) and often worked without fluoroscopy. The radiologic variant with percutaneous catheterization of the vein (see Chapter 3, Catheterization of the Subclavian Vein, p. 79) and fluoroscopic guidance for correct placement of the catheter therefore represents a genuine advance. Today this method has become the treatment of choice even among surgeons.

Even those radiologists who, like most, do not implant the port themselves may occasionally be asked to correct the position of a catheter that was introduced via the subclavian vein and whose end lies in the internal jugular vein. It is usually fairly easy to hook the errant catheter with a

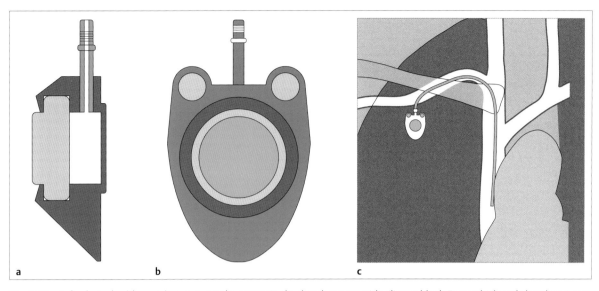

Fig. 7.11 Infraclavicular (thoracic) port. Example: BARD single-chamber port with silicone block 5 mm thick and chamber 4 mm deep.
a Lateral view of port.
b Coronal view of port.
c Position of the port within the chest.

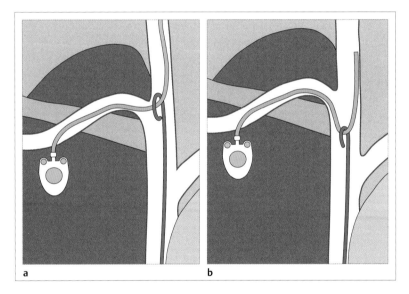

Fig. 7.12 The port catheter is drawn out of the internal jugular vein and into the superior vena cava with a pigtail catheter.
a Hooking the port catheter with the pigtail catheter.
b Pulling it down into the superior vena cava.

long pigtail catheter introduced via the right femoral vein and pull it back into the superior vena cava (**Fig. 7.12**).

> ▽ When one has injected contrast to evaluate a port, one should flush it afterward with 10 mL of heparinized saline solution.

References

Baum S. Arteriographic diagnosis and treatment of gastrointestinal bleeding. In: Baum S, Pentecost MJ, eds. Abrams Angiography Interventional Radiology. 2nd ed. Philadelphia, PA: Lippincott Williams & Wilkins: 2006:487–515

Görich J. Therapie arterieller Blutungen. In: Görich J, Brambs HJ, eds. Interventionelle minimal-invasive Radiologie. Stuttgart, New York: Thieme; 2001:308–354

Hoppe H, Kaufman JA. Inferior vena cava filters. In: Kandarpa K, ed. Peripheral Vascular Interventions. Philadelphia, PA: Lippincott Williams & Wilkins; 2008:401–415

Mathias K. Perkutane transluminale Katheterbehandlung supra-aortaler Arterienobstruktionen. Angio 1981;3:47–50

Ohki T, Malas MB. Endovascular treatment of abdominal and thoracic aortic aneurysms. In: Casserly IP, Sachar R, Yadav JS, eds. Manual of Peripheral Vascular Intervention. Philadelphia, PA: Lippincott Williams & Wilkins; 2005:183–213

Reiner E, Pollak J, White RJ. Gonadal embolotherapy. In: Kandarpa K, ed. Peripheral Vascular Interventions. Philadelphia, PA: Lippincott Williams & Wilkins; 2008:427–435

8 Complications

Even minimally invasive interventional radiology involves certain risks (**Table 8.1**). One must be thoroughly familiar with them, weigh them against the expected benefit, and discuss them with the patient. The risks involve the access site, the site and type of treatment (percutaneous transluminal angioplasty, stent placement, etc.), and the entire body (systemic complications). When minor complications such as hematoma are included, then the overall rate is ~ 10%.

The number and severity of all complications can be influenced by careful action (Cragen and Heuser 2008). The high number of local complications at the vascular access site can largely be attributed to errors in puncture, catheterization, and aftercare.

Complications at the Arterial Access Site

Pseudoaneurysm

A pseudoaneurysm usually occurs in the absence of a buttressing structure during compression. It is essentially caused by performing the puncture too far distal. Compression applied at the wrong place (to the superficial cannula track without compression of the wound in the vessel wall) is also conducive to pseudoaneurysm (see Chapter 3, Retrograde Catheterization of the Common Femoral Artery, p. 42 and Chapter 3, Treatment of the Access Site, p. 66). The risk also increases with the diameter of the sheath, the length of time the sheath remains in place, and impaired coagulation, and when the patient gets out of bed too soon.

Table 8.1 Incidence of complications according to Pentecost et al[a] and Matsi and Manninen[b]

	Complication rate (%)	
	Pentecost et al (1994)	Matsi and Manninen (1998)
Complications at the arterial access site		
Bleeding or hematoma	3.4	5.4
Pseudoaneurysm	0.1	1.2
Arteriovenous fistula	0.1	0.5
Retroperitoneal hematoma		0.5
Local infection		0.5
Complications at the percutaneous transluminal angiography or stent site		
Thrombosis	3.2	1.4
Rupture or perforation	0.3	
Distal embolization	2.3	2.2
Dissection	0.4	
Systemic complications		
Renal failure	0.2	
Myocardial infarction	0.2	
Cerebral insult	0.55	
Mortality	0.2	

[a]Retrospective study of 3,784 interventions.
[b]Prospective study of 410 interventions.

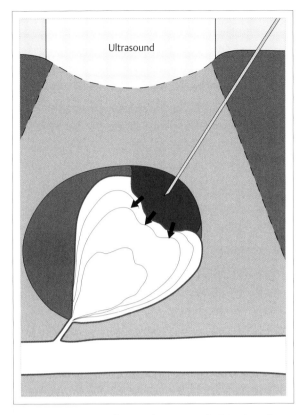

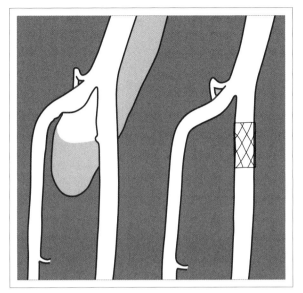

Fig. 8.2 Seventy-six-year-old woman with severe heart failure: arteriovenous fistula between the superficial femoral artery and the femoral vein (secondary to superficial femoral artery puncture). The treatment with a covered stent shown here is the exception and is reserved for patients who are unable to undergo surgery.

Fig. 8.1 Treatment of a pseudoaneurysm by injection of thrombin. During the slow injection, the color Doppler scan shows how the thrombus grows and fills the aneurysm within seconds. The flow signals disappear. **Important:** No thrombin must enter the artery!

There are two options for treating pseudoaneurysm:
- **Precise compression with the ultrasound probe:** This has the advantage of directly visualizing the effect of compression: blockage of the track to the artery with the disappearance of flow signals. However, this can take 1 to 2 hours and is very painful for the patient. For the physician it is invariably strenuous and often unsuccessful.
- **Ultrasound-guided injection of bovine thrombin into the pseudoaneurysm** (**Fig. 8.1**). This is an elegant method with success rates as high as 100%. It is important to use ultrasound visualization to ensure that the injection is ended as soon as the pseudoaneurysm is thrombosed. Absolute sterility is required for the thrombin injection!

> **Caution:** Thrombin entering the artery can cause acute arterial thrombosis in the entire leg. Emergency treatment involves immediate local thrombolysis.

Surgery is indicated wherever the pseudoaneurysm expands too quickly, leads to distal ischemia or neuropathy, or becomes infected.

Arteriovenous Fistulas

Arteriovenous fistulas can only occur where both the anterior and the posterior walls of the artery are punctured and where the puncture of the posterior arterial wall also passes through the anterior wall of a vein. Small fistulas often resolve spontaneously. Larger fistulas can occur where a sheath is introduced through the artery and into a vein. These tend to grow and eventually lead to a volume load on the heart. Treatment is invariably surgical. Treatment with a short covered stent is indicated only in patients who are unable to undergo surgery (**Fig. 8.2**).

Retroperitoneal Hematoma

The most dangerous complication arising directly from the arterial access site is the retroperitoneal hematoma. This occurs only where the **puncture is too far proximal**. There is no suitable buttressing structure for effective compression there and the blood finds its way through the sparse tissue into the retroperitoneum. The symptoms can be unspecific: decreased blood pressure and increased pulse rate, nausea, and occasionally back pain. Order a computed tomographic scan if there is the slightest doubt!

The most important thing here is to **avoid incorrect puncture technique** that can cause a retroperitoneal hematoma. If it is suspected that the cannula may have entered the artery above the inguinal ligament, remove it, compress the site for 5 minutes, and perform the puncture again.

Important: Do not hesitate to again apply local anesthesia for a new skin incision and to perform a second puncture farther distal!

The error may be discovered only at the conclusion of the intervention. In that case, use a vascular closure system (which some authors think is wrong) because the only alternative would be compression, for which a suitable buttressing structure is lacking.

Occasionally blood from a puncture wound too far proximal that cannot be effectively compressed will find its way into the **abdominal wall** instead of the retroperitoneum. There it is less dangerous because it will more likely be tamponed and because it is painful: It will not be overlooked.

Infection of the Access Site

With a prevalence of 0.12%, infections, thankfully, are rare occurrences. It is obvious that insufficient hygiene measures (skin disinfection, sterile draping, surgical hand disinfection, mask) can cause a dramatic increase in these numbers at any time. Germs on the skin are usually the cause of the infection. A stab incision that is large enough will help one to avoid transporting such bacteria on particles of skin through the cannula or sheath into the deep layer.

Complications at the Angioplasty Site

Local thrombosis is generally a sequela of the trauma to the vessel wall. This risk can be minimized by precisely matching the size of the balloon to the width of the vessel and then slowly inflating the balloon. Appropriate ancillary medication also plays a role: heparin at the beginning of the intervention and preparation with aspirin and clopidogrel (see also Chapter 1, Preparing the Patient, p. 5).

Peripheral emboli may be expected in large numbers when acutely thrombosed vascular segments are catheterized, when they are catheterized several times, and when local thrombi form. The latter can be avoided by observing the rules already discussed.

Systemic Reactions

Anaphylactic Reaction to Contrast Agent

Adverse reactions to contrast agents are not entirely avoidable. When they occur, they must be treated by giving the patient plenty of fluids and, where indicated, intravenous epinephrine and corticosteroids (see also Chapter 2, Prophylaxis and Treatment of Reactions to Contrast Agents, p. 38). The important thing is the **prophylactic treatment** of patients who have experienced adverse reactions during previous interventions. Because the anaphylactic reaction occurs in response to the organic carrier molecule and not the iodine, the first step is to use a different agent than in the previous examination. This will greatly reduce the likelihood of another reaction. Nonetheless, every patient with such a history should be given an oral corticosteroid 12 to 24 hours before the intervention and should receive intravenous antihistamines at the time of the intervention.

Contrast-Induced Nephropathy

Contrast-induced nephropathy must be assumed where creatinine clearance drops by at least 25% during the first 2 days. Prophylactic steps must be taken with every patient confirmed or suspected to have impaired kidney function:

- Hydration (1 mL of isotonic saline solution per kg body weight per hour 12 hours before and 12 hours after contrast administration)
- Administration of acetylcysteine in applicable cases
- Above all, sparing use of contrast (see Chapter 3, Angiography, p. 80).

The preservation of kidney function justifies every imaginable effort in this regard. One can also use CO_2 as a contrast agent for all or part of the procedure (see Chapter 2, CO_2 as a Contrast Agent, p. 36).

Myocardial Infarction

The risk of a myocardial infarction is of course greatest in patients with known coronary insufficiency. For these patients, be sure to consult with the attending internist or cardiologist. If it is decided to perform the procedure, do everything possible to spare the patient emotional stress. When talking to the patient, make an effort to gain the patient's trust and confidence. Spare the patient any avoidable pain (slow, careful local anesthesia) and administer mild sedation if necessary. Here, too, the contrast burden must be kept to a minimum.

Vasovagal Syncope

Vasovagal syncope is the most common systemic complication:

- The patient yawns,
- breaks out in sweat,
- becomes bradycardic, and
- suffers a drop in blood pressure.

When observing these signs, have an assistant raise the patient's legs, give the patient 0.5 mg of IV atropine (diluted to 10 mL so that it will not remain in the veins), and administer isotonic saline solution intravenously. The patient will usually recover within a few minutes.

> ◣ **Important:** Do not hesitate to call in an anesthesiologist at the first signs of serious complications. Every serious complication should be immediately documented and discussed candidly with the patient.

The numbers quoted earlier come from large studies and series of patients in the 1980s and 1990s. Since then a lot has been learned collectively. We are now more aware of all of the errors that can lead to complications. And certain material conditions have improved decisively:

- The hazardous dissections are securely managed with stents.
- Treatment with aspirin and clopidogrel as aggregation inhibitors, now standard practice, only gained widespread acceptance in the late 1990s.
- Many systems have become more slender, creating a correspondingly smaller access wound in the vascular wall.
- CO_2 as a contrast agent and the general use of nonionic contrast agents are advances of the 1980s and 1990s.

This gives hope that current and future complication rates will be lower.

References

Cragen DT, Heuser HH. Complications of peripheral interventions. In: Heuser RR, Henry M, eds. Textbook of Peripheral Vascular Interventions. 2nd ed. London: Informa UK; 2008:791–798

Matsi PJ, Manninen HI. Complications of lower-limb percutaneous transluminal angioplasty: a prospective analysis of 410 procedures on 295 consecutive patients. Cardiovasc Intervent Radiol 1998;21(5):361–366

Pentecost MJ, Criqui MH, Dorros G, et al. Guidelines for peripheral percutaneous transluminal angioplasty of the abdominal aorta and lower extremity vessels. A statement for health professionals from a special writing group of the Councils on Cardiovascular Radiology, Arteriosclerosis, Cardio-Thoracic and Vascular Surgery, Clinical Cardiology, and Epidemiology and Prevention, the American Heart Association. Circulation 1994;89(1):511–531

9 Recurrent Stenosis

Pathogenesis

The risk that recurrent stenosis (restenosis) may develop is the most important weakness of endovascular interventions. Local deposition of thrombocytes and an inflammatory reaction occur as a consequence of mechanical injury to the vessel wall occurring during treatment. Together they induce intimal hyperplasia. Most recurrent stenoses occur within 6 months of the intervention. Gradual resolution of the intimal hyperplasia at the stent site has been observed in patients after more than 12 months since the intervention.

Muscular arteries (permitting active vessel diameter changes in response to end-organ need) such as the coronary, arm, and leg arteries are at greatest risk. This makes sense when one considers that an essential component of intimal hyperplasia is the migration and proliferation of smooth muscle cells. The recurrence rate for vascular occlusion is generally higher than for stenosis. Diabetes mellitus increases the risk of recurrent stenosis.

Recurrent stenoses have been observed in up to 53% of cases in the legs, whereas the rate for the carotid arteries is only 5 to 8%. The rates of restenosis in the subclavian artery are equally low at 5 to 7%. In the iliac arteries, a restenosis rate of only 6% was observed after placement of a nitinol stent. Renal arteries treated for arteriosclerotic stenosis with stent placement show a restenosis rate of 14 to 25%. The recurrence rates in renal arteries less than 4 mm in diameter and in smokers are higher (Kedhi et al 2008).

Prophylaxis against Recurrence

Platelet Aggregation Inhibitors

Aspirin and clopidogrel play an important role in prophylaxis against recurrence. This is because the initial reaction to the trauma of intervention is the deposition of thrombocytes. Via growth factors, these thrombocytes stimulate the proliferation of smooth muscle cells and their migration into the neointima.

Avoidance of Unnecessary Injuries to the Vessel Wall

Because the recurrent stenosis is a reaction to the trauma of intervention, the first logical step in prophylaxis is to meticulously avoid unnecessary injuries to the vessel wall during dilation. This means precisely matching the balloon to the width of the vessel, carefully dilating with slowly increasing pressure, avoiding excessive expansion, and not dilating unaffected segments.

Active Prophylaxis against Recurrence

All concepts of active prophylaxis against recurrence are based on the premise that recurrent stenoses are manifestations of an excessive reaction of the inner layers of the vessel wall to the mechanical trauma of dilation and possibly to the permanent mechanical irritation by the stent. Therefore these concepts seek to reduce the proliferative ability of the inner layers of the wall by applying topical noxious agents:

- Ionizing radiation (brachytherapy)
- Cytostatic agents and immunosuppressants
- Cold

Brachytherapy

Endoluminal irradiation with **afterloading** is performed via a special catheter introduced after dilation. An alternative to this is the **placement of stents** coated with radioactive phosphorus-32 (a β emitter, range in water 8 mm, half-life 14.3 days). **Percutaneous irradiation** has also been attempted, with therapy divided among several sessions. The best results were those with a focal dose of 14 Gy.

All three methods are expensive and not available at every facility. The results achieved were mostly positive, although not always uniformly so (Waksman 2008).

Cytostatic Agents and Immunosuppressants

Cytostatic agents and immunosuppressants intended to reduce the growth potential of the intima are usually introduced on drug-eluting stents. These are stents coated with a carrier layer that gives off the active ingredient over an extended period of time (Levi 2006). Here, too, the results achieved were mostly positive, for example, a reduction in recurrent stenosis from 14 to 7%. Apparently there are differences in the action of the various medications used. This method has not become established in daily clinical practice. One reason for this is its significantly higher cost.

Recent experience has shown that even a single application of a cytostatic agent (paclitaxel) to the vascular wall can have a positive effect in avoiding recurrent stenosis. For this purpose, balloons are used whose **surface is coated with the cytostatic agent** (Kedhi and Bilodeau 2008, Tepe et al 2010). One advantage over drug-eluting stents is that the balloon applies the medication to the entire surface of the stenotic area and not only where the stent is in contact with the vessel wall.

Cryoplasty
Filling the percutaneous transluminal angioplasty balloon with liquid nitrogen oxide instead of contrast agent will suddenly cool the inner layers of the wall to about $-10°C$. This causes intracellular water to freeze (Kedhi and Bilodeau 2008). According to the results available to date, this reduces the rate of recurrent stenosis (Das et al 2009).

Reduction of Plaque Mass
Atherectomy and excimer laser treatment have been successfully used to reduce the mass of plaque with the intent of decreasing the probability of recurrent stenosis (Kedhi und Bilodeau 2008).

Finally, remember that **regular follow-up** is crucial in preventing a recurrent stenosis from progressing to a vascular occlusion.

References
Das TS, McNamara T, Gray B, et al. Primary cryoplasty therapy provides durable support for limb salvage in critical limb ischemia patients with infrapopliteal lesions: 12-month follow-up results from the BTK Chill Trial. J Endovasc Ther 2009;16(2, Suppl 2)II19–30

Kedhi E, Bilodeau L. Interventional therapies: new approaches. In: Heuser RR, Henry M, eds. Textbook of Peripheral Vascular Interventions. 2nd ed. London: Informa UK; 2008:770–775

Kedhi E, Tanguay JF, Bilodeau L. Pathophysiology of restenosis. In: Heuser RR, Henry M, eds. Textbook of Peripheral Vascular Interventions. 2nd ed. London: Informa UK; 2008:763–769

Levi E. Vascular stents. In: Baum S, Pentecost MJ, eds. Abrams Angiography Interventional Radiology. 2nd ed. Philadelphia, PA: Lippincott Williams & Wilkins; 2006:205–219

Tepe G, Zeller T, Albrecht T, et al. Lokale Applikation von Paclitaxel zur Prävention der Restenose bei peripherer arterieller Verschlusskrankheit. Persistierender Effekt der medikamentenbeschichteten Ballons auch nach zwei Jahren. Berlin: Deutscher Röntgenkongress; 2010

Waksman R. Update on peripheral vascular brachytherapy. In: Heuser RR, Henry M, eds. Textbook of Peripheral Vascular Interventions. 2nd ed. London: Informa UK; 2008:776–781

10 Documentation and Postprocessing

Once the patient is back in bed after the intervention and the access site has been treated, evaluate the angiographic documentation (**Table 10.1**): Select the most important images, perform the necessary postprocessing (contrast adjustment, sharpness, and definitive measurement of stenosis grades, see below), and compile a preliminary report for the ward:

- Mark the findings and treatment results in a schematic diagram of the vascular tree (**Fig. 10.1**).
- Give preliminary evaluation of treatment results.
- List type and quantity of contrast agent.
- List type of treatment of vascular access site.
- List other aftercare (bed rest).

For this purpose, copy the diagram of the vascular tree shown in **Fig. 10.3**. Paste the name of the department over the top right-hand corner. Paste the name of the preparation used over "Local anesthetic." Then copy the diagram.

Visit every inpatient on afternoon rounds. Check the access site and the results of treatment. Discuss the results and any additional measures with the patient.

Image Postprocessing

Some operators delegate the task of postprocessing images to coworkers. Even if they are very good at this, it is not the best solution because certain details are only visualized during postprocessing with optimized window settings and contrast enhancement. Only you can really decide how much of this is important and should be documented. Remember that the quality of your images, in terms of both their information content and their aesthetic appeal, will define your own image among your colleagues in allied disciplines!

Subtraction very often requires improvement. There will almost always be several pre-contrast images. The one of these that is closest to the first contrast-filled image will be the most suitable mask. Selecting a different image as a mask has an advantage over pixel shift in that it compensates for even complex motions. Only when one brings together the most suitable mask with the most high-contrast filling image may one start the pixel shift function if necessary.

The rule is that the window setting must be wide enough so that not only the outer contours of the vessel can be evaluated with hard black and white contrast. On the contrary, details within the vessel should be discernible as different gray scale values (**Fig. 10.2**), and all important details of this sort should be emphasized by contrast enhancement. The angiographic image is only two-dimensional. Information about the third dimension is provided only by the gray scale visualization.

The relationship to bony landmarks is very helpful in many places. What is often missed is visualization of the femoral artery bifurcation and the femoral head on a single image. This can be decisive for selecting the optimal access site in subsequent interventions.

Table 10.1 The physician's most important tasks after completing the intervention

Image postprocessing
Preliminary report of findings for the ward
Visit during afternoon
Discussion of findings with vascular surgeons

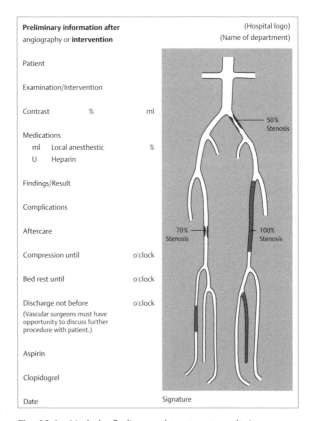

Fig. 10.1 Mark the findings and treatment results in a diagram.

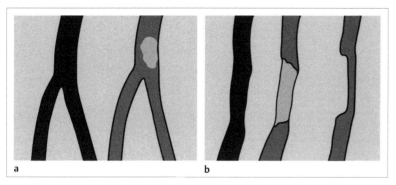

Fig. 10.2 Only a wide window reveals important findings in the imaged vessel.
a Plaque in the common femoral artery.
b Eccentric residual stenosis in the superficial femoral artery. Right: second plane.

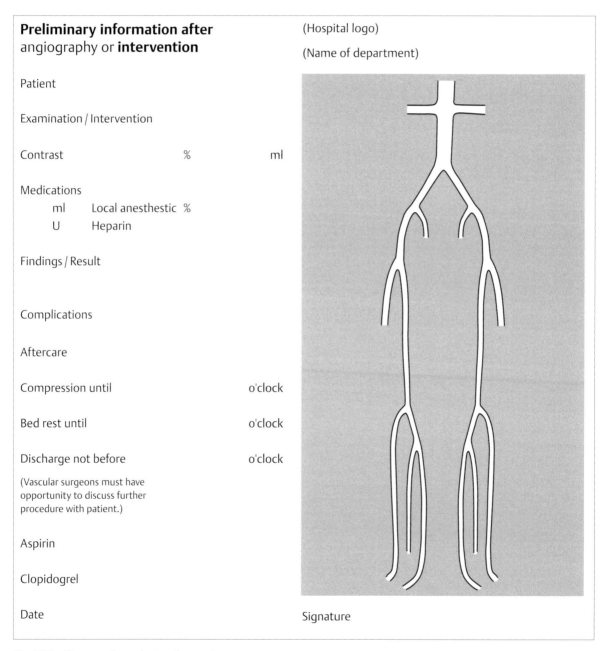

Preliminary information after angiography or **intervention**

(Hospital logo)

(Name of department)

Patient

Examination / Intervention

Contrast   %   ml

Medications
     ml   Local anesthestic %
     U   Heparin

Findings / Result

Complications

Aftercare

Compression until   o'clock

Bed rest until   o'clock

Discharge not before   o'clock

(Vascular surgeons must have opportunity to discuss further procedure with patient.)

Aspirin

Clopidogrel

Date   Signature

Fig. 10.3   Diagram of vascular tree for copying

Index

Illustrations are comprehensively referred to from the text. Therefore, significant material in illustrations and tables have usually only been given a page reference in the absence of their concomitant mention in the text referring to that figure.